Lecture Notes of the Institute for Computer Sciences, Social Informatics and Telecommunications Engineering 524

The LNICST series publishes ICST's conferences, symposia and workshops.

LNICST reports state-of-the-art results in areas related to the scope of the Institute.
The type of material published includes

- Proceedings (published in time for the respective event)
- Other edited monographs (such as project reports or invited volumes)

LNICST topics span the following areas:

- General Computer Science
- E-Economy
- E-Medicine
- Knowledge Management
- Multimedia
- Operations, Management and Policy
- Social Informatics
- Systems

Marouan Mizmizi · Maurizio Magarini ·
Prabhat Kumar Upadhyay ·
Massimiliano Pierobon
Editors

Body Area Networks

Smart IoT and Big Data for Intelligent Health Management

18th EAI International Conference, BODYNETS 2024-A
Milan, Italy, February 5-6, 2024
Proceedings

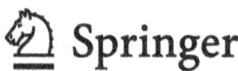 Springer

Editors
Marouan Mizmizi ⓘ
The Polytechnic University of Milan
Milan, Italy

Maurizio Magarini
The Polytechnic University of Milan
Milan, Italy

Prabhat Kumar Upadhyay ⓘ
Indian Institute of Technology Indore
Indore, Madhya Pradesh, India

Massimiliano Pierobon ⓘ
University of Nebraska-Lincoln
Lincoln, NE, USA

ISSN 1867-8211   ISSN 1867-822X (electronic)
Lecture Notes of the Institute for Computer Sciences, Social Informatics
and Telecommunications Engineering
ISBN 978-3-031-72523-4   ISBN 978-3-031-72524-1 (eBook)
https://doi.org/10.1007/978-3-031-72524-1

This Springer imprint is published by the registered company Springer Nature Switzerland AG
The registered company address is: Gewerbestrasse 11, 6330 Cham, Switzerland

If disposing of this product, please recycle the paper.

Preface

We are delighted to introduce the proceedings of the European Alliance for Innovation (EAI) 18th EAI International Conference on Body Area Networks (BODYNETS 2024-A): Intelligent Edge Cloud for Dependable Globally Connected BAN. BODYNETS 2024-A was an international conference that brought together researchers, scientists, and practitioners from around the world who are developing and deploying smart body technologies. The 18th edition of Bodynets was originally scheduled to take place in 2023 but was postponed until 2024.

The technical program of BODYNETS 2024-A consisted of 20 papers framed within a diverse range of tracks, each focusing on a critical aspect of body area networks:

- **Implantable devices and in-body communication:** This track explored topics surrounding implantable devices and their communication channels within the body.
- **Body Area Networks and Transmission Technologies:** This track focused on the vital issue of data transmission for implanted devices.
- **Smart Healthcare Applications:** This track showcased the vast potential of smart body technologies in various healthcare and real-time monitoring applications.
- **Privacy and Security in Wireless Body Area Networks:** Recognizing the criticality of data security in body area networks, this track addressed emerging challenges.

In addition to the high-quality technical paper presentations, the technical program also featured 2 keynote speeches.

We are grateful to the steering chairs and the organizing committee for their hard work in making BODYNETS 2024-A a success. We are also grateful to the Technical Program Committee for their work in reviewing the papers. Finally, we would like to thank all of the authors who submitted papers to BODYNETS 2024-A.

We believe that BODYNETS 2024-A provided a valuable forum for researchers, developers, and practitioners to discuss all science and technology aspects that are relevant to body area network technologies. We hope that the proceedings will be a valuable resource for all those interested in this field.

Maurizio Magarini
Massimiliano Pierobon
Marouan Mizmizi
Prabhat Kumar Upadhyay

Organization

Steering Committee

Imrich Chlamtac   University of Trento, Italy

Organizing Committee

General Chair

Maurizio Magarini   Politecnico di Milano, Italy

General Co-chair

Tahar Kechadi   University College Dublin, Ireland

TPC Chairs and Co-chairs

Massimiliano Pierobon   University of Nebraska-Lincoln, USA
Prabhat Kumar Upadhyay   Indian Institute of Technology Indore, India
Anna Vizziello   Università di Pavia, Italy
Liming Chen   Ulster University, UK

Publications Chair

Marouan Mizmizi   Politecnico di Milano, Italy

Publicity and Social Media Chair

Luca Barletta   Politecnico di Milano, Italy

Web Chair

Stefano Caputo   University of Florence, Italy

Local Chair

Francesco Linsalata   Politecnico di Milano, Italy

Technical Program Committee

Ahmed Khorshid	University of California, Irvine, USA
Allen Huang	University of Ottawa, Canada
Attaphongse Taparussanagorn	Asian Institute of Technology, Thailand
Chika Sugimoto	Yokohama National University, Japan
Claire Goursaud	INSA de Lyon, France
Eryk Dutkiewicz	University of Technology Sydney, Australia
Giancarlo Fortino	University of Calabria, Italy
Hamed Farhadi	Harvard University, USA
Heikki Karvonen	University of Oulu, Finland
Hirokazu Tanaka	Hiroshima City University, Japan
Huan-Bang Li	National Institute of Information and Communications Technology, Japan
Ilangko Balasingham	Oslo University Hospital, Norway
Jianqing Wang	Nagoya Institute of Technology, Japan
John Farserotu	CSEM, Switzerland
Juha Petäjäjärvi	University of Oulu, Finland
Kamran Sayrafien	National Institute of Standards and Technology, USA
Kamya Yekeh Yazdandoost	Aalto University, Finland
Kimmo Kansanen	Norwegian University of Science and Technology, Norway
Kohei Ohno	Meiji University, Japan
Ladislau Matekovits	Politecnico di Torino, Italy
Lin Wang	Xiamen University, China
Luca De Nardis	University of Rome La Sapienza, Italy
Marc Girod-Genet	Institut Mines-Télécom – Télécom SudParis, France
Marcos Katz	University of Oulu, Finland
Mariella Särestöniemi	University of Oulu, Finland
Mehmet Yuce	Monash University, Australia
Michael Heimlich	Macquarie University, Australia
Minseok Kim	Niigata University, Japan
Mohammed Ghavami	London South Bank University, UK
Omid Dehzangi	University of Michigan-Dearborn, USA
Qiong Wang	Technische Universität Dresden, Germany

Contents

Implantable devices and In-Body Communication

A Study on the Implant Interface of Brain-Computer Interface Technology in the THz Band

Marco Hernandez$^{(\boxtimes)}$ and Matti Hämäläinen

Center of Wireless Communications, University of Oulu, Pentti Kaiteran katu 1, 90570 Oulu, Finland
Marco.Hernandez@oulu.fi

Abstract. ETSI SmartBAN defines the basic access of an ad hoc personal wireless network for wearables around the human body. SmartBAN provides a communication interface for such wearables and a monitoring station known as the hub. In the next phase of development for SmartBAN, new use cases are explored. In particular Brain-Computer Interface (BCI) with implant devices. Recording neural activity with high spatial and temporal resolution has been elusive as it requires bulky and expensive equipment or highly invasive implants with limited throughput. To overcome such limitations, the use of THz technology is studied as it enables a small form factor and very high throughput. The paper presents an initial study on this promising technology for in-body applications and in particular the next generation of BCI systems.

Keywords: Brain Computer Interface · Body Area Networks · SmartBAN

1 Introduction

The paper explores the use cases of BCI (Brain Computer Interface) targeting the development of innovative neural technologies to advance the resolution of neural recording and stimulation toward the dynamic mapping of brain activity and neural processing with potential use in the THz band.

This study gives an overview of the state of the art in brain-based electronics and how this technology in the THz range may be used and developed. Hence, we summarize technologies for sampling, processing, and transmitting brain signals that have recently appeared in the literature.

These advanced neuro-technologies will enable new studies and experiments to advance the current understanding of the brain. Hence, enabling advances in diagnosis and treatment opportunities over a broad range of neurological diseases and disorders, as well as commercial applications.

© ICST Institute for Computer Sciences, Social Informatics and Telecommunications Engineering 2024
Published by Springer Nature Switzerland AG 2024. All Rights Reserved
M. Mizmizi et al. (Eds.): BodyNets 2024, LNICST 524, pp. 3–16, 2024.
https://doi.org/10.1007/978-3-031-72524-1_1

2   State of Art in Neural Recording

Studying the dynamics and connectivity of the brain requires a wide range of technologies to address temporal and spatial resolutions. In [1], the authors condensed the most relevant technologies. Figure 1 shows such spatial and temporal resolutions in the function of various brain monitoring technologies that are currently available: noninvasive methods such as Magnetic Resonance Imaging (MRI), Functional Magnetic Resonance Imaging (fMRI), Magneto-Encephalon-Graphy (MEG), and Positron Emission Tomography (PET) provide whole-brain spatial coverage. A summary of these technologies [1–5] is as follows:

- fMRI provides high spatial resolution (around 1 mm), but its temporal resolution is limited (1 to 10 s) for the system measuring neural activity [1].
- MEG provides higher temporal resolution (0.01 to 0.1 s) at the expense of spatial resolution (1 cm) [1].
- PET offers molecular selectivity in functional imaging at the expense of lower spatial (1 cm) and temporal (10 to 100 s) resolutions. However, neither fMRI, MEG or PET are suitable for wearable or portable applications, as they all require very large, expensive, and high-power equipment to support the sensors, as well as extensively shielded environments [1].

In contrast, electrophysiology methods that directly measure electrical signals from the neurons' activity, offer superior temporal resolution. They have been extensively used to monitor brain activity due to their ability to capture a wide range of brain activities from the subcellular level to the whole brain oscillation level as shown in Fig. 1 [1, 9–11].

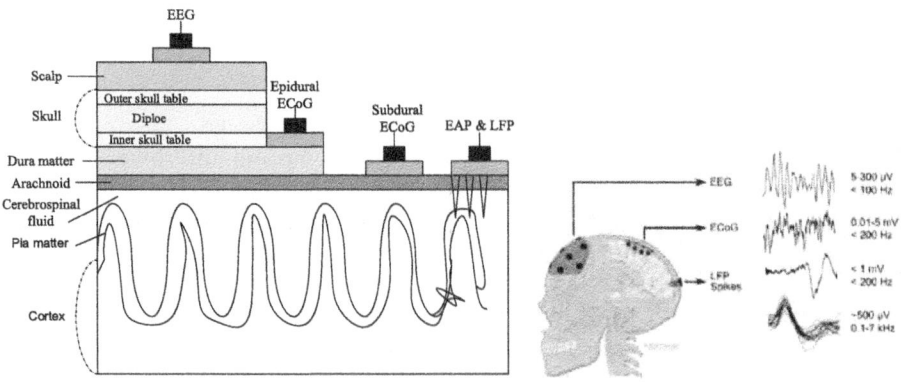

Fig. 1. Illustration of electrophysiology methods.

Due to recent advances in electrode and integrated circuit technologies, electrophysiological monitoring methods became portable with wearable or implantable configurations for BCI. In particular, Electro-encephalography

(EEG) records the electrical activity on the scalp resulting from volume con-
duction of neural activity across the brain, as shown in Fig. 1. Moreover, EEG
recording is noninvasive, but its spatiotemporal resolution is limited to about
1 cm and 100 Hz due to the electrical properties of diverse layers of head and
brain tissues, particularly the skull (between the brain and the scalp) [1,9–12].

In contrast, microelectrode technology such as Extracellular Action Potentials (EAPs) and Local Field Potentials (LFPs) enable recording from multiple neurons across multiple cortical areas and layers. Those can achieve much
higher resolution because of the closer proximity to individual neurons. Hence,
EAP+LFP techniques are widely used for brain research and BCI applications
[1,9,10]. On the other hand, microelectrodes may suffer from tissue damage
during insertion, and susceptibility to signal degradation due to electrode displacement with the time and immune response reaction against the electrodes.
Because of these issues, penetrating microelectrodes in humans is not yet viable
[1,9–12].

A practical alternative is an electrocorticography (ECoG), or intracra-
nial/intraoperative EEG (iEEG) [1], which records synchronized postsynaptic
potentials at locations much closer to the cortical surface, as illustrated in Fig. 1
[1,9–12].

ECoG has a higher spatial resolution than EEG, a higher signal-to-noise
ratio, broader bandwidth, and much less susceptibility to displacement. Furthermore, ECoG does not penetrate the cortex, does not scar, and can have superior
long-term signal stability recording. Furthermore, advances in integrated circuits enable high channel count and wireless operation, ECoG has become an
important tool not only for more effective treatment of neurological disorders,
like epilepsy, but also for investigating other types of brain activity across the
cortical surface, and its applications to BCI systems. ECoG recording provides
stable brain activity recording at a mesoscopic spatiotemporal resolution with a
large spatial coverage or at least a significant area of the brain [1,9–12]. Figure 2
shows the deployment of ECoG devices, illustrating the high spatial resolution
[11,12].

Advanced and miniaturized electrode arrays have reached a spatial resolution
of less than 1 mm, enabling monitoring of large-scale brain activity with greater
accuracy. Moreover, wireless implantable microsystems based on flexible technology can record more closely to the cortical surface while enabling coverage
along the natural curvature of the cortex without penetration as shown in Fig. 3
[1,9–12].

This ECoG technology, labeled as μECoG, enables even higher spatial resolution than conventional ECoG systems and is beginning to enable next-generation
brain mapping, therapeutic stimulation, and sophisticated BCI systems. Therefore, recording with modern implementations of ECoG arrays falls into one of
two categories [1,12]:

1) Medium-size brain regions (about 80 mm × 80 mm) at low spatial resolution
   10 mm electrode spacing): conventional ECoG [1,9–12].

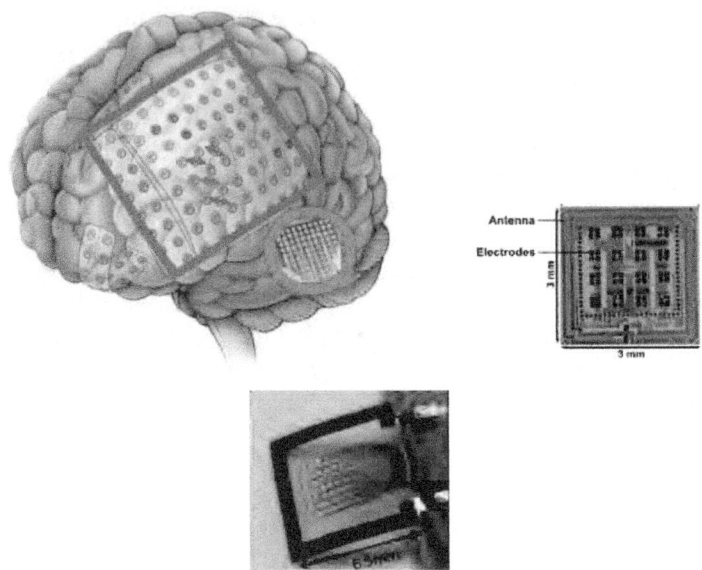

Fig. 2. Illustration of ECoG deployed in the brain.

2) Small brain regions (10 mm × 10 mm) at high spatial resolution (0.5–1mm electrode spacing): µECoG [1, 9–12].

The paper discusses the potential and feasibility of a wireless interface for the next generation of µECoG electrode arrays, illustrated in Fig. 2, including recording, stimulation of large regions of the brain at a high spatial resolution, as well as energy harvesting, power management, and data communications processing in the THz band. This is a hot topic of research with references in literature, although none in the THz band region. We indicate significant and illustrative implementations.

3   Brain Computer Interface Wireless Node

Neural data acquisition with a high spatial resolution requires a high channel density of µECoG arrays and, consequently, smaller electrode size. If the area overhead of the application-specific integrated circuits (ASIC) should be kept small, then the area dedicated to the functions illustrated in Fig. 4 [1, 12–19].

On the other hand, a denser array of amplifiers in the Analog front-ends (AFE), will dissipate more power and generates more heat [1, 19]. Thus, the power of each AFE must be reduced to meet thermal regulatory limits.

Unfortunately, As the signal power decreases, the signal-to-noise ratio (SNR) also decreases, affecting the transmission or reception performance requirements for wireless signals. However, a higher channel count requires higher communication throughput, increasing the power consumption and heat dissipation of the

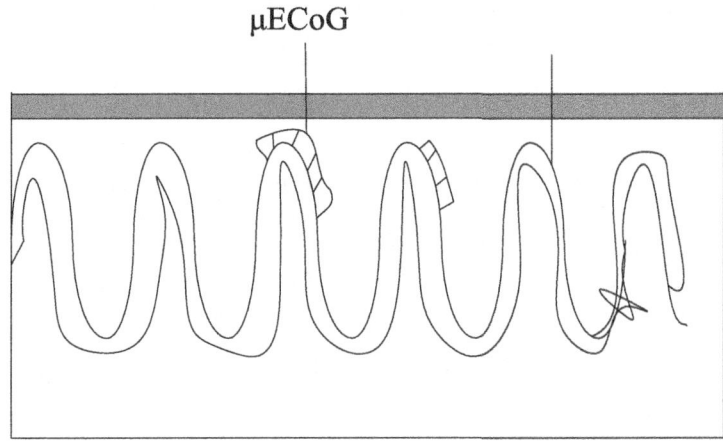

Fig. 3. Implantable μECoG on flexible substrate.

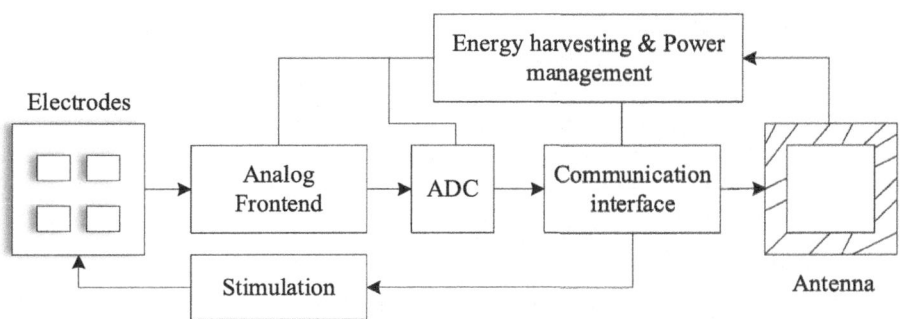

Fig. 4. Schematic diagram of functional blocks for BCI node.

communication interface. All these requirements are interrelated and trade-off with each other. Also, there are several circuit designs challenges, like difficulty in using external components such as inductors or capacitors [1,12–19].

3.1   Energy Source Subsystem

The constrained environment around the brain presents an energy source challenge. Indeed, one of the mayor challenges on implantable μECoG arrays for BCI nodes is how to power such implantable devices. Even logistically, it is an issue. For example, the electrode array is placed on the cortex, while the other components are placed under the scalp connected with lead wires or better mounted over a titanium plaque that replaced part of the skull by a craniotomy, eliminating the risk of infection by the lead wires. Regardless of placement, the constrained environment around the brain presents a energy source challenge. There are three primary methods for powering an implanted device 1) use a battery,

2) harvesting energy from the environment, 3) delivering power transcutaneous via a wireless power transmitter [1, 12, 19].

3.1.1 Battery

Popular medical implant application such as pacemakers has used batteries extensively. However, it makes sense to use a battery in a pacemaker, because the required power is relatively small (microwatts) and there is a large physical area available such that a battery can last around 10 years.

In contrast, the power consumption in high-density neural recording and stimulation applications is typically much larger (milliwatts), and the physical volume available for a large battery is very small, making it unfit [1, 17, 18].

Another important aspect is that going through surgical re-implantation to replace a battery is unacceptable to most patients. The medical risks of regular brain surgery and recovery disqualify batteries from being employed in high-density neural applications [1, 17, 18], [?].

3.1.2 Energy Harvesting

Harvesting energy from ambient sources in local environments is a potential power source option. Although theoretically attractive for implant neural devices, the limited area available near the brain and the stochastic nature of many energy harvesting sources result in a power source that is too small and too variable to operate multi-channel neural technologies [1, 18].

3.1.3 Wireless Power Transfer

The most promising means to power an implanted device with higher power requirements than pacemakers is to deliver energy wirelessly via a transcutaneous link, also known as wireless power transfer (WPT) [1, 6, 15–19].

A transcutaneous link may use electromagnetic waves (typically near-infrared light), acoustics (typically at ultrasound frequencies), or radio waves (obviously not in the light range). Each method can deliver up to mW of energy power. However, such delivered energy varies according to the geometry, material, implant depth, and alignment of the implanted device.

- On the other hand, WPT via infrared light has a short penetration depth (around mm), confining its benefit to subcutaneous applications [1, 6].
- Ultrasound can penetrate deeper into tissues. However, it is known that ultrasound hardly penetrate bone, reducing the energy transfer to implants from outside the skull.
- Radio waves are generally considered the most efficient and practical WPT method to implant devices on brain tissues (inside the skull) [1, 6, 15–19]. Therefore, the most promising transcutaneous power delivery approach utilizes electromagnetic waves.

However, WPT with radio waves to in-body implants has challenges. Conductivity and losses in tissues and bone depend on the radio frequency. Moreover, the usage of a given radio spectrum is constrained by government regulations. For medical devices additional regulations limit the amount of dissipated energy over tissues for safety reasons. For example, the FCC sets a specific absorption rate (SAR) of less than 1.6 W/kg in the USA. For these reasons WPT to in-body implant devices using radio waves should be carefully designed.

Technology-wise, recent advances microelectronics, sensors, and antennas with small form factor show that WPT would perform better at higher frequencies, while operating with low tissue heat-up under regulatory limits [1,6,15–19].

Consequently, in a next step on research, we will investigate implementations of electronics in the THz band and its effect on human tissues and bone.

3.1.4 Communication Interface

Sophisticated in-body implant devices, such as µECoG, shall transmit the data from sensors to an external controller or access point (AP) via a wireless link, where the information can be processed and monitored for diverse healthcare applications.

In contrast to conventional star topologies for wireless networks, the external controller or AP must support more traffic data from implant devices to the AP, known as the uplink, than the other way around (downlink).

Depending on the number of aggregated data links from sensors (also known as channels), the overall uplink aggregated data rate can be significantly high (in the order of Mb/s or higher) and that will require high power consumption. However, in-body implanted devices are subject to hard power consumption constraints. Reconciling the technologies required to power such devices such as WPT and the amount of transmitted data to an AP is incredibly challenging.

On another note, the radio waves for the uplink may be in the near-field or far-field, depending on the application. Assuming the AP is mounted on goggles or headband, the radio link is in the near field, while if the AP is over 1 m, the radio link is in the far field. SmartBAN was designed to work in the far field. However, it will not require much modification to the MAC layer but will require a new PHY to cope with near-field and far-field protocols for communication and WPT in the THz band. The current state-of-the-art of wearable radios, like Bluetooth Low Energy, require more than 1 nJ/bit [1,19], which is larger than what a typical µECoG device uses. Hence, the design problem is divided into two categories: research directions in THz spectrum, and a transition phase.

An intermediate transition phase assumes one fusion center mounted on a titanium plaque implanted on the skull (part of the skull is removed to fit the titanium plaque). Such a fusion center can connect µECoG devices implanted in the brain tissues via small cables. The wireless interface is in the fusion center to connect to an external AP. In that manner, the aggregated throughput is centralized in one unit, which is not close to the brain tissue and consequently can tolerate heat-up.

A candidate is UWB technology. UWB enables low power consumption (around pJ/bit). However, due to government regulatory constraints, the allocated UWB band varies from country to country, and it is not possible to operate a system in the range of 3.1 to 10 GHz anymore. However, the THz band allows operation with the potential high bandwidth required to operate BCI wireless links.

Next, we describe the potential technologies for a wireless interface in the THz band.

3.2 Backscatter Communications

Near-field communications operate at distances about one wavelength of the carrier frequency. Hence, it is suitable when the AP is located on the head, for instance, on virtual reality goggles, headbands, or the titanium plaque on the skull.

Regarding the WPT interface for the downlink (AP to the implanted device), the backscattering method is one of the most popular. Backscattering is a technique to transfer power wirelessly from a transmitter to a receiver by modulating the impedance of the receiver's antenna such that the carrier signal from the transmitter gets more absorbed at the receiver's antenna or more reflected to the transmitter. The principle is that the reflected carrier signal from the receiver modulates the information bits using a switch. In that manner, the power consumption on the μECoG's communication interface is minimal (around pJ/bit) [1,6,15].

However, the data reception of the reflected carrier signal at the transmitter depends on the power of such backscattered signal, which in turn depends on the system design and distance between transmitter and receiver. Backscattering is best suited for applications where low to moderate power transfer is sufficient and energy efficiency and passive operation in the implanted devices are priorities. That is the case for BCI applications with implanted devices.

3.2.1 ECoG Wireless Links

BCI applications with implanted μECoG lead toward short-range wireless links, where the processing power, power consumption, and size of μECoG devices are significantly constrained. We are addressing potential applications where μECoG devices typically have a depth of a few cm and high-throughput neural recording. Hence, WPT seems the best candidate as the primary mode of power supply due to its efficiency and robustness in comparison to ultrasound and energy scavenging [1,6,15].

Over the years, several methods of WPT have been proposed. The case of inductive power transfer has been the focus of studies resulting in the development of efficient designs and methodologies. Moreover, near-field communication (NFC) using inductive links is a low-cost solution [1,6,15–19] (Fig. 5).

On another note, μECoG devices may be arranged with three configurations: a device placed on the cortex, an electrode array placed on the cortex with a cable interface to the fusion center in the skull, or placed under the scalp [1,6,15], [16–19]. Figure 6 shows the first two cases. In these configurations, the location of such devices results in a challenge for WPT and data communication.

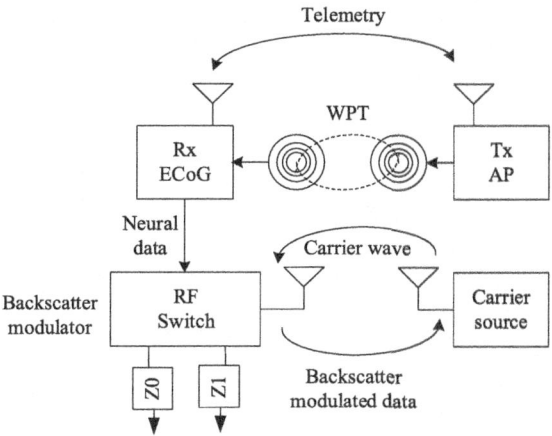

Fig. 5. Schematic diagram of backscatter communication.

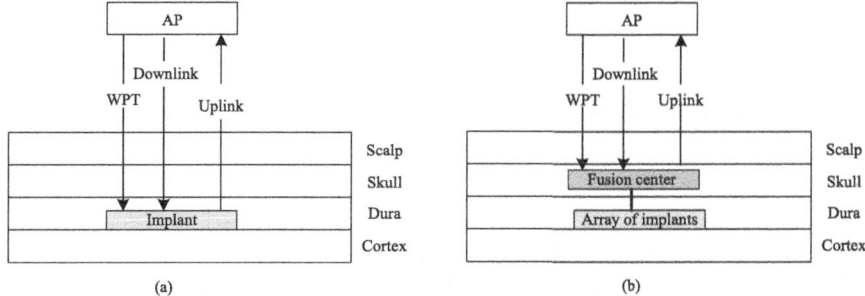

Fig. 6. Illustration of WPT and data communication links of an μECoG (a) and array of μECoG or electrodes to a fusion center (b).

To have an idea of the throughput requirements and design parameters, let us assume an example of μECoG recording with 1024 channels with a sampling rate of 600 samples/s per channel and a data resolution of 10 bits. The digital recording requires 6.15 Mb/s. Similarly, 64-channel recording with 10,000 samples/s and 10-bit resolution requires 6.4 Mb/s. That is to increase the brain area of the recording at a moderate sampling rate (losing resolution) or to increase the resolution in a smaller area [1, 6, 15].

The point is that for the transmission of this data rate figure, advanced implementations of implant devices transmitting at these data rates, typically consume mW []. Moreover, the position of the antenna's implant device on brain tissue has an impact on the WPT and communication link requirements. Implementations for transmitting and receiving radio waves may be based on coil designs or using printed antennas [1, 6, 15].

The use of THz frequencies would enable a small antenna form factor and electronics and consequently decrease the power consumption requirements while maintaining high throughput. Figure 7 shows reported configurations for implementation [1, 6, 15–19].

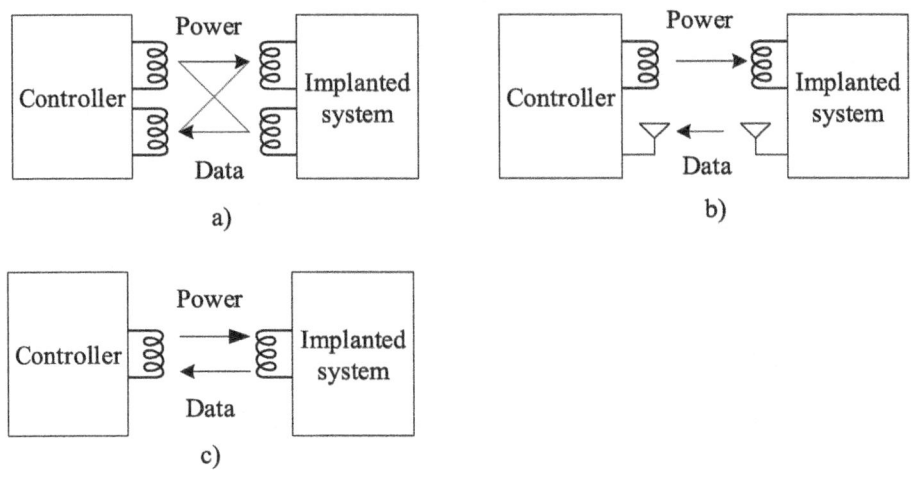

Fig. 7. Radio interfaces for WPT and data communication.

1) Using two inductive links for WPT and data communication, respectively, are shown in Fig. 7(a). The links are optimized to achieve a high data rate while maintaining high power transfer efficiency. However, this approach experiences cross-talk [1, 6, 15].
2) Using two different carrier signals as shown in Fig. 7(b). The scheme can achieve the required data rate. However, it requires more energy for data communications and increased antenna configuration complexity [1, 6, 15].
3) The simplest configuration approach using one inductive link for WPT and data communications is illustrated in Fig. 7(c). In this case, backscattering is used for passive data communication [1, 6, 15].

4   Body Terahertz Networks

Covering significant portions of the brain with an adequate sampling resolution will require a high throughput to be handled adequately for one central unit with significant processing and power constraints.

Therefore, we research the use of THz technology for WPT and data communication due to the recent advances in the field.

Figure 8 shows classifications of the THz band. From the RF spectrum perspective, THz frequencies start at 100 GHz (0.1 THz), while from an optical communication perspective, the THz band is below 10 THz (the far-infrared spectrum). Most publications are within this spectrum range, and according to

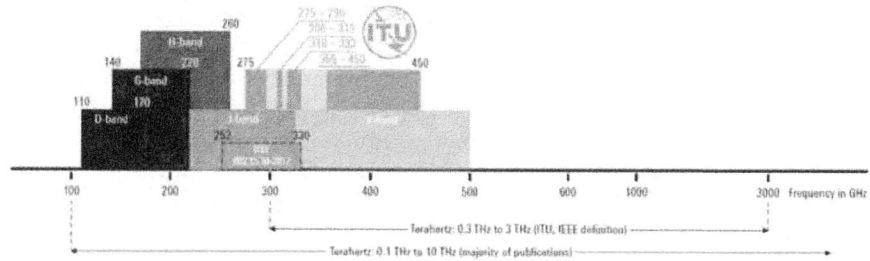

Fig. 8. THz frequency bands.

the ETSI Industry Specification Group THz. Other standardization body, IEEE 802.15.3-2023 specifies the range 252.72 GHz to 425.52 GHz.

Some medical applications use already the THz band, such as in oncology, and medical imaging. Due to the short-range connectivity, small form factor, and wide available bandwidth, the THz band enables connectivity of in-body wireless networks. Moreover, THz radiation is relatively safe on biological tissues []. Hence, the THz spectrum can improve the performance of existing Body Area networks, enabling various medical applications. In particular, a THz-based network can operate inside the human body in real time for health monitoring and medical implant communication. Therefore, THz technology is very attractive for the next generation of BCI systems.

On another vein, THz systems have been associated with the operation of nano-machines and interaction with so-called molecular communications. However, the paper does not consider these applications, but rather the potential use of radio interfaces for WPT (source power) and communication of high data throughput in a small form factor, power-efficient, and safe for human tissue, which are closer to practical implementations.

Indeed, the proposed BCI use case and the use of THz bands may be seen as part of the key enablers for 6G next generation of wireless communications, as it enables E-health for all, fully merged virtual worlds, mixed reality and immersive events, like sports, entertainment, gaming, work, social networks.

4.1   Enhancements to Channel Modeling

THz technologies still face various challenges. Among others, propagation characteristics of THz channels. Indeed, describing THz channel measurements and modeling indicate:

1) Path loss and shadowing (large scale) parameters in THz bands exhibit specific features compared to frequencies below 100 GHz. THz waves suffer much higher free space path loss when compared to mm-wave and lower frequencies. Moreover, its properties of penetration, diffraction, and scattering are different.

2) Similarly, small-scale (fast-fading) parameters are also unique to the THz band [i.9].
3) Furthermore, molecular absorption and the effect of changing ambient conditions, like humidity, cannot be neglected in the case of THz channels [i.9].
4) THz wavelengths are small compared to mm-wave wavelengths, resulting in a reduction of the effective aperture antenna. Hence, a THz antenna array would be attractive to implement in the uplink receiver. However, this means that the Rayleigh distance (the conventional boundary between the near field and far field) may be larger than the communication range, and then spherical wave modeling is required [i.9].
5) The spatial non-stationarity (antenna elements at different spatial positions may capture different multipath characteristics) may need to be modeled for the THz bands as the antenna array aperture may be larger relative to the wavelength [i.9].

4.2   Electronic and Photonic Technologies

Electronic sources have advanced in the past years, especially with the refinement of various semiconductor materials. For example, frequency multiplier chains with resonant tunneling diodes (RTD). However, they still have certain limitations in bandwidth and efficiency. There are two methods of generating THz radiation using photonic devices:

1) Direct THz generation with optical sources includes the quantum cascade laser (QCL) or nonlinear optics that directly generate THz radiation. Reasonable power levels can be reached with QCL, but the efficiency is still limited as they operate at cryogenic temperatures.
2) Indirect THz generation involves one or more devices oscillating at a much higher frequency (typically infrared or optical) along with a nonlinear mixing device. For example, the output of two continuous wave single-mode lasers with closely spaced emission frequencies, v_1, and v_2, respectively, are mixed in an ultrafast photodetector inducing a photocurrent-modulated at the optical frequency of $v = v_1 - v_2$ in the THz region. The photo mixing technique has the advantage that tuning the lasers is relatively easy with current technology, and consequently, the difference frequency can be varied over a broad spectral range, or highly tunable THz radiation.

5   Conclusions

THz bands are promising candidates for future radio systems due to potential applications beyond high data rate capacity such as integrated sensing and imaging. In particular, THz technology enables in-body networking that for the case of BCI supports high spatial and temporal resolution for neuro recording. The paper highlights the promising THz technologies for the next generation of BCI. In a future publication, the authors will address implementations.

Acknowledgement. This work is partially funded by Academy of Finland.

References

1. Ha, S., et al.: High-Density Integrated Electrocortical Neural Interfaces Low-Noise Low-Power System-on-Chip Design Methodology. Academic Press (2019)
2. Steinmetz, N.A., et al.: Challenges and opportunities for large-scale electrophysiology with Neuropixels probes. Science Direct (2018). https://doi.org/10.1016/j.conb.2018.01.009
3. Gutruf, P., et al.: Implantable, wireless device platforms for neuroscience research. Science Direct (2017). https://doi.org/10.1016/j.conb.2017.12.007
4. Ghosh, S., et al.: Probing the brain with molecular fMRI. Science Direct (2018). https://doi.org/10.1016/j.conb.2018.03.009
5. Seo, D., et al.: Neural dust: an ultrasonic, low power solution for chronic brain machine interfaces. In: The Future of the Brain: Essays by the World's Leading Neuroscientists. Princeton University Press (2015). https://doi.org/10.2307/j.ctt9qh0x7
6. Costello, J.T., et al.: A low-power communication scheme for wireless, 1000 channel brain-machine interfaces. J. Neural Eng. **19**, 036037 (2022). https://doi.org/10.1088/1741-2552/ac7352/pdf
7. Lee, A.-H., et al.: A distributed ensemble of wireless intracortical microdevices for charge-balanced photovoltaic current stimulation. In: International IEEE/EMBS Conference on Neural Engineering (2021)
8. St. Amant, R.: 2018 BioElectronic medicine roadmap. Semiconductor Research Corporation. https://www.src.org/program/bem/bem-roadmap-2018-final-1st-edition.pdf
9. Laiwalla, F., et al.: A distributed wireless network of implantable sub-mm cortical microstimulators for brain-computer interfaces. In: 41st Annual International Conference of the IEEE Engineering in Medicine and Biology Society (EMBC) (2019)
10. Mahmood, M., et al.: Wireless soft scalp electronics and virtual reality system for motor imagery-based brain-machine interfaces. Adv. Sci. (2021). https://doi.org/10.1002/advs.202101129
11. Lee, J., et al.: Distributed wireless networks of microimplants for neural recording and stimulation. IEEE Brain Newsl. (2022). https://brain.ieee.org/newsletter/2022-issue-1/distributed-wireless-networks-of-microimplants-for-neural-recording-and-stimulation
12. Seymour, J.P.: State-of-the-art MEMS and microsystem tools for brain research. Microsyst. Nanoeng. (2017). https://www.nature.com/articles/micronano201666#Abs1
13. Brodnick, S.K., et al.: μECoG recordings through a thinned skull. Front. Neurosci. (2019). https://doi.org/10.3389/fnins.2019.01017/full
14. Keramatzadeh, K., et al.: Wireless, miniaturized, semi-implantable electrocorticography microsystem validated in vivo. Sci. Rep. (2020). https://doi.org/10.1038/s41598-020-77953-8
15. Park, Y.-G., et al.: Recent progress in wireless sensors for wearable electronics. Sensors **19**(20), 4353 (2019). https://doi.org/10.3390/s19204353
16. Muller, R.: A minimally invasive 64-channel wireless μECoG implant. IEEE J. Solid-State Circuits **50**(1) (2015)
17. Song, Y.-K.: A neural recording microimplants with wireless data and energy transfer link. In: 6th International Conference on Brain-Computer Interface (BCI) (2018)

18. Leung, V.W., et al.: Distributed microscale brain implants with wireless power transfer and MBPS bi-directional networked communications. In: 2019 IEEE Custom Integrated Circuits Conference (CICC) (2019)
19. Ture, K., et al.: Wireless Power Transfer and Data Communication for Intracranial Neural Recording Applications. Springer, Cham (2020)
20. Han, C., et al.: Terahertz wireless channels: a holistic survey on measurement, modeling, and analysis. IEEE Commun. Surv. Tutor. **24**(3) (2022)
21. Ericsson. Microwave backhaul beyond 100 GHz. Ericsson Technology Review (2017)
22. Nagatsuma, T., et al.: Advances in terahertz communications accelerated by photonics. Nat. Photon. **10**, 371–379 (2016)
23. Liebermeister, L., et al.: Optoelectronic frequency-modulated continuous-wave terahertz spectroscopy with 4 THz bandwidth. Nat. Commun. **12**, 1071 (2021)
24. Ishibashi, T., Ito, H.: Uni-traveling carrier photodiodes: development and prospects. IEEE J. Sel. Top. Quantum Electron. **28**(2), 1–6 (2022)
25. Castro, C., et al.: 32 GBd 16QAM wireless transmission in the 300 GHz band using a PIN diode for THz upconversion. In: Optical Fiber Communications Conference and Exhibition (OFC), pp. 1–3 (2019)
26. Dan, I., Ducournau, G., Kalfass, I., et al.: A 300-GHz wireless link employing a photonic transmitter and an active electronic receiver with a transmission bandwidth of 54 GHz. IEEE Trans. Terahertz Sci. Technol. **10**(3), 271–281 (2020)
27. Gashi, B., et al.: Broadband 400-GHz InGaAs mHEMT transmitter and receiver S-MMICs. IEEE Trans. Terahertz Sci. Technol. **11**(6), 660–675 (2021)
28. Reilly, R.B.: Neurology: central nervous system. In: Webster, J.G. (ed.) The Physiological Measurement Handbook. CRC Press, New York (2014)
29. Muller, R., et al.: A minimally invasive 64-channel wireless μECoG implant. IEEE J. Solid-State Circuits **50**(1) (2015)
30. Ahn, D., et al.: Optimal design of wireless power transmission links for millimeter-sized biomedical implants. IEEE Trans. Biomed. Circuits Syst. **10**(1) (2016)
31. Mercier, P.P., Chandrakasan, A.P. (eds.): Ultra-Low-Power Short-Range Radios. Springer, Cham (2015)

Implant and In-Body Communications: The ETSI SmartBAN Vision

Daisuke Anzai[1], Takahiro Ito[2], Hirokazu Tanaka[2], Matti Hämäläinen[3], Marco Hernandez[3], Tuomas Paso[3], and Lorenzo Mucchi[4(✉)]

[1] Nagoya Institute of Technology, Nagoya, Japan
`anzai@nitech.ac.jp`
[2] Hiroshima City University, Hiroshima, Japan
`{ito-t,hitanaka}@hiroshima-cu.ac.jp`
[3] University of Oulu, Oulu, Finland
`{matti.hamalainen,marco.hernandez,tuomas.paso}@oulu.fi`
[4] University of Florence, CNIT and CNR, Firenze, Italy
`lorenzo.mucchi@unifi.it`

Abstract. In this review, we envisioned how the new ETSI Smart-BAN wireless technology for smart body area networks can be utilised in implant and in-body communications. The use cases can be links, for example, between in-body medical devices (IMDs) such as wireless capsule endoscopes and their on-body counterpart, or between smart implants, in general. First, we briefly introduced the current trends of implant and in-body communications and showed some application examples of IMDs utilised in in-body wireless communications. The advantage of in-body ultra wideband communications was then discussed to highlight the ETSI SmartBAN approach for in-body communications standardisation.

Keywords: in-body · UWB · implantable medical devices

1 Introduction

To realise future personal wireless networks, a body area network (BAN), which can transmit healthcare/medical data around a human body, is one of the promising wireless communication technologies. The standardisation related to

Supported partially by the European Union's Horizon 2020 programme under the Marie Skłodowska-Curie grant agreements No. 346208 and No. 872752, the Research Council of Finland via 6G Flagship (grant 318927), Infotech Oulu, JST Moonshot R&D Grant Number JPMJMS2214-06, and JSPS KAKENHI Grant Number 21H01325.

body area communications was established in 2013 via the Technical Committee (TC) SmartBAN in The European Telecommunications Standards Institute (ETSI) [1]. In the field of wireless BANs, medical/healthcare-related applications, including vital data monitoring, sports, and entertainment, have been proposed and discussed. Wireless BANs can typically be divided to two classifications: on-body (wearable) BANs and in-body (implant) BANs. Main applications of on-body BANs includes vital data sensing and health condition monitoring. On the other hand, implantable or in-body medical devices (IMDs) in general have been included as one of the in-body BAN applications. As an example, a wireless capsule endoscope (WCE), which is used in gastrointestinal track studies, consists of a radio frequency (RF) communication circuit and an ultra-small camera inside a small swallowable pill-type device. Videos and images obtained by a WCE can be delivered to an external receiver to aid in the diagnosis of gastrointestinal disorders. In this review, we pay attention to IMD applications either using implanted or ingestible devices. Low-energy wireless connectivity should be required in such healthcare and medical applications to extend the device's lifetime to provide high trustability.

From these backgrounds, in addition to narrowband on-body physical layer solution [1], ultra wideband (UWB) technology is also focused in the ETSI TC SmartBAN to achieve reliability and low power consumption in in-body communications. In in-body communications, especially in UWB communications at higher UWB frequencies, the wireless signal suffers from significant attenuation, which may lead to undesired performance degradation. On the other hand, the wide spectrum UWB is utilising, still provides frequency diversity which helps to obtain better performance at the signal reception. Therefore, it is important to consider suitable communications systems to ensure the transmission quality. Therefore, we need to optimise modulation and detection schemes for UWB communications for IMDs. Additionally, this review introduces multiple-input multiple-output (MIMO) techniques to further improve the quality of in-body UWB communications. As a realisation example of implant UWB-MIMO transmission, this review also presents a design of implant-side diversity antennas and discusses the basic performance through electromagnetic simulations and experiments.

In this paper, as a literature review, we briefly introduce the current trends of implant and in-body communications systems, and show some application examples of IMDs utilised in in-body wireless communications. Then, the advantage of in-body UWB communications is discussed. To highlight the ETSI SmartBAN approach for the in-body communications standardisation, performance evaluation results with UWB-impulse radio (IR) scheme and energy detection solution are demonstrated. Also, this paper discusses the impact of MIMO-UWB systems on performance improvement for in-body UWB communications.

2   Literature Review on Implant Communications

2.1   Current Trends of Implant and in-Body Communications

Implant communications refer to the wireless communications between implanted medical devices as well as between smart implants and external, typically on-body devices. Figure 1 shows an example of system realisation with in-body communications. In-body communications extends this approach to ingestible or other non-implanted in-body devices. This technology plays a crucial role in various medical applications, including health monitoring, disease diagnosis, and treatment [2,3]. Regulatory bodies, i.e., the US Federal Communications Commission (FCC) and ETSI, define the frequency range for IMD communications [2]. The Medical Implants Communication Services (MICS) band, which operates at 402–405 MHz, is commonly used for implantable medical device communications [2,4].

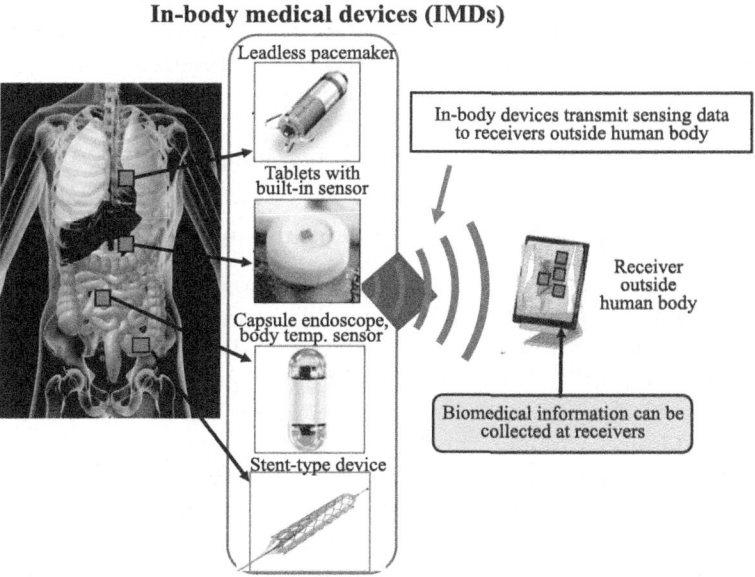

Fig. 1. In-body communication system example

Wireless communications in implantable and ingestible devices can be achieved through various methods. One approach is to use non-metallic or non-conductive biocompatible materials to package the wireless chip, which allows successful wireless communications [5]. Another method is to utilise the conductive properties of the body for wireless communications [5]. However, these methods have limitations in terms of transmission efficiency and miniaturisation [5]. Cooperative diversity has been proposed as a important approach to improve the performance of IMD communications schemes, improving implant lifetime and communications link reliability [6].

Implantable medical devices can also communicate with the body via molecules, enabling a symbiotic relationship between the device and the body [7]. Enzymes implanted in animals have been successfully used to establish a long-term communications with the body [7]. However, challenges, such as sterile inflammatory response, encapsulation, and degradation, need to be addressed for the long-term success of implanted devices [7]. This is valid also for ingestible medical devices. When developing IMDs for in-body applications, it is important to take biocompatibility into consideration.

2.2   Neural Implants

Neural implants target to develop and utilise novel applications of innovative neural technologies to advance the resolution of neural recording, and stimulation towards the dynamic mapping of the brain activity and neural processing. These advanced neuro-technologies will enable new studies and experiments to advance the current understanding of the brain. Hence, enabling advances in diagnosis and treatment opportunities over a broad range of neurological diseases and disorders, as well as commercial applications will open new ways for personalised healthcare. Due to the recent advances in electrode and integrated circuit technologies, new electrophysiological monitoring methods became portable with wearable or implantable configurations. ETSI SmartBAN will provide a reliable wireless connectivity to make this approach becoming a reality.

2.3   Advantage of in-Body UWB Communications

As described before, due to the existing regulation to realise the implant communications, commercially available IMDs usually select the 2.4 GHz and 400 MHz bands. For example, the 2.4 GHz and 400 MHz bands are used for wake up control and data transmission, respectively, in typical implant communication chip for cardiac pacemaker. However, in these frequency bands, data rates are only a few hundred kbps. Although this kind of data rate is sufficient for typical use cases, in view of the implant or novel in-body communications applications, such as WCE, data rate of more than 1 Mbps to provide reliable real-time image and video transmission is required, thus UWB is a good candidate [8].

UWB technology holds promise for implant and in-body communications. [9] highlights the advantages of UWB interfaces in terms of higher data transmission rates, although path losses may be higher. The authors of [10] support that UWB can establish reliable short-distance IMD communications with lower power consumption. Authors in [11] demonstrate the use of an energy detector as a receiver concept for UWB communications through human tissues. A compact UWB antenna design suitable for implant-to-air communications is presented in [12]. These findings collectively indicate that UWB technology can be effective for implant and in general, in-body communications, offering higher data rates and lower power consumption than the corresponding narrowband solutions. One benefit is also very low transmitted power spectral density, which makes the use of UWB safe for a human.

3   The ETSI SmartBAN Approach

In order to satisfy the requirements for implant and in-body communications to support next-generation IMDs, ETSI SmartBAN approach utilises UWB communications. Among the existing UWB modulation methods, UWB-impulse radio (IR) is a technology that repeatedly transmits extremely short pulses in nanoseconds per bit. Therefore, it has the advantage of low power consumption. Moreover, coherent detection (in other words, correlation detection) can be considered as one good suitable demodulation scheme for the receiver side. In the aid of the generation of a template signal in the coherent detection, the reliability is generally superior to that of non-coherent receiver.

Here, an example of UWB-IR implant communications system is presented. Figure 2(a) demonstrates one example of the transmitter structure. As a modulation scheme, a multi pulse position modulation (MPPM) is employed, which can control the data rate and the reliability based on the assignment of the number of UWB pulses to a modulation symbol. We can see that there is no carrier signal generator in the IR-type transmitter structure, which supports the realisation of low-power consumption at the transmitter side. On the other hand, Fig. 2(b) shows a realisation example of the receiver structure. In correlation detection, the binary MPPM selects one of two symbol mappings based on the calculation of the two different energies of the corresponding pulse assignment from the received signals. Also, the receiver does not require a threshold for detection. Synchronisation of the symbol timing is achieved by a pilot signal sent by the transmitter.

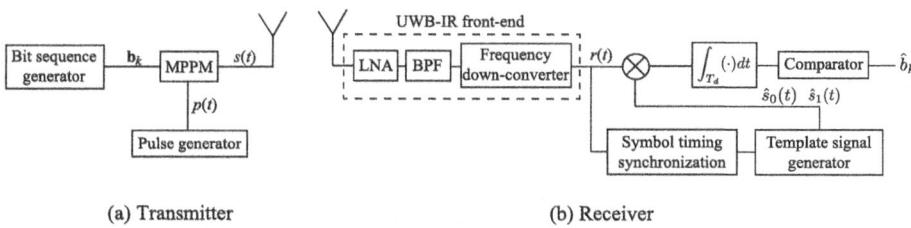

(a) Transmitter   (b) Receiver

Fig. 2. In-body transmitter and receiver structures.

Then, we discuss the fundamental performance of the in-body UWB-IR communications. In order to demonstrate the basic properties of in-body UWB communications, we conducted a measurement experiment using a liquid phantom. As a on-body receive antenna put on the liquid phantom surface with 1 cm-spacing, a helical-type antenna was used. Considering a transmit antenna inside the liquid phantom, a one-wavelength loop antenna was employed. To prevent direct touch from the transmit antenna to the liquid phantom, the transmit antenna, including the feeding point, was covered with glue. The relative permittivity and conductivity of the liquid phantom were set to those of muscle

tissue of a human body at the UWB band. For measuring the path loss characteristics, namely, S_{21} measurement, we used a vector network analyser (VNA)
connecting the transmit and receive antennas with coaxial cables. We beforehand
measured the S21 performance at a frequency of 4 GHz against the transceiver
distance. Figure 3 shows the measurement results in terms of the path loss characteristics over the distance between the transmit and receive antennas. From
these results, the path loss is around 80 dB at a depth of around 70 mm from
the body surface. It is possible to establish an implant wireless connection under
such a path loss level in present UWB techniques [8].

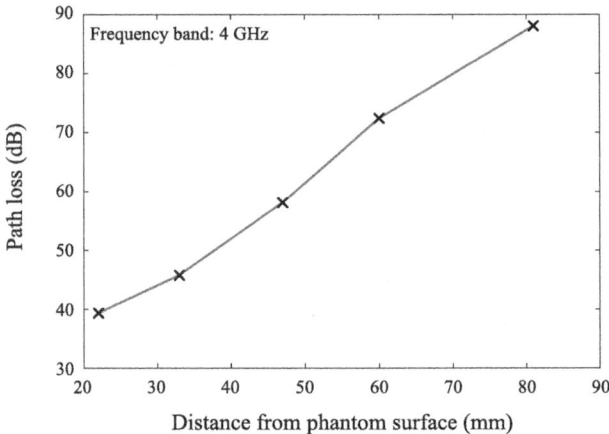

Fig. 3. Path loss measurement in phantom environment.

To introduce a multiple antenna system for in-body communications, this
paper assumes a polarisation diversity antenna at an in-body transmitter. In
order to accomplish the implantable polarisation diversity antenna, we developed an implant-side diversity antenna that contains two planar loop antennas.
Additionally, each antenna element was established to realise the polarisation
diversity in the UWB low band (from 3.4 GHz to 4.8 GHz) with a low reflection
coefficient and low coupling effect [13]. Figure 4(a) and (b) show the structure
of the one element and the overview of the developed implant diversity antenna,
respectively. The average path loss characteristics of the developed UWB diversity antenna were evaluated through a living animal experiment. Figure 4 shows
the measurement results. The path loss characteristics in two cases of excitation at either Port one or two are shown in Fig. 4(b). It should be noted that
we achieved a path loss of below 80 dB in the experimental environment. More
experiment details can be found in [14].

Next, let us discuss the improvement of the communications performance
using the implant (in-body in general) side diversity system. Figure 5 shows the
developed system model operating at the UWB low-band. As the transmitter
side, a UWB impulse radio (UWB-IR) scheme was employed. The On-Off Keying

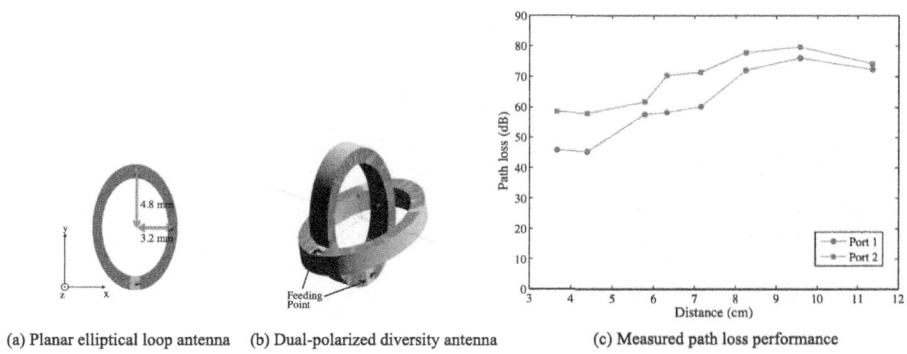

(a) Planar elliptical loop antenna   (b) Dual-polarized diversity antenna   (c) Measured path loss performance

Fig. 4. In-body diversity antenna performance.

(OOK) modulation with a pulse rate of 66 MHz was used. We adopted a selection diversity method with two implant antennas. On the other hand, the receiver used an equal gain combining (EGC) method with four receive antennas. After combining the signals received at each antenna, the receiver demodulates the signals with a non-coherent detection. We then carried out an experiment using the liquid phantom. In the experiment, we put the transmitter inside the liquid phantom, and the receiver antennas were put on the phantom's surface. We used a loop antenna shown in Fig. 4(a) and an imbalanced dipole antenna as the transmit and receive antennas, respectively. Note that both antennas satisfy the reflection coefficient S_{11} below -10 dB in the UWB low-band. Finally, Fig. 6 demonstrates the bit error rate (BER) performance for the developed UWB-MIMO system at each transmission point. As seen from the results, the MIMO transmission can increase the available transmission points (distance), where the BER of 10^{-2} is accomplished if compared with the single antenna case [15].

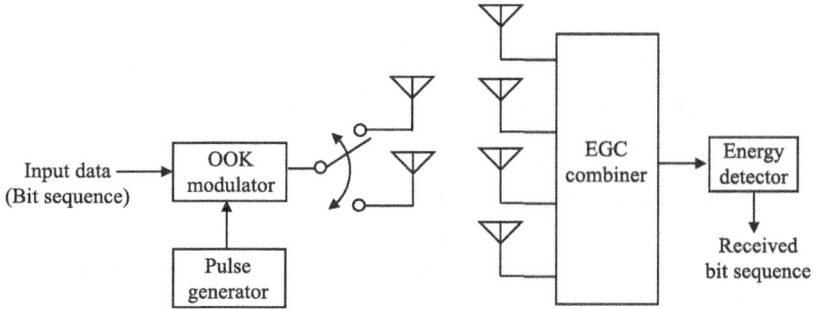

Fig. 5. Development of UWB-MIMO communication system.

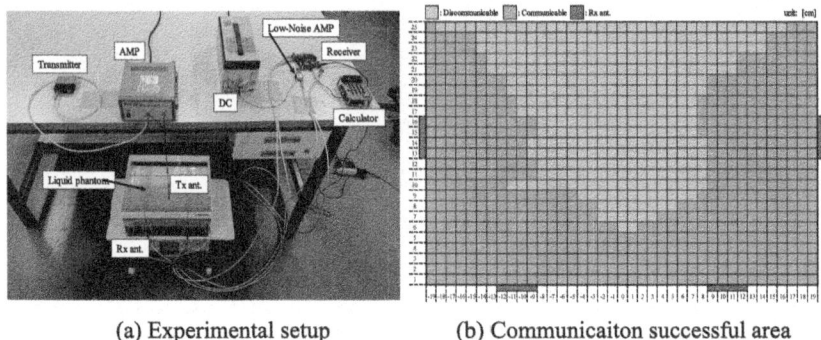

(a) Experimental setup   (b) Communicaiton successful area

Fig. 6. Performance evaluation on the developed UWB-MIMO communications.

4   Conclusions and Future Directions

In this paper, we have explored the potential of the UWB technology as a promising communications method for IMDs. Our findings and analysis have shed light on the numerous advantages that UWB offers in the context of IMDs, including high data rates, low power consumption, and robustness to interference. The utilisation of UWB for IMDs has the potential to revolutionise the field of medical implantable and in-body devices, offering improved performance and new capabilities for patient monitoring and treatment.

One of the key advantages of UWB technology is its ability to support high data rates, which is essential for transmitting a wide range of medical data from IMDs to external devices located on the body. This enables real-time monitoring of patient health and the collection of comprehensive data that can aid in early diagnosis and treatment adjustments. Moreover, the low power consumption of UWB devices ensures that IMDs can operate for extended periods without the need for frequent battery replacement or recharging, reducing patient inconvenience and healthcare costs.

Another notable benefit of UWB communications for IMDs is its resistance to interference. The ability to coexist with other wireless technologies in the crowded spectrum ensures reliable and secure communications between IMDs and external devices. This is particularly critical in healthcare settings where multiple co-located devices may be in operation simultaneously, and interference can have life-threatening consequences. Furthermore, UWB's fine time resolution and ability to operate in challenging environments make it suitable for a wide range of medical applications, including precise localisation of implanted and ingestible devices and effective communications through biological tissues. These capabilities open up new possibilities for targeted therapies and interventions that can improve patient recovery.

Notably, this paper gives the fundamentals of the ETSI SmartBAN approach to standardisation of UWB for IMDs. However, it is important to acknowledge that there are still challenges to address, such as global regulatory approvals, standardisation, and the development of compatible hardware and software ecosystems.

Acknowledgements. This work was supported in part by the Italian Ministry of Foreign Affairs and International Cooperation, grant number US23GR04 (CUP: D43C23000350001). We would like to thank the European Telecommunications Standards Institute's (ETSI) SmartBAN Technical Committee for given the opportunity to perform the studies towards ETSI standard.

References

1. Hmlinen, M., et al.: ETSI Smartban architecture: the global vision for smart body area networks. IEEE Access **8**, 150 611–150 625 (2020). https://ieeexplore.ieee.org/document/9167215
2. Joung, Y.H.: Development of implantable medical devices: from an engineering perspective. Int. Neurourol. J. **17**, 98 (2013). https://www.ncbi.nlm.nih.gov/pmc/articles/PMC3797898/
3. Li, P., Lee, G.A., Kim, S.W., Kwon, S.Y., Kim, H., Park, S.: From diagnosis to treatment: recent advances in patient-friendly biosensors and implantable devices. ACS Nano **15**, 1960–2004 (2021)
4. Islam, M.N., Khan, J.Y., Yuce, M.R.: A MAC protocol for implanted devices communication in the MICS band. In: 2013 IEEE International Conference on Body Sensor Networks (2013)
5. Ferguson, J., Redish, A.D.: Wireless communication with implanted medical devices using the conductive properties of the body. Expert Rev. Med. Devices **8**, 427–433 (2011)
6. Hegyi, B., Levendovszky, J.: Enhancing the performance of medical implant communication systems through cooperative diversity. Int. J. Telemed. Appl. **2010**, 1–10 (2010)
7. Alcaraz, J., Cinquin, P., Martin, D.C.: Tackling the concept of symbiotic implantable medical devices with nanobiotechnologies. Biotechnol. J. **13**, 1800102 (2018)
8. Anzai, D., Katsu, K., Chavez-Santiago, R., Wang, Q., Plettemeier, D., Wang, J., Balasingham, I.: Experimental evaluation of implant UWB-IR transmission with living animal for body area networks. IEEE Trans. Microw. Theory Tech. **62**(1), 183–192 (2014)
9. Garcia-Pardo, C., Chavez-Santiago, R., Cardona, N., Balasingham, I.: Experimental UWB frequency analysis for implant communications. 2015 37th Annual International Conference of the IEEE Engineering in Medicine and Biology Society (EMBC). IEEE (2015). https://doi.org/10.1109/embc.2015.7319626
10. Ghildiyal, A., Godara, B., Amara, K., Dalmolin, R., Amara, A.: UWB for low power, short range, in-body medical implants. In: 2010 IEEE International Conference on Wireless Information Technology and Systems. IEEE (2010). https://doi.org/10.1109/icwits.2010.5611844
11. Leib, M., Mach, T., Schleicher, B., Ulusoy, C., Menzel, W., Schumacher, H.: Demonstration of UWB communication for implants using an energy detector. In: German Microwave Conference Digest of Papers, pp. 158–161 (2010). https://api.semanticscholar.org/CorpusID:32206709
12. Dissanayake, T., Yuce, M., Ho, C.: Design and evaluation of a compact antenna for implant-to-air UWB communication. IEEE Antennas Wirel. Propag. Lett. **8**, 153–156 (2009). https://doi.org/10.1109/lawp.2009.2013370
13. Qorvo. Getting back to basics with ultra-wideband (UWB). White Paper (2021). https://www.qorvo.com/search?key=getting&mode=1&search-value=1

14. Shimizu, Y., Anzai, D., Chavez-Santiago, R., Floor, P.A., Balasingham, I., Wang, J.: Performance evaluation of an ultra-wideband transmit diversity in a living animal experiment. IEEE Trans. Microw. Theory Tech. **65**(7), 2596–2606 (2017)
15. Anzai, D., Ohta, M., Shimizu, Y., Balasingham, I., Wang, J.: Development and experimental evaluation on implant UWB-MIMO transmission. In: 2017 39th Annual International Conference of the IEEE Engineering in Medicine and Biology Society (EMBC) (2017)

Experimental Evaluation of Initial Connection Time with Interference in Body Area Network

Tatsuki Hiramatsu[1]([envelope]) [ID], Takahiro Ito[1] [ID], Daisuke Anzai[2] [ID], and Hirokazu Tanaka[1] [ID]

[1] Graduate School of Information Sciences, Hiroshima City University, 3-4-1 Ozuka-Higashi, Asaminami-ku, Hiroshima 731-3194, Japan
hiramatsu.tatsuki@mict.info.hiroshima-cu.ac.jp, {ito-t, hitanaka}@hiroshima-cu.ac.jp

[2] Graduate School of Engineering, Nagoya Institute of Technology, Gokiso-cho, Showa-ku, Nagoya 466-8555, Japan
anzai@nitech.ac.jp

Abstract. In recent years, demand for healthcare IoT including daily healthcare monitoring has been increasing. Body area network (BAN) is expected to be a core technology to realize such healthcare IoT. In particular, SmartBAN, a BAN technology standardized by the European Telecommunications Standards Institute (ETSI) and the International Electrotechnical Commission (IEC), is attracting attention. SmartBAN uses the 2.4 GHz ISM band, which may receive interference from various electronic devices such as wireless LAN and Bluetooth. In this paper, the influence of radio wave interference during the initial connection process of SmartBAN is experimentally evaluated by generating radio interference using devices that simulate an adaptive frequency hopping for Bluetooth. We measured the initial connection time when changing the hopping frequency and transmission timing of the interference wave sources and evaluated the effects of interference on the initial connection procedure of SmartBAN. The evaluation results revealed that although the connection time when there is interference may become slightly longer, it does not significantly affect the establishment of the initial connection.

Keywords: Body Area Network · SmartBAN · Radio interference

1 Introduction

Active Assisted Living (AAL) is attracting attention as an application field of healthcare IoT. AAL provides autonomous support to elderly people using ICT. Demand for AAL is expected to increase in the future in countries with aging populations, particularly in developed countries. A typical AAL service is a monitoring service that utilizes vital information, environmental information, location information, etc. obtained from various sensors and wearable devices attached on the body and placed in the surrounding area.

M. Mizmizi et al. (Eds.): BodyNets 2024, LNICST 524, pp. 27–34, 2024.
https://doi.org/10.1007/978-3-031-72524-1_3

One of the essential technologies to realize such healthcare IoT is Body Area Network (BAN). This paper focuses on Smart Body Area Network (SmartBAN). SmartBAN was first standardized by the European Telecommunication Standards Institute (ETSI) and later became an international standard by the International Electrotechnical Commission (IEC) in 2022. SmartBAN is a seamless IoT data collection technology characterized by four technical requirements: MAC protocol for low power consumption at the node, optimal QoS control, coexistence with other systems using the same frequency band, and a quick initial connection [1–3].

Among these technical features, this paper focuses on the initial connection procedure. Since SmartBAN uses the 2.4 GHz band, the signals transmitted from devices using the same frequency bands such as wireless LAN and Bluetooth may interfere with each other. To ensure a quick initial connection even with interference, the effects of interference on the initial connection need to be investigated. It is evaluated that the effect of radio interference on the initial connection procedure of SmartBAN by creating interference wave sources simulating Bluetooth frequency hopping and its hopping parameters.

2   Initial Connection Procedure of SmartBAN

The network based on SmartBAN consists of a hub and one or more nodes and employs a star topology. Figure 1 shows the channel structure of SmartBAN. SmartBAN allocates 40 channels in the 2.4 GHz band and each channel has 2 MHz bandwidth. Among the 40 channels, two types of channel configurations exist; three control channels (C-ch) and 37 data channels (D-ch). The control channel beacon (C-beacon) via C-ch provides information of the hub address, slot length, and data channel number. The data channel beacon (D-beacon) through D-ch acts as the communication timing trigger between the hub and nodes. The period between a D-beacon and the subsequent D-beacon, named Inter Beacon Interval (IBI), contains some timeslots for the node to transmit data packets.

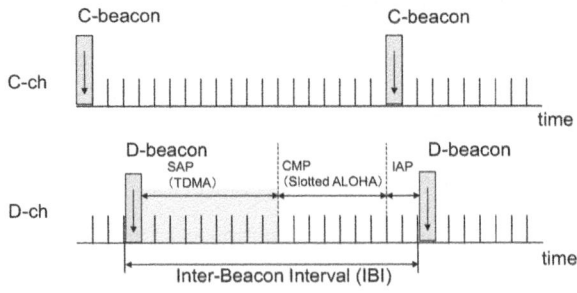

Fig. 1. Channel structure of SmartBAN

In SmartBAN, the IBI is divided into three periods: Scheduled Access period (SAP), Control & Management period (CMP), and Inactive period (IAP). In the SAP, transmission and reception are performed by time division multiple access (TDMA), and in the CMP, transmission and reception are performed by slotted ALOHA. The IAP does not send or receive data. The length information of these three kinds of periods are broad-casted through the D-beacon from the hub. The length of the IAP can be set to zero minimally.

Figure 2 illustrates the initial connection procedure. First, a node obtains the current D-ch number from the C-beacon transmitted by the hub via three C-ch. Next, the node starts to listen to the D-beacon on the designated D-ch. Upon receiving the D-beacon, the node attempts to transmit a connection request (C-req) towards the hub. If the hub successfully receives the C-req, an acknowledgement (ACK) is sent to the node in response. The hub then assigns an exclusive timeslot among the unassigned timeslots for data transmission and returns a Connection Assignment (C-Ass). The ACK for C-Ass is also sent back from the node to the hub. Theoretically, the initial connection completes within 3 times of IBI.

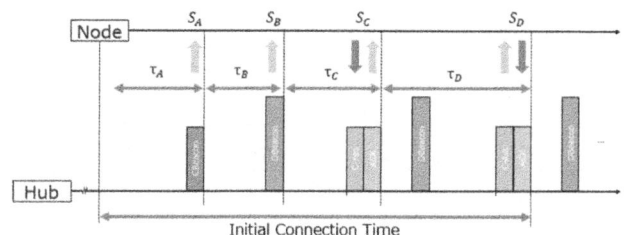

Fig. 2. Initial connection procedure

3 Experimental Evaluations

3.1 Evaluation Parameters

The initial connection procedure, as shown in Fig. 2, is divided into four phases. First, τ_A is the duration time from the node's startup to the receipt of C-beacon. Next, τ_B represents the duration between the node's receiving C-beacon and D-beacon. τ_C is from the end of receiving D-beacon to node's receipt of the ACK for C-req. Finally, τ_D is the remaining time until the end of the initial connection. The initial connection time is the total of all phases. Each phase consists of several timeslots, so the length of each phase is calculated by subtraction of finish timeslot number from start timeslot. For example, (τ_B) is calculated by the following equation.

$$\tau_B = T_s \times (S_B - S_A - 1) + e \tag{1}$$

Here T_s, S_A, S_B and e are the duration of a timeslot, the timeslot number of receiving C-beacon, the timeslot number of the acquisition of D-beacon and time synchronization error, respectively.

Table 1. Parameters of implemented transceivers

Frequency (C-Beacon)	2402/2426/2480MHz
Frequency (D-Beacon, C-req, C-Ass)	2440 MHz
IBI	16 slots (1280ms)
Slot length (T_s)	80ms
Modulation	GFSK
Number of Bits (C-Beacon)	120 bits
Number of Bits (D-Beacon)	144 bits
Number of Bits (C-req)	212 bits
Number of Bits (C-Ass)	184 bits

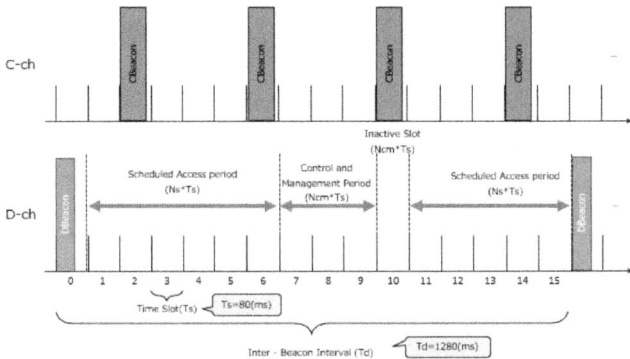

Fig. 3. Channel Structure of SmartBAN in experiment

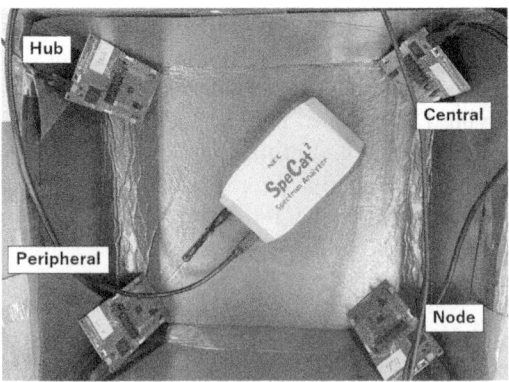

Fig. 4. Experimental environment

3.2 Experimental Conditions and Procedure

In this experiment, the SmartBAN hub and node were implemented using CC2650 evaluation boards. Table 1 shows the parameters of the devices. Figure 3 illustrates the channel structure of SmartBAN in this experiment. The hub periodically broadcasts C-beacon and D-beacon. The C-beacon is broadcasted via C-ch in order of control channel number (0, 12 and 39). The node starts the initial connection immediately after startup. The IBI consists of 16 time slots. The node receives C-beacon using only the C-ch number of 0 in this experiment due to time constraints and data collection.

Figure 4 illustrates the experimental environment. The hub and node are placed on the corner of a box (360 × 340 × 190 mm). This experiment was conducted in the box covered by the radio wave absorption sheet to reduce interference from other systems. Note that the spectrum analyzer is also located in the center of the box for monitoring the emitted wave strength. Two types of interference wave sources are implemented and placed in the vicinity of the SmartBAN system. In order to prevent measurement bias, the initial connection was started after waiting some moments, which was randomly selected between 0 to 1280 ms. The duration time of each phase is measured with repeating the initial connection procedure.

Table 2. Parameters of Interference wave sources

Frequency (Advertising channel)	2402/2426/2480 MHz
Frequency (Data channel initial value)	2404/2414 MHz
Advertising Interval	300 ms
Hop increment	6
Modulation	GFSK
Number of Bits (ADV_IND)	64 bits
Number of Bits (CONNECT_IND)	204 bits
Number of Bits (DATA)	816 bits

3.3 Interference Wave Source

The Central and Peripheral in Fig. 4 are implemented assuming Bluetooth [4]. The Central is a coordinator device in Bluetooth like hub in SmartBAN. The Peripheral is a device for collecting and transmitting information in Bluetooth like node in Smart-BAN. Table 2 shows the parameters of interference wave sources. Figure 5 illustrates the channel structure of interference wave sources. Bluetooth which is mainly used for wearable sensors allocates 40 channels in the 2.4 GHz band and each channel has 2 MHz bandwidth. Among the 40 channels, two types of channel configurations exist; 3 advertising physical channels and 37 data physical channels. These configurations are almost same with SmartBAN, so the advertising physical channels and the data physical channels may interfere with C-ch and D-ch in SmartBAN respectively. The Central observes

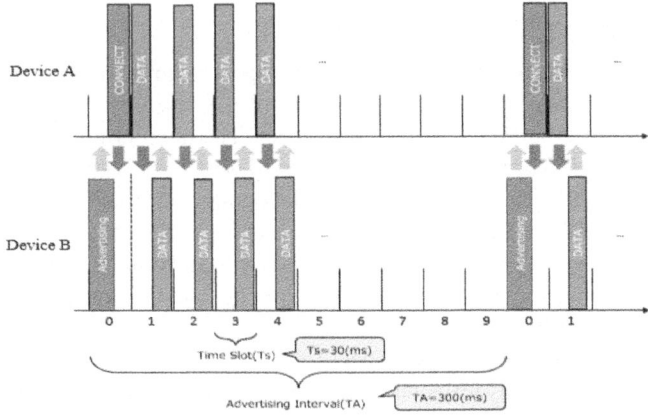

Fig. 5. Channel Structure of Interference wave source

the RSSI of each data channel after startup to create a channel map and waits until it receives the advertising packets from Peripheral. On the other hand, the Peripheral broadcasts advertising packets every 300 ms using the advertising physical channel. As with the SmartBAN hub, the advertising physical channels (37, 38, and 39) are used in turn for advertisement. When the Central receives an advertising packet, it immediately becomes the connected state by sending a connection request frame and changes the channel for data transmission based on the channel map. In this study, these devices repeatedly connect and disconnect to generate radio interference in both the C-ch and the D-ch in SmartBAN. Two situations are assumed in this experiment. As case A, the Peripheral broadcasts the adverting packet using 3 advertising physical channels, then, the Central uses only 39th channel to transmit and receive the connection request. The channel map is set to avoid the same data channel as SmartBAN. As case B, the Peripheral also broadcasts advertising packet using 3 channels, however, the Central uses 37th channels, which is same to the control channel in SmartBAN. The channel map in case B is set to use the same data channel as SmartBAN as one of the candidate channels use. Therefore, in case A, only the advertising interferes with the initial connection in SmartBAN. In addition, adverting, connection request and data transmission affect the initial connection time of SmartBAN in case B.

4   Evaluation Results

Table 3, 4 and 5 show the duration of each phase in the case of SmartBAN transceiver only, with case A, and with case B, respectively. From Table 3, the maximum of total initial connection time is 3505 ms. The IBI length is 1280 ms, so that the hub and node could complete the initial connection within the duration of 3 times of IBI. This result indicates that the packets were successfully sent and received at each phase. However, in the case of existing interference wave sources, Tables 4 and 5 show that the maximum values of total time become longer than the duration of 3 times of IBI, which indicates that packets may not be received at the proper timing due to radio interference. Comparing the results, the maximum of the initial connection time in Table 4 is longer for 809 ms than that in Table 3, moreover, the maximum of the initial connection time in Table 5 is longer for 1368 ms than that in Table 3. This means that the differences among them is whether the connection request and data transmission interfere with the initial connection in SmartBAN.

Figure 6 shows the histogram of the total initial connection time. From the result, the stronger interference, the longer initial connection time. The number of samples in case B over 3000 milliseconds increases compared with the others. This causes the significant increase of the standard deviation of total initial connection time in Table 5.

Table 3. Result without interference

	τ_A	τ_B	τ_C	τ_D	Total
Sample	288	288	288	288	288
Average (ms)	268	537	559	1296	2659
Maximum (ms)	851	800	560	1297	3505
Minimum (ms)	5	159	558	1295	2022
Std. Dev. (ms)	161	254	0.58	0.63	362

Table 4. Result with weak interference (case A)

	τ_A	τ_B	τ_C	τ_D	Total
Sample	289	289	289	289	289
Average (ms)	344	504	559	1296	2703
Maximum (ms)	1340	1120	560	1297	4314
Minimum (ms)	7	159	557	1295	2021
Std. Dev. (ms)	270	232	0.58	0.67	412

Table 5. Result with strong interference (case B)

	τ_A	τ_B	τ_C	τ_D	Total
Sample	287	287	287	287	287
Average (ms)	369	617	559	1296	2840
Maximum (ms)	1898	1760	560	1297	4873
Minimum (ms)	4	160	557	1295	2019
Std. Dev. (ms)	321	256	0.56	0.60	519

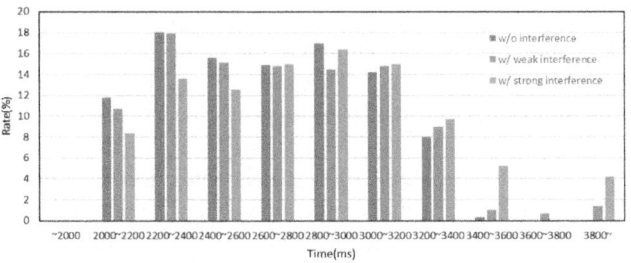

Fig. 6. Distribution of total initial connection time

5   Conclusions

In this paper, we evaluated the initial connection performance of SmartBAN hub and node using interference wave sources assuming Bluetooth devices. As a result, it was found that SmartBAN transceivers can complete the initial connection within three times of IBI in the case of without interference. In addition, they can still complete the initial connection within the duration of 4 times IBI even if the interference wave sources are communicating near the hub and node. One of the future works is to conduct more experiments using the interference wave sources with various conditions assuming realistic environments.

Acknowledgments. This work was supported by JSPS KAKENHI Grant Number 21H01325.

References

1. IEC 63203-801-1:2022. Wearable electronic devices and technologies - Part 801-1: Smart body area network (SmartBAN) - Enhanced ultra-low-power physical layer Nov. N (2022)
2. IEC 63203-801-2:2022. Wearable electronic devices and technologies - Part 801-2: Smart body area network (SmartBAN) - Low complexity medium access control (MAC) for SmartBAN (2022)
3. Tanaka, H., Hatakeyama, Y., Komori, T., Matsukuma, T.: Next generation body area network for healthcare application, SmartBAN. In: Proceedings on the 39th Annual International Conference of the IEEE Engineering in Medicine and Biology Society (EMBC 2017). FrBT4.2 (2017)
4. Bluetooth CORE SPECIFICATION Version 5.4. https://www.bluetooth.com/ja-jp/specifica tions/specs. Accessed 12 Nov 2023

Performance Improvement in Channel-Estimated Implant Communication by Spatial Transmit Diversity and Signal Pre-emphasis Technique

Lijia Liu$^{(\boxtimes)}$ ⓘ and Jianqing Wang

Nagoya Institute of Technology, Nagoya, Aichi 466-8555, Japan
`l.liu.103@stn.nitech.ac.jp`

Abstract. Human body communication (HBC) technology in the 10–60 MHz band offers ample possibilities for high-speed and deep-implanted communications with data rates over 10 Mb/s. However, signals transmitted within the human body undergo power decay and waveform distortion, while different orientations of the implant antenna can further decrease communication performance. This study proposes a spatial transmit diversity combined with a signal pre-emphasis technique to improve bit error rate (BER) performance. First, a two-branch spatial transmit diversity is established by an anatomical human body model and MHz-band small helix/spiral antennas. Then, a signal pre-processing method is applied to the on-body transmitter to counteract the channel fading and distortion. It extracts the channel response through channel estimation and adaptively alters the transmitted signal waveform, consequently deriving received signals optimized for demodulation. Finally, the effect of spatial diversity and signal pre-emphasis is evaluated by calculating the BER performance in a maximal ratio combining (MRC) simulation. The results indicate that applying pre-emphasis significantly improves the BER performance while implementing spatial transmit diversity can further enhance the signal-to-noise ratio (SNR) by 2–5 dB when the BER equals 10^{-3} at 20 Mb/s.

Keywords: Implant communication · Spatial transmit diversity · Channel estimation · Signal pre-emphasis technique

1 Introduction

Advancements in implantable medical technology are pushing wireless communication speeds within the human body from Kb/s-level to Mb/s-level. For

ⓒ ICST Institute for Computer Sciences, Social Informatics and Telecommunications Engineering 2024
Published by Springer Nature Switzerland AG 2024. All Rights Reserved
M. Mizmizi et al. (Eds.): BodyNets 2024, LNICST 524, pp. 35–41, 2024.
https://doi.org/10.1007/978-3-031-72524-1_4

instance, high-quality in-vivo image transmission by capsule endoscopes and
real-time control of a large number of micro-motors by implant surgical robots
require data rates of up to tens of Mb/s. However, the frequency-dependent
dielectric properties of human tissues can lead to severe signal attenuation and
waveform distortion, especially at a higher frequency band. The human body
communication (HBC) technique operating at tens of MHz band is a promising
option for deep-implanted communications due to its available wide bandwidth
and low power consumption. However, the long wavelength within this frequency
band poses a challenge for antenna miniaturization, consequently limiting the
communication bandwidth and transmission speed. Therefore, implementing a
spatial transmit diversity is expected to improve communication performance,
and the combination of a signal-processing method can further address channel
fading and distortion issues. By weighting the amplitude and correcting the phase
of transmitted signals, the impact of maximal ratio combining (MRC) diversity
can be directly applied at the in-body receiver. Additionally, the signal pre-
emphasis technique pre-processes the transmitted signal based on the channel
response to obtain an optimal received signal. In this paper, to clarify the effectiveness of spatial diversity and pre-emphasis technique, the bit error rate (BER)
performance is evaluated through computer simulations in the HBC band. The
enhanced signal-to-noise ratio (SNR) facilitates high-speed signal transmission
from on-body to in-body at a data rate of 20 Mb/s.

2   Spatial Transmit Diversity

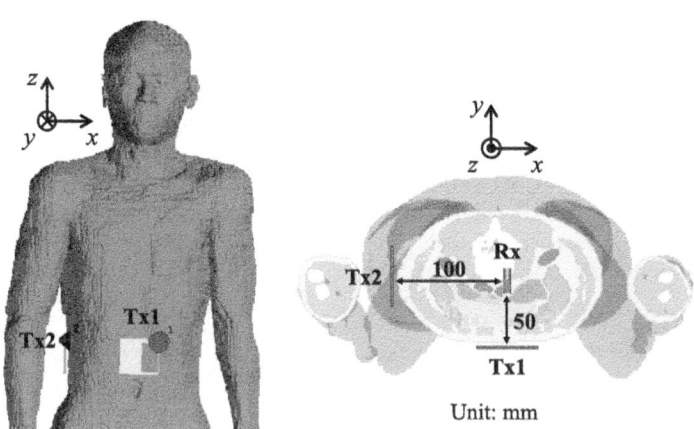

Fig. 1. Spatial transmit diversity model using a human body model and miniaturized
helix/spiral antennas. (Tx: transmitting antenna, Rx: receiving antenna)

As shown in Fig. 1, the spatial transmit diversity is modelled using an anatomical
human body model [1] and miniaturized helix/spiral antennas working in the 10–
60 MHz band [2]. The realistic human body model of an adult male features a

spatial resolution of 2 mm and incorporates 51 types of tissues, ensuring high-precision numerical simulations. The human body model used in the simulation indicates a lossy medium, with its frequency-dependent dielectric properties in the 10–60 MHz band producing a frequency-selective fading channel. Meanwhile, the antennas employed include a miniaturized helical implant antenna with a hollow cylindrical shape and two matched wearable antennas with spiral planar structures, for assessing the effects of spatial diversity and signal pre-emphasis technique.

To implement a two-branch spatial transmit diversity, two transmitting antennas (Tx1 and Tx2) are arranged on the frontal and lateral surfaces of the abdomen respectively, while a receiving antenna (Rx) is implanted within the small intestine at the same height. Specifically, the in-body Rx is positioned at a 5-cm distance from Tx1 and a 10-cm distance from Tx2, with its cylindrical axis aligned perpendicularly to Tx1 (an arrangement proved to have the maximum coupling strength) and parallel to Tx2. The two Tx antennas are excited to transmit the impulse signal with a pulse width of about 50 ns and a frequency component covering the 10–60 MHz band. Then, two sub-channels generate a correlation between the two received signals, and the correlation coefficient needs to be calculated to confirm the possibility of spatial diversity:

$$\rho(i,j) = \frac{\sum_{m=1}^{M} \left(U_{ri,m} - \overline{U_{ri}}\right) \left(U_{rj,m} - \overline{U_{rj}}\right)}{\sqrt{\sum_{m=1}^{M} \left(U_{ri,m} - \overline{U_{ri}}\right)^2 \sum_{m=1}^{M} \left(U_{rj,m} - \overline{U_{rj}}\right)^2}} \tag{1}$$

where $M = 2$ indicates two branches in the spatial transmit diversity, $U_{ri,m}$ and $U_{rj,m}$ are the instant received energies, and $\overline{U_{ri}}$, $\overline{U_{rj}}$ are their average values respectively. As a result, the calculated correlation coefficient between the two-branch received signals is 0.291, which is below 0.5, indicating the feasibility of spatial transmit diversity in this scheme [3].

3   Signal Pre-emphasis Technique

As shown in Fig. 2a, the diversity communication system comprises a diversity transmitter equipped with two Tx antennas and a receiver with a single Rx antenna. Pilot-based channel estimation is employed to derive the sub-channel responses $h_1(t)$ and $h_2(t)$, by transmitting a pilot signal from the receiver to the diversity transmitter. This attempt enables the amplitude weighting and phase correction of the two-branch transmitted pulse signals at the transmitter. To obtain an MRC diversity impact at the receiver, the amplitude of each transmitted pulse signal $s(t)$ needs to be weighted according to a weighting factor:

$$w_m = \frac{|v_m|}{\sqrt{\sum_{m=1}^{M} |v_m|^2}} e^{-j\phi_m} \tag{2}$$

$$\sum_{m=1}^{M} |w_m|^2 = 1 \tag{3}$$

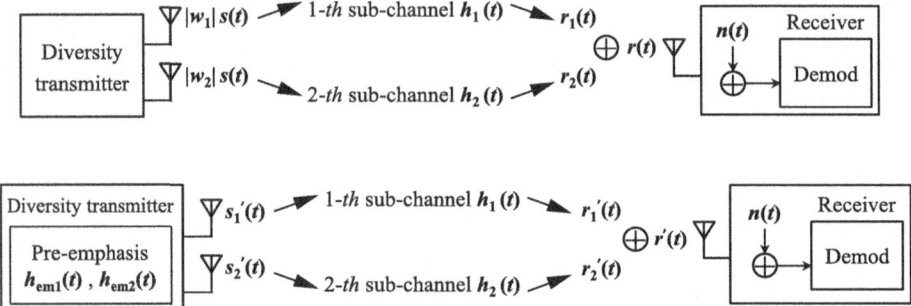

Fig. 2. Communication system model composed of two diversity branches (sub-channels). (a) Diversity transmitter without pre-emphasis. (b) Diversity transmitter with pre-emphasis.

where v_m represents the received signal magnitude from the m-th branch when sending a pilot signal from the receiver, and ϕ_m indicates the signal phases. As a result, the diversity weights $|w_1|$ and $|w_2|$ for the two branches are calculated as 0.988 and 0.103, respectively. Subsequently, the input power to each sub-channel is allocated by $|w_m|^2$, while the amplitude of each transmitted signal is adjusted according to $|w_m|$, respectively.

Based on the channel response derived by channel estimation, a signal pre-emphasis technique is implemented at the diversity transmitter to improve communication performance, as depicted in Fig. 2b. This pre-emphasis operates as a signal-processing method, effectively mitigating signal attenuation and waveform distortion induced by the frequency-selective channel fading in the simulation. It is characterized by a time response denoted as $h_{em}(t)$ and adaptively modifies the transmitted signal waveform before transmission to the channel. The frequency response of pre-emphasis is $1/H(f)$ which corresponds to the inverse of the channel frequency response $H(f)$. As a result, assuming in the time domain, based on two sub-channel impulse responses $h_1(t)$ and $h_2(t)$, the pre-emphasis reproduces two distinct transmitted signals $s_1'(t)$ and $s_2'(t)$:

$$s_1'(t) = |w_1|\, s(t) \otimes h_{em_1}(t) \tag{4}$$
$$s_2'(t) = |w_2|\, s(t) \otimes h_{em_2}(t) \tag{5}$$

where the $h_{em_1}(t)$ and $h_{em_2}(t)$ indicate the distinct time responses of pre-emphasis for two branches. Then, two optimized received signals are obtained and a combined received signal is derived for demodulation:

$$r_1'(t) = s_1'(t) \otimes h_1(t) = |w_1|\, s(t) \tag{6}$$
$$r_2'(t) = s_2'(t) \otimes h_2(t) = |w_2|\, s(t) \tag{7}$$

$$\begin{aligned} r'(t) &= r_1'(t) + r_2'(t) + n(t) \\ &= (|w_1| + |w_2|)s(t) + n(t) \end{aligned} \tag{8}$$

where $n(t)$ represents the thermal noise introduced at the receiver front end. As a result, since $|w_1| + |w_2|$ is greater than 1, the amplitude of the diversity-combined received signal exceeds that of the signal received without applying diversity. Meanwhile, with the removal of the channel effect from the received signals, effective mitigation of signal decay and waveform distortion can be achieved through the application of signal pre-emphasis technique.

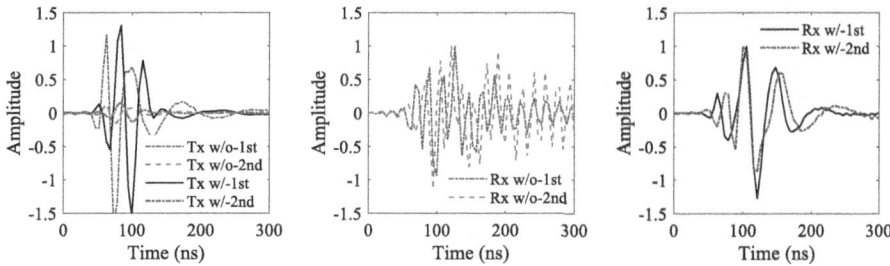

Fig. 3. Signal time waveforms. (a) Transmitted signals to two branches without and with pre-emphasis. (b) Normalized received signals from two branches without pre-emphasis. (c) Normalized received signals from two branches with pre-emphasis (after phase shift). (w/o: without pre-emphasis, w/: with pre-emphasis, 1st: the first branch in diversity, 2nd: the second branch in diversity).

Figure 3 shows the signal time waveforms, where the amplitudes of received signals are normalized to a maximum value of 1. The amplitudes of two-branch transmitted signals in Fig. 3a are adjusted respectively according to the weighting factor. As can be seen from Fig. 3b, the existence of two distinct sub-channels introduces a delay τ in the arrival time between two received signals. Transmit diversity typically removes time delays by integrating a phase detector and shifter in the transmitter. In this study, the time delay τ is determined through pilot-based channel estimation. Subsequently, the phases of transmitted signals are corrected to include a time difference in diversity transmitted signals, ensuring consistent arrival time between two received signals. As a result, the delay in arrival time between two received signals can be effectively eliminated, as shown in Fig. 3c, leading to an enhancement in the combined received power. Furthermore, in comparison to the signals depicted in Fig. 3b, the received signals employing pre-emphasis (depicted in Fig. 3c) exhibit a reduced time duration for optimizing demodulation at the receiver. The signal waveform distortion can also be mitigated apparently.

4   BER Performance in MRC Diversity

In channel-weighted transmit diversity, the amplitude weighting and phase correction of transmitted signals are performed at the transmitter, so that an MRC diversity effect can be achieved at the receiver. The received signals from two branches are directly combined at the receiver:

$$r_{MRC} = \sqrt{\sum_{m=1}^{M} |r_m|^2} \qquad (9)$$

where r_m indicates the root of received power from the m-th branch. (When applying pre-emphasis, it transforms into r'_m.) The MRC diversity presents an optimal combined SNR in comparison to other diversity schemes, in which the SNR can be maximized over the two branches:

$$\gamma_{MRC} = \frac{\sum_{m=1}^{M} |r_m|^2}{N} = \sum_{m=1}^{M} \gamma_m \qquad (10)$$

where N denotes the power of thermal noise introduced at the receiver front end:

$$N = kT_0 N_F B \qquad (11)$$

where $k = 1.38 \times 10^{-23}$ J/K is the Boltzmann constant, $T_0 = 300$ K is the environment temperature, $N_F = 5$ dB is the noise figure of the receiver, and B is the transmission bandwidth of 50 MHz.

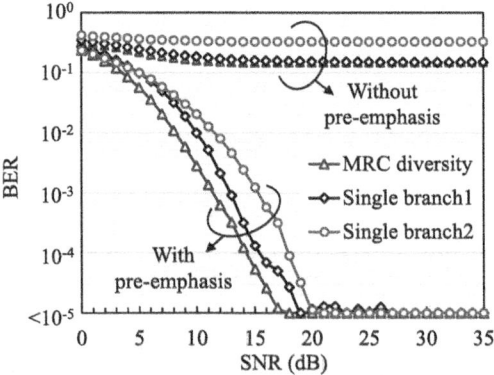

Fig. 4. BER performance without and with pre-emphasis for MRC diversity and single branches 1, 2.

As a consequence, the BER performance is evaluated for MRC diversity both with and without pre-emphasis at a data rate of 20 Mb/s, applying envelope detection for demodulation. As shown in Fig. 4, the BER equals 10^{-3} is taken as an index in the physical layer. Without the use of pre-emphasis, neither the single branch nor the MRC diversity can support communication at a data rate of 20 Mb/s. Applying the pre-emphasis, however, significantly improves the BER performance in both schemes of single branch and MRC diversity. Furthermore, the MRC diversity ($\rho = 0.291$) exhibits an SNR enhancement of approximately 2 dB and 5 dB compared to the single branch 1 and branch 2, respectively, when the BER equals 10^{-3}.

5   Conclusion

In this study, two-branch spatial transmit diversity combined with a signal pre-emphasis technique is proposed to achieve reliable implant communication at a data rate of 20 Mb/s. On one hand, the channel-weighted transmit diversity is employed at the transmitter through amplitude weighting and phase correction, allowing for a direct application of MRC diversity on the receiver side. On the other hand, the signal pre-emphasis indicates a signal pre-processing method operating at the transmitter, which alters the transmitted signal waveform adaptively to obtain a received signal optimized for demodulation. To illustrate the effect of spatial diversity and the pre-emphasis technique, BER performance is evaluated through computer simulations in the HBC band. The results demonstrate that the proposed signal pre-emphasis technique is an effective means to improve communication performance, and spatial transmit diversity can further enhance the SNR for implant communications. Increasing the number of diverse branches and investigating communication performance under various antenna orientations will be considered in future works.

References

1. Nagaoka, T., et al.: Development of realistic high-resolution whole-body voxel models of Japanese adult males and females of average height and weight, and application of models to radio-frequency electromagnetic-field dosimetry. Phys. Med. Biol. **49**(1), 1–15 (2003)
2. Shi, J., et al.: Miniaturized dual-resonant helix/spiral antenna system at MHz-band for FSK impulse radio intrabody communications. IEEE Trans. Antennas Propag. **68**(9), 6566–6579 (2020). https://doi.org/10.1109/TAP.2020.2993149
3. Shimizu, Y., Anzai, D., Chavez-Santiago, R., Floor, P.A., Balasingham, I., Wang, J.: Performance evaluation of an ultra-wideband transmit diversity in a living animal experiment. IEEE Trans. Microw. Theory Tech. **65**(7), 2596–2606 (2017). https://doi.org/10.1109/TMTT.2017.2669039

Body Area Networks and Transmission Technologies

Wireless Data Transfer for Implanted Real-Time Peripheral Nerve Interfaces

Chiara Quartana[1], Antonio Coviello[1], Paolo Motto Ros[2], Fabiana Del Bono[2], Danilo Demarchi[2], Umberto Spagnolini[1], and Maurizio Magarini[1(✉)]

[1] Department of Electronics, Information and Bioengineering, Politecnico di Milano, Piazza L. Da Vinci 32, 20133 Milan, Italy
chiara.quartana@mail.polimi.it,
{antonio.coviello,maurizio.magarini}@polimi.it
[2] Department of Electronics and Telecommunications, Politecnico di Torino, Corso Duca Degli Abruzzi 24, 10129 Turin, Italy

Abstract. Rapid technological advancements have opened up exciting possibilities for incorporating electronic devices in medical applications, providing solutions to problems and diseases that were previously challenging to address using traditional treatments. This paper presents an optimization of the wireless communication between microcontrollers in the context of a biomedical application. Specifically, the research explores the utilization of Nordic Semiconductor© microcontrollers to establish reliable and efficient communication in real-time between an implanted device and an external unit, leveraging Bluetooth Low Energy (BLE) 5 protocol. To achieve a fast data transmission, careful consideration was given to selecting the optimal parameters for the BLE stack. Two distinct sets of tests were conducted to evaluate the wireless communication performance. Initially, offline tests were carried out, involving the transmission of a small amount of data. This allowed for assessing the coherence and reliability of the received data at close proximity. Subsequently, continuous streaming tests were performed to simulate real-time data transmission scenarios. Furthermore, the analysis encompassed an assessment of the implications arising from varying the distance between the two devices and the influence of biological tissues incorporated within the wireless communication system. These conditions were crucial in assessing the system's robustness and ability to overcome potential obstacles in a medical environment.

Keywords: Implanted Device · Firmware · Bluetooth Low Energy (BLE) · Performance Evaluation

1 Introduction

Peripheral nerve injuries, resulting from various medical conditions and traumatic events, are increasingly affecting the global population. Their rising prevalence demands urgent and innovative solutions due to the range of debilitating

---

C. Quartana and A. Coviello—Both authors contributed equally to this research.

© ICST Institute for Computer Sciences, Social Informatics and Telecommunications Engineering 2024
Published by Springer Nature Switzerland AG 2024. All Rights Reserved
M. Mizmizi et al. (Eds.): BodyNets 2024, LNICST 524, pp. 45–63, 2024.
https://doi.org/10.1007/978-3-031-72524-1_5

symptoms they cause. These symptoms, which include loss or alteration of sensation and motor control, lead to significant dysfunction and disability, impacting both physical well-being and quality of life [4].

In traditional medicine, there are three different approaches to managing peripheral nerve injuries [7]:

- **Microsurgical Techniques:** These involve re-establishing nerve connections to facilitate neuronal regeneration.
- **Implantation of Grafts:** This method employs grafts to guide and support the correct regeneration of nerves, which can be enhanced by combining with drug delivery techniques.

However, these traditional approaches often face limitations in effectively addressing the complexities of such clinical issues. This gap has led to the emergence of non-traditional medicine techniques, notably in the field of neuroscience. A key development in this area is the advent of Peripheral Nerve Interfaces (PNIs), an example diagram is shown in Fig. 1. These implanted devices are designed to interface directly with the peripheral nervous system (PNS), offering new hope in situations where nerve damages are involved. PNIs function by bypassing injury sites to facilitate the flow of neural information, essential for restoring lost functionalities [22]. They achieve this by recording Electroneurographic (ENG) signals from downstream of nerve lesions and transmitting these signals to an external unit for detailed analysis and classification. This process is crucial for deciphering the types of information transmitted through nerves and determining appropriate stimuli for feedback to the PNS [10,24].

The effectiveness of PNIs heavily relies on the efficiency and reliability of the communication system employed. This is critical as implanted devices, equipped with microcontrollers for signal recording, have inherent limitations in terms of processing power, storage capacity, and power consumption [9]. Therefore, optimizing this communication channel is key to maximizing the functional efficacy of PNIs. In addressing these communication needs, wireless systems have emerged as the superior choice over wired systems. Wired systems, while providing reliable data transmission, pose limitations such as reduced mobility, infection risks, and potential movement-induced noise [6,15]. Wireless systems, on the other hand, enhance user mobility, reduce infection and skin complications, and are less conspicuous, improving both psychological well-being and the user's quality of life and optimizing patient comfort in real-world applications [14]. Despite challenges like limited battery life and potential signal interference, advancements in wireless technologies have made significant strides in addressing these issues.

An example of a case study that tries to implement a solution for a PNI is the SenseBack device [25]. This implantable system is semi-flexible and bidirectional designed to remain inside the body for up to six months. It is capable of both sensing and stimulating ENG signals, thereby creating an effective neural bypass. The device uses a wireless Bluetooth Low Energy (BLE) 5 communication for the bidirectional data transfer with an external unit where the analysis is conducted. The preprocessing and the classification can be performed in many different ways such as the one present in [10,24].

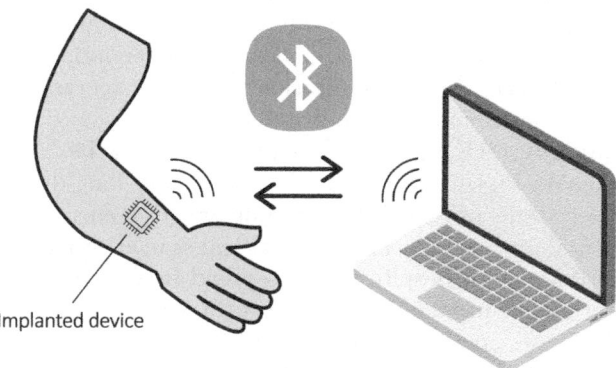

Fig. 1. Schematic idea behind a PNI using a wireless communication system. The implanted device records data from the nerve and sends it to the external unit through a wireless communication system

This paper focuses on leveraging BLE 5 technology for PNIs, this choice has been driven by the considerations made in Sects. 2 and 3. Although BLE 5 has recently garnered increasing interest in the realm of PNIs as in [20, 25], the realization of real-time communication and the optimization of its data transfer rate present significant challenges. Addressing these challenges to fully exploit the capabilities of BLE 5 in the context of PNIs is the primary objective of this work.

The structure of the paper is organized as follows: Sect. 2 provides an overview of potential wireless communication systems, Sect. 3 introduces BLE 5, Sect. 4 describes the experimental setup, and then in Sect. 5, the firmware loaded on the device is detailed. Finally, Sects. 6, 7, and 8 present the results along with the corresponding discussions.

2   Communication Systems in Peripheral Nerve Interfaces

In the development of PNIs, various communication systems have been considered, each with distinct characteristics. This section offers a comparison of these systems, leading to the rationale behind selecting BLE 5 for this project.

- **Inductive Link:** Utilizes inductive coupling for data transmission and wireless power transfer. While efficient and non-invasive, challenges include design constraints, safety considerations at high data rates, and signal quality affected by tissue interference and coil misalignment [16].
- **Optical Systems:** Employs optogenetics and light-sensitive proteins for data transmission. These systems offer high data rates and are immune to electromagnetic interference. However, they face challenges such as tissue absorption and scattering, limited penetration depth, and long-term biocompatibility concerns [13].

- **Ultrasound Systems:** Uses ultrasonic waves for communication, offering excellent spatial resolution and minimal energy attenuation in tissues. However, ultrasound systems have limitations in terms of range and potential interference with surrounding tissues [8, 17, 21].
- **Radio Frequency (RF):** RF systems, particularly in the 2.4 GHz ISM band (encompassing Wi-Fi, Bluetooth, and Zigbee), enable long-distance communication. These systems provide flexibility but are often energy-intensive, prone to environmental interference, and face challenges in effective miniaturization. The 2.4GHz ISM band, despite its widespread use, can suffer from congestion and interference in high-activity areas [18]. Among these, BLE 5 stands out due to its lower power consumption and compact form factor, making it particularly suited for implantable medical devices.

3   BLE 5

Among the available communication systems, Bluetooth, and specifically BLE 5, stands out as an attractive choice for PNIs applications, [20, 25], owing to several compelling reasons. Firstly, BLE 5 adheres to established industry standards and it is already integrated into many different devices. It is readily accessible in the market, especially in compact devices and offers a cost-effective solution. Moreover, it keeps the radio off as much as possible when no data has to be sent offering a lower power consumption.

BLE 5 employs radio frequency technology operating in the 2.4 GHz Industrial, Scientific, and Medical (ISM) band, segmented into 2 MHz channels, which corresponds to the raw data rate of this protocol [2]. This characteristic does impose limitations on the achievable maximum throughput, a challenge addressed in this work to optimize this communication protocol; a crucial step toward achieving real-time communication capabilities for PNIs. In this kind of system, it is important to keep in mind that Bluetooth technology is founded on a master-slave concept, in fact, the communication primarily involves two key roles [1]:

- *Peripheral* (Slave): advertises its presence and responds to central devices.
- *Central* (Master): scans for advertising packets and can initiate connections and establish the parameters that control the communication.

During a connection, central devices send connection requests to peripherals, and then a predetermined schedule is followed to synchronize frequencies, implement security, and exchange data. This communication utilizes a dynamic channel allocation, called Adaptive Frequency Hopping (AFH), across the 2.4 GHz ISM band to minimize interference [3]. To maintain the connection, both devices regularly exchange packets at least at every Connection Event (CE), Fig. 2. These packets could include application data or BLE control data that correspond to the communication payload. In contrast, in the absence of these data, the devices send "empty packets" without any payload, [5]. As in Fig. 2, multiple consecutive packet exchanges can occur within a CE serving to exchange data and maintain

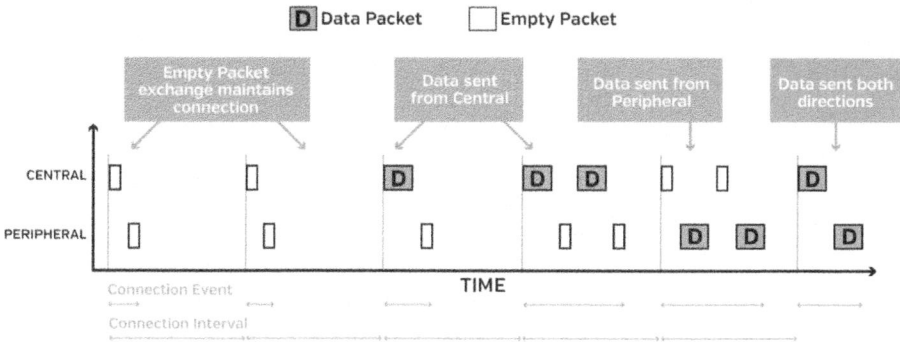

Fig. 2. Flow of what could happen in a connection [5].

the connection. The interval between CEs, known as the Connection Interval (CI), will influence the throughput analysis as will be shown in Sect. 6.

The BLE protocol stack, based on the Open Systems Interconnection (OSI) model, comprises several layers with different functions [23]. The important layers to understand the developed firmware presented in this work are [1]:

– *Generic Access Profile* (GAP), that manages advertisements, connection establishment and device security.
– *Generic Attribute Profile* (GATT), which defines data exchange format and access procedures.
– *Physical layer* (PHY), responsible for data transfer in the radio. Channel bandwidth can be 1 Mbps or 2 Mbps, starting from Bluetooth version 5.0.

3.1   BLE Throughput

The data throughput in BLE is primarily determined by the data rate of the PHY that is the bandwidth, which governs the transmission speed of the radio. From BLE 5 and beyond, this value depends on the operating mode and PHY selection. It can either be set to 1 Mbps or achieve an enhanced 2 Mbps when utilizing the high-speed feature. However, achieving these maximum data rates in real-world applications is influenced by several factors:

– *Packet overhead*: Various protocol layers introduce bytes of overhead. Reducing this overhead by maximizing the data payload in each packet is essential for efficient data transfer, Table 1.
– *CI*: The CI affects the number of packets sent within a CE and the time gaps between consecutive CEs.
– *Data Length Extension* (DLE): Enabling DLE allows for larger payloads in packets, up to 251 bytes.
– *Attribute Maximum Transmission Unit* (ATT MTU): Setting the ATT MTU to 247 bytes (accounting for the L2CAP header) allows all ATT data to fit into a single packet.

Table 1. Table captions should be placed above the tables.

Preamble	Access Address	PDU (2–257 bytes)						CRC
1 byte (1M PHY) 2 bytes (2M PHY)	4 bytes	**LL Header**	**Payload** (0–251 bytes)				**MIC** (Optional)	3 bytes
		2 bytes	**L2CAP Header**	**ATT Data** (0–247 bytes)				
			4 bytes	**ATT Header**		**ATT Payload**		
				OpCode	**Attribute Handle**	Up to 244 bytes		
				1 byte	2 bytes			

– *Operation type*: These can be different, however, Notifications, which do not require acknowledgement packets, are preferred for fast data transfer.

Considering these parameters, a simple connection between one peripheral and one central, and assuming that only the peripheral transmits data continuously as Notifications while the central sends back just empty packets as shown in Fig. 3, the theoretical throughput can be calculated following the subsequent steps:

1. Set the PHY to 2 Mbps.
2. Set the payload of a data packet as 244 bytes through the DLE and the ATT MTU parameters. This leads to a $size(data\ type[bits])_{ATTPayload}$ equal to 1952 bits.
3. Calculate the transmission time for the single data packet and the empty packet, accounting for PHY speed, Inter Frame Space (IFS) of 150 μs between every packet in the air, and packet structure.
4. Determine the maximum number of packets that can be transmitted within a CI for instance of 50 ms.

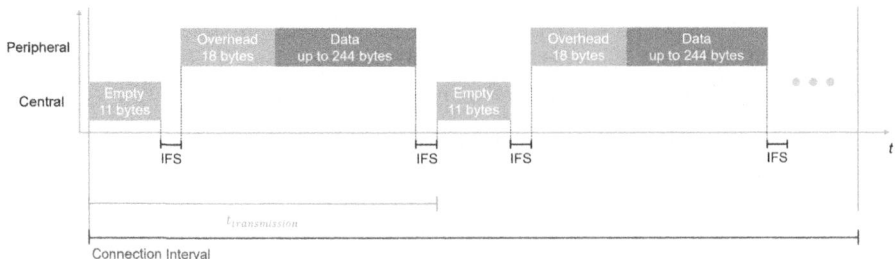

Fig. 3. Example of the communication simulated in this work

Then using Eq. 1, the **theoretical throughput (Thr) of BLE 5** can reach 1.366 Mbps.

$$Thr = \frac{\#Packets_{perCI} \cdot size(data\ type[bits])_{ATTPayload}}{CI} \tag{1}$$

Section 3.2 details the analysis of the throughput necessary for real-time data transmission in an implantable device functioning as a PNI. This analysis is crucial to determine whether BLE can meet the specific requirements of this application.

3.2 Throughput Requirement for a PNI

To determine the required data rate Thr_r needed to meet real-time requirements in such systems, various factors must be taken into account:

- *Sampling frequency* f_s that is imposed by the characteristics of the ENG signal [12, 19]. In particular, since its energy is concentrated between 0.5 and 2.5 kHz, a $f_s \geq 5$ kHz can be used without losing information.
- *Number of electrodes* n that are used for the recording, supposed equal to 16.
- $size(data\ type[bits])$ is the bit representation of the data to be transmitted. It depends on the digitalization of the recorded signal and the unit of information of the communication protocol. It can be hypothesized to be 16 bits (2 bytes).

$$Thr_r = f_s \cdot n \cdot size(data\ type[bits]) \tag{2}$$

Considering these hypothetical values, using the Eq. 2 the Thr_r is equal to 1.28 Mbps. This value is lower than the theoretical value reachable with BLE of 1.366 Mbps, as seen in Sect. 3.1, meaning that BLE if accurately optimized could be suitable for these systems. In this context, this project aims to develop and optimize the firmware for wireless communication using this protocol.

3.3 Packet Error Rate (PER)

Besides the optimization of the transmission rate, it is also important to account for the number of retransmitted packets over the total transmitted ones. In this way, it is important to assess the performance of the communication.

Let

$$r = [r_1, r_2, ..., r_n] \tag{3}$$

be the vector of n retransmissions that occurred during a test and

$$p = [p_1, p_2, ..., p_m] \tag{4}$$

be the vector of the total transmissions that occurred during the same test. With these two values, it is possible to calculate the PER as:

$$PER = \frac{n}{m} \tag{5}$$

As will be seen in Sect. 6, in BLE, increased PER does not significantly impact throughput due to several key features of the protocol. One such feature is adaptive frequency hopping (AFH), which significantly reduces interference-related errors. This technique involves dynamically switching communication channels to avoid interference-prone frequencies. Since BLE operates in the 2.4 GHz ISM band, which is crowded with various other wireless signals like Wi-Fi and other BLE devices, AFH helps in identifying and avoiding channels with high interference. By rapidly shifting across frequencies, BLE minimizes the likelihood of collision and interference from other devices, thereby enhancing the overall reliability and reducing further packet errors. Furthermore, BLE employs efficient retransmission protocols that utilize a stop-and-wait flow control mechanism based on cumulative acknowledgements for error recovery. Each data packet header contains Sequence Number (SN) and Next Expected Sequence Number (NESN) fields to manage packet identification and acknowledgement. This system ensures quick recovery of lost data by resending packets as needed, which minimizes throughput degradation [11].

4   Experimental Setup

This section details the experimental setup designed to simulate a realistic scenario involving implanted medical devices communicating with an external unit via BLE. Our primary objective was to assess the reliability and efficiency of BLE communication in conditions that closely mimic implanted environments. To achieve this, we utilized a single transmitter and a single receiver setup, as depicted in Fig. 4, employing nRF52832 development kits from Nordic Semiconductor©.

Additionally, to gain deeper insights into the intricacies of the BLE communication process, we employed a nRF52840 Dongle, also from Nordic Semiconductor©, as a packet sniffer. This setup allowed us to monitor and analyze the communication flow during the tests using Wireshark software in conjunction with the nRF Sniffer Tool. The role of Matlab in our setup was twofold: firstly, it served to facilitate the transmission of commands from the receiver to the transmitter over BLE, and secondly, in our offline data transmission tests, it was instrumental in evaluating the communication reliability by computing the discrepancies between the received and expected data.

Following the establishment of our experimental setup, we configured the BLE stack parameters used in the BLE communication tests. The specific parameters chosen were as follows:

– PHY Layer Rate: 2Mbps, to facilitate high data rate transmission.
– DLE: Enabled, allowing for extended data packet length.
– ATT MTU: Set to 247, maximizing the data payload per packet and minimizing the overall communication overhead.
– Operation Type: Notifications, suitable for continuous data transfer.

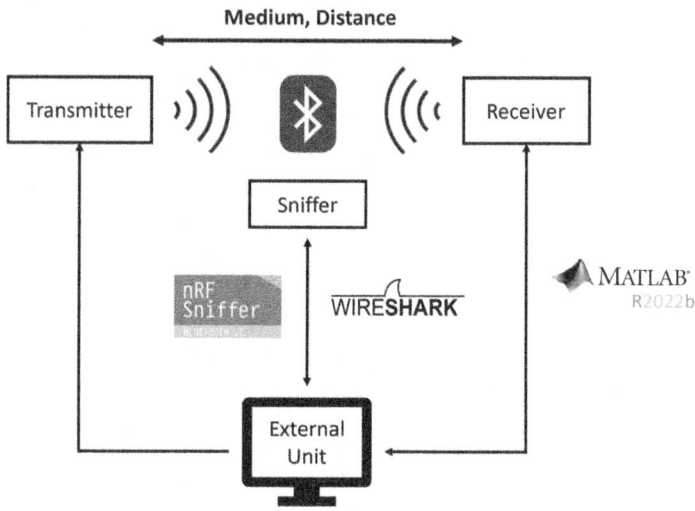

Fig. 4. Diagram of the experimental setup.

It is important to note that these parameters align closely with those employed in the theoretical throughput calculations for BLE 5, except for the CI. The latter impacts the overall throughput, and this was a key focus of our investigation. In addition to this technical parameter, our tests were designed to explore the system's robustness in various environmental conditions. This approach was crucial to replicate the diverse scenarios likely to be encountered in implanted settings. Our tests aimed to provide comprehensive insights into the transmission system's capabilities and limitations in real-world applications by varying environmental factors and analysing the system's performance under these conditions.

In particular, our experimental design included two primary sets of tests:

- **Distance Variation Tests:** The first set focused on the impact of varying distances between the transmitter and receiver. We selected distances of 0 cm, 10 cm, and 50 cm to simulate possible proximities between a subject with an implanted device and the external unit. This range was chosen based on the hypothesis that the external unit is a wearable device.
- **Transmission Medium Tests:** The second set examined the transmission medium's influence on communication efficacy. To emulate the internal body environment, tissue samples of approximately 10 mm thickness were placed atop the transmitter. This setup, with the transmitter 50 cm from the receiver, allowed us to test under conditions mimicking those encountered by implanted devices. We used two types of tissue samples, high ($> 30 \, \text{kg/m}^2$) and low ($< 18.5 \, \text{kg/m}^2$) Body Mass Index (BMI), to evaluate the system's adaptability to varying tissue compositions. The chosen tissue thickness mirrors real-world

considerations such as skin thickness, implantation depth variability, and the presence of fibrotic capsules around implants.

To derive robust conclusions from these setups, two distinct types of tests were conducted:

1. *Offline Data Transmission Test:* This test involved the offline transmission of a predetermined data volume over the BLE connection. Critical to this test was the analysis of factors affecting throughput, such as BLE connection parameters (packet size and CI), signal generation rate, and data consistency. The primary objective was to evaluate the system's reliability and identify the maximum data rate achievable in an offline application.
2. *Online Data Transmission Test:* Building upon the offline test setup, these tests involved continuous data streaming for a duration of 4 min. The focus here was on evaluating the performance and stability of data transmission in continuous applications, under the various environmental conditions established in our experimental framework.

Each of these tests was meticulously designed to address specific hypotheses about the BLE communication system, contributing significantly to our understanding of its potential and limitations in medical applications.

5   Firmware

A crucial aspect of testing the communication system outlined in Sect. 4 involves the development of specialized firmware for the microcontrollers and the appropriate configuration of auxiliary programs.

5.1   Transmitter

The transmitter operates as a Finite State Machine (FSM), taking on the role of a Peripheral device in the BLE connection. Its operation can be delineated into several key states:

- **OFF State:** The initial dormant state.
- **ON State:** Activates the device and initializes the system.
- **ADVertising State:** In this phase, the transmitter broadcasts advertising packets and awaits a connection.
- **CONNection State:** This state is entered upon successful pairing.
- **TX State:** Triggered by a START command received over BLE, the transmitter mimics data reception from an FPGA at a rate of 80 kHz, which comes from 16 channels of ENG at 5 kHz of sampling rate. For simplicity, the data was emulated as a stair-step signal pattern, illustrated in Fig. 5. After completing data transmission or receiving a STOP command, it reverts to the CONNection state.

5.2   Receiver

Similarly, the receiver board is designed as a FSM and functions as a Central device in the BLE setup. Its state transitions are as follows:

- **OFF State:** The initial state before activation.
- **ON State:** Starts up and prepares the device for operation.
- **SCANning State:** Here, it listens for advertising packets and searches for the Nordic UART Service (NUS) used by the transmitter to send data over BLE.
- **CONNection State:** Entered upon locating the service of the transmitter, and at this point the Central and the Peripheral negotiate the specific parameters of the communication.
- **RX State:** Upon receiving a START command from a Matlab script, it begins data reception, buffering the data, and forwarding it to a computer via UART protocol. On receiving a STOP signal, it calculates throughput using the formula in Eq. 6.

$$Thr = \frac{bits_{received}}{t_{elapsed}} \tag{6}$$

5.3   Dongle

The nRF52840 Dongle, in conjunction with Wireshark and the nRF Sniffer firmware, serves as a critical tool for BLE network analysis. It captures data

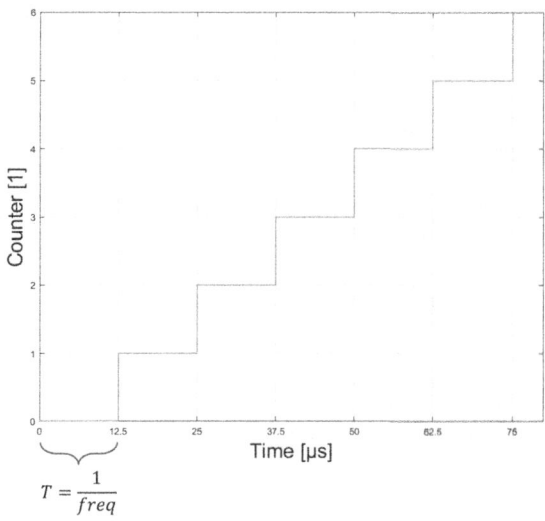

Fig. 5. Signal sent over the BLE communication simulating the correct frequency of the ENG signal to send. This signal was generated using just a counter incremented at 80 kHz.

packets during transmission, enabling us to analyze the PER. This is achieved by counting the number of retransmissions and transmitted packets that occurred during a specific test, followed by the calculation of PER using Eq. 5.

5.4 Matlab Script

Two distinct Matlab scripts were developed for the offline and online tests. During offline tests, the script manages transmission initiation and data reception for reliability analysis, comparing expected and received data to calculate errors. For online tests, due to the memory constraints of the receiver and the slower data rate of the UART connection with the computer, the script primarily handles the transmission of "START\n" and "STOP\n" commands.

6   Results

6.1   Ideal Case Analysis

In our examination of an ideal scenario, where the devices are positioned at a distance of 0 cm from each other with only air as the transmission medium, we conducted both offline and online data transmission tests. The findings, illustrated in Fig. 6, reveal a significant disparity in throughput between these two modes. Specifically, the offline transmission achieved a maximum throughput of approximately 1.4 Mbps, whereas the online transmission was limited to around 1.07 Mbps. This variance primarily stems from the operational dynamics of the CI.

In offline streaming scenarios, particularly when the CI is approximately 200 ms or higher, all transmitted data fit within a single CE, as depicted in Fig. 7.

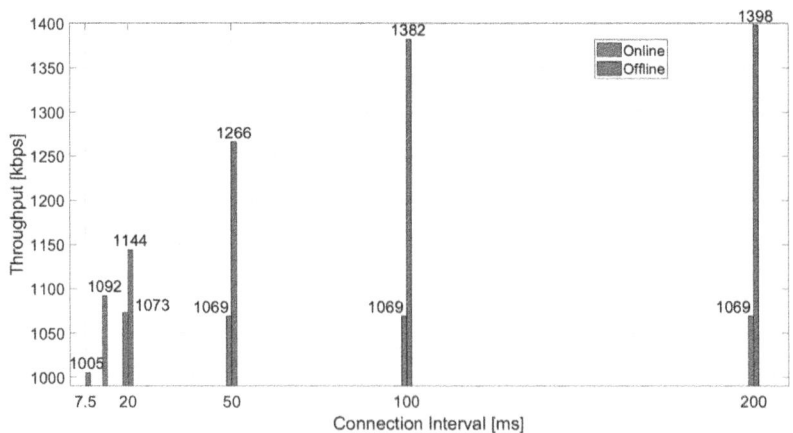

Fig. 6. Comparison of Offline-Online tests in the ideal configuration.

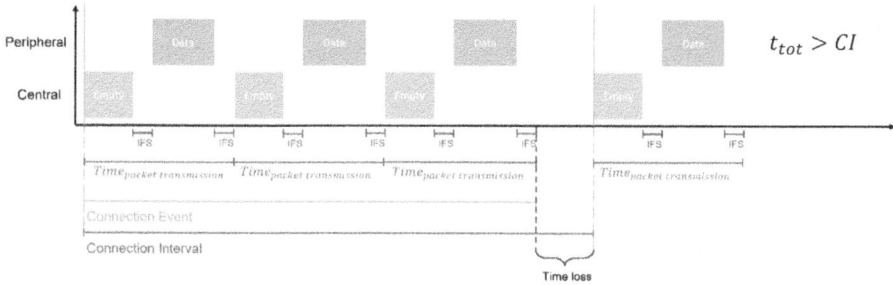

Fig. 7. When $t_{tot} < CI$, there is no time delay between the packets sent.

Conversely, in online streaming or scenarios where the CI is shorter than the total time required for data transmission, there is a noticeable latency between the transmission of the last packet in one CE and the commencement of the next as reported in Fig. 8. This interval contributes to a reduction in throughput. Additionally, in the streaming case, as the throughput decreases, the delay caused by data buffering within the transmitter is worsened, leading to a further reduction in throughput. These observations underscore the need for optimization in the firmware of the transmitter. Specifically, a refinement in the buffering and transmission strategy could minimize the impact on throughput, enhancing the system's efficiency, especially in applications where continuous data streaming is critical.

Importantly, in offline tests, the receiver consistently obtained the correct data sent by the transmitter, showcasing the reliability of the BLE communication. This reliability was quantitatively assessed using a Matlab-based error calculation, which consistently yielded a zero error rate. The same result was confirmed across various experimental setups, ensuring consistency in the system's performance. Acknowledging these findings, alongside the practical significance

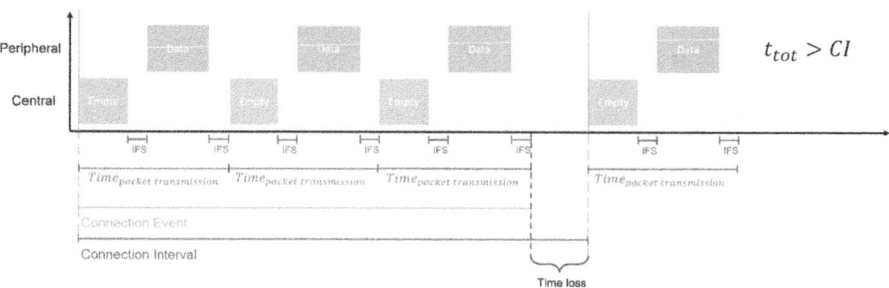

Fig. 8. When $t_{tot} > CI$, a noticeable latency occurs between the end of one CE's last packet transmission and the start of the next.

of online data transmission in real-world applications, the subsequent sections of this paper will shift focus exclusively to the examination of online tests.

6.2 Distance Analysis

The analysis of distance effects on transmission, as depicted in Fig. 9, indicates that distances up to 50 cm have a minimal impact on the transmission rate. This finding underscores the suitability of our communication system for medical scenarios where devices operate in close proximity. However, the influence of high CI values on system performance warrants careful consideration. Our tests suggest that excessively high CIs, especially in conjunction with a higher PER observed at distances of 50 cm, might have been suboptimal. This combination can potentially lead to diminished transmission rates and an increased risk of data loss. The higher PER at this distance (reaching 0.15%–0.20%) implies a greater likelihood of packet errors. Combined with a longer CI, this can delay the detection and retransmission of erroneous packets, exacerbating the risk of data loss. That's why for the case of 50 cm the results are shown for values of the CI just up to 100ms. In fact, in this scenario, a data loss was experienced, with not all data being received on the receiver side.

Notably, even with these higher PER values, the system maintained stable throughput and robust data transfer capabilities as in the tests at shorter distances (10 cm and 0 cm) with nearly 0% PER. This resilience is attributed to the system's effective error correction and retransmission mechanisms, which mitigate the impact of errors and ensure data integrity. However, the combined effect of higher PER and longer CI at 50 cm impacts the permissible CI values. This could be because the higher amount of packet errors necessitates more frequent retransmissions, making shorter CIs more effective in maintaining data integrity and throughput.

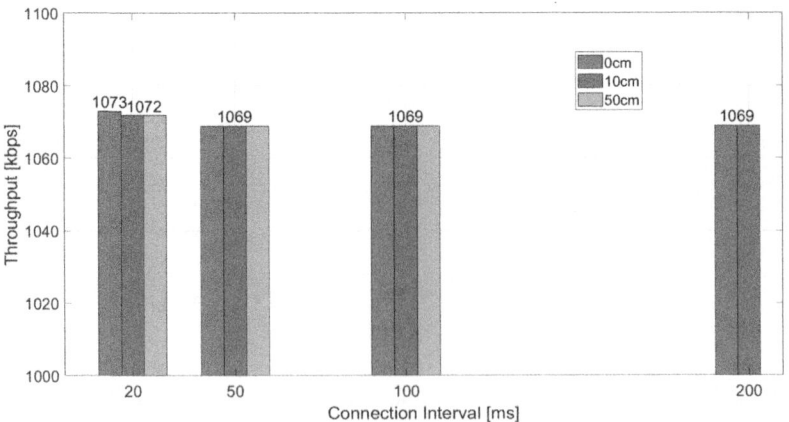

Fig. 9. Results of the Online tests using different distances.

These findings provide crucial insights for the practical deployment of our communication system, laying the groundwork for its application and further enhancement in diverse real-world scenarios.

6.3   Medium Analysis

The impact of different tissue samples on throughput and acceptable CIs was analyzed in Fig. 10. Tissues corresponding to high BMI significantly constrained the viable CIs to a narrow range of 20 ms–50 ms, mirroring the constraints observed at a distance of 50 cm. This observation underscores the importance of considering the characteristics of the medium for ensuring reliable data transmission. The influence of tissues with varying BMI on PER was noteworthy, with higher PER values in comparison to scenarios where air was the sole medium. Specifically, tissues representative of high BMI exhibited a PER of around 1%, while those indicative of low BMI showed a PER between 0.7%–0.9%. This disparity in PER associated with different BMI categories indicates a direct relationship between tissue composition and the effectiveness of data transmission.

The increased PER in tissues representative of high BMI, similar to the trend observed at longer distances, highlights the need for adapting both CI and error correction strategies to the specific challenges posed by these mediums. The increased PER requires a careful choice of CIs and improved error handling to reduce data loss and maintain strong data reliability. In practical applications, particularly in medical device contexts involving varied BMI tissues, these insights are crucial for devising communication solutions that are responsive to the unique challenges of the medium, thereby improving the system's reliability and performance.

These findings emphasize the necessity for customized solutions and optimization strategies that account for medium variability, such as different BMI

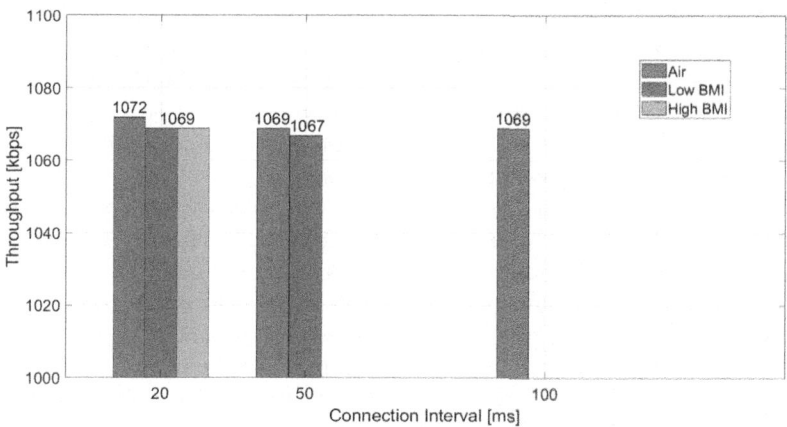

Fig. 10. Results of the Online tests using different mediums.

tissues, to advance communication in real-world scenarios involving biological tissues.

7 Discussion

Our comprehensive testing has yielded critical insights into the reliability and efficiency of our transmission mechanism. The minimal PER and consistent error-free data reception across various scenarios affirm the robustness of our approach.

Offline tests performed under ideal conditions showcased the system's maximum achievable data rate with the selected parameters, enabling efficient and high-speed data transmission. This outcome holds particular significance for scenarios involving asynchronous downlink of packets, such as in nerve stimulation applications. Assuming the same setup as discussed in this paper and considering only the data direction where stimulation is transmitted from the central to the peripheral unit, we anticipate achieving the same data throughput as calculated in Sect. 3.1 and observed in the offline tests. Given that this involves sending a single packet of 244 bytes, we estimate the transmission time for this packet to be less than 2ms. This rapid transmission capability presents a compelling avenue for further investigation, particularly in the development of a complete nerve bypass system.

On the other hand, the online tests provided valuable insights into the system's performance for real-time applications. These tests demonstrated the system's ability to maintain stable and consistent data delivery, despite a slightly lower throughput than ideal for real-time needs. The factors contributing to this, including delays in packet transmission, CI optimization, and buffering time, emerge as key areas for further development. Overcoming these challenges is critical for boosting real-time transmission capabilities.

Particularly noteworthy is the system's performance at short distances, up to 50 cm, where the transmission rate remains largely unaffected. This finding is encouraging for implanted settings. However, our tests indicate the need for firmware optimization to enhance transmission efficiency at a proper CI. Moreover, the system demonstrated commendable resilience in the face of higher PERs, particularly at extended distances. The effective error correction and retransmission strategies in place were instrumental in maintaining reliable data transfer, underscoring the system's robustness.

The exploration of data transmission in the presence of biological tissues, representing varying BMI, brought to light some challenges. It highlighted the critical need for solutions and optimization strategies tailored to these specific mediums. This aspect of our research paves the way for enhanced system performance and reliability in complex biological environments.

In summary, this analysis paints a comprehensive picture of our system's current capabilities and areas of potential improvement. By addressing the identified challenges and fine-tuning the system, we aim to significantly enhance the practical utility and dependability of our communication system, especially in the demanding realm of real-time medical applications.

8   Conclusions and Future Developments

This research successfully demonstrates the efficacy of the BLE 5 protocol in achieving efficient, reliable, and robust wireless communication, particularly tailored for biomedical applications. Through extensive experimentation, we optimized the system's firmware, achieving data rates of up to 1.4 Mbps in offline tests and approximately 1.07 Mbps in online scenarios. Although the online test results show a slightly lower data rate than the generation rate of the data, leading to minor transmission delays due to buffering, these results are still highly promising for practical applications.

A critical aspect of our study was the assessment of communication performance in the face of varying distances and the presence of biological tissues. These findings underscore the system's applicability and potential effectiveness in implanted settings, where such factors are prevalent.

The robustness and flexibility of the firmware established in this study lay a strong foundation for its implementation in a wide range of biomedical applications. Looking ahead, there are several key areas for further research that we have identified. Understanding the nuances of the delay introduced during transmission and optimising the firmware to minimize this delay. Moreover, it is important to investigate other critical parameters like power consumption, data encapsulation, security measures, and compression techniques are essential. These factors must be examined thoroughly to ensure the safety, functionality, and optimal throughput of the system in biomedical applications.

In conclusion, this study not only demonstrates the practical viability and reliability of our proposed communication system for real-time medical applications but also provides invaluable insights into the realm of wireless data transmission in implanted settings. The groundwork laid here paves the way for future advancements in this field, promising enhanced data transmission capabilities in diverse medical scenarios.

Acknowledgment. This work was supported by the Italian Ministry of Foreign Affairs and International Cooperation, grant number US23GR04 (CUP: D43C23000350001).

References

1. Bluetooth low energy: a primer. https://interrupt.memfault.com/blog/bluetooth-low-energy-a-primer. Accessed 05 June 2023
2. Bluetooth low energy (BLE): A complete guide. https://novelbits.io/bluetooth-low-energy-ble-complete-guide/. Accessed 05 June 2023
3. How bluetooth technology uses adaptive frequency hopping to over-come packet interference. https://www.bluetooth.com/blog/how-bluetooth-technology-uses-adaptive-frequency-hopping-to-overcome-packet-interference/. . Accessed 05 June 2023
4. Peripheral nerve injuries market size & share report (2030). https://www.grandviewresearch.com/industry-analysis/peripheral-nerve-injuries-market-report. Accessed 30 July 2023

5. Ultimate guide to managing your BLE connection. https://punchthrough.com/manage-ble-connection/. Accessed 05 June 2023

6. Barua, N., et al: Intermittent convection-enhanced delivery to the brain through a novel transcutaneous bone-anchored port. J. Neurosci. Methods **214**(2), 223–232 (2013). https://doi.org/10.1016/j.jneumeth.2013.02.007, https://www.sciencedirect.com/science/article/pii/S0165027013000733

7. Caillaud, M., Richard, L., Vallat, J.M., Desmoulière, A., Billet, F.: Peripheral nerve regeneration and intraneural revascularization. Neural Regen. Res. **14**(1), 24 (2019)

8. Charthad, J., Weber, M.J., Chang, T.C., Arbabian, A.: A mm-sized implantable medical device (IMD) with ultrasonic power transfer and a hybrid bi-directional data link. IEEE J. Solid-State Circuits **50**(8), 1741–1753 (2015). https://doi.org/10.1109/JSSC.2015.2427336

9. Coviello, A., et al.: Comparison of data compression methods for implanted real-time peripheral nervous system. In: IEEE MetroXRAINE 2023 Proceedings, pp. 110–115 (2023)

10. Coviello, A., Porta, F., Magarini, M., Spagnolini, U.: Neural network-based classification of ENG recordings in response to naturally evoked stimulation. In: Proceedings of the 9th ACM International Conference on Nanoscale Computing and Communication, pp. 1–7 (2022)

11. Gomez, C., Oller, J., Paradells, J.: Overview and evaluation of bluetooth low energy: an emerging low-power wireless technology. Sensors **12**(9), 11734–11753 (2012). https://doi.org/10.3390/s120911734, https://www.mdpi.com/1424-8220/12/9/11734

12. Hoffer, J., Kallesoe, K.: How to use nerve cuffs to stimulate, record or modulate neural activity (2000)

13. Jeong, J.W., et al.: Wireless optofluidic systems for programmable in-vivo pharmacology and optogenetics. Cell **162**(3), 662–674 (2015). https://doi.org/10.1016/j.cell.2015.06.058, https://www.sciencedirect.com/science/article/pii/S0092867415008284

14. Kim, H., Rigo, B., Wong, G., Lee, Y.J.: Advances in wireless, batteryless, implantable electronics for real-time, continuous physiological monitoring. Nano-Micro Lett. **16** (2023). https://doi.org/10.1007/s40820-023-01272-6

15. Koch, J., Schuettler, M., Pasluosta, C., Stieglitz, T.: Electrical connectors for neural implants: design, state of the art and future challenges of an underestimated component. J. Neural Eng. **16**(6), 061002 (2019). https://doi.org/10.1088/1741-2552/ab36df

16. Lee, B., Ghovanloo, M.: An overview of data telemetry in inductively powered implantable biomedical devices. IEEE Commun. Mag. **57**(2), 74–80 (2019). https://doi.org/10.1109/MCOM.2018.1800052

17. Meng, H., Sahin, M.: An electroacoustic recording device for wireless sensing of neural signals. In: 2013 Conference Proceedings: ... Annual International Conference of the IEEE Engineering in Medicine and Biology Society. IEEE Engineering in Medicine and Biology Society, pp. 3086–3088 (2013). https://doi.org/10.1109/EMBC.2013.6610193

18. Nelson, B., Karipott, S., Wang, Y., Ong, K.: Wireless technologies for implantable devices. Sensors **20**, 4604 (2020). https://doi.org/10.3390/s20164604

19. Raspopovic, S., Carpaneto, J., Udina, E., Navarro, X., Micera, S.: On the identification of sensory information from mixed nerves by using single-channel cuff electrodes. J. Neuroeng. Rehabil. (2010)

20. Schnle, P., et al.: A wireless system with stimulation and recording capabilities for interfacing peripheral nerves in rodents. In: 2016 38th Annual International Conference of the IEEE Engineering in Medicine and Biology Society (EMBC), pp. 4439–4442 (2016). https://doi.org/10.1109/EMBC.2016.7591712
21. Seo, D., Carmena, J., Rabaey, J., Alon, E., Maharbiz, M.: Neural dust: an ultrasonic, low power solution for chronic brain-machine interfaces. ArXiv.org/abs/1307.2196 (2013)
22. Shahriari, D., Rosenfeld, D., Anikeeva, P.: Emerging frontier of peripheral nerve and organ interfaces. Neuron **108**(2), 270–285 (2020). https://doi.org/10.1016/j.neuron.2020.09.025
23. Tanenbaum, A., Wetherall, D.: Computer Networks, 5th edn. (2011)
24. Vasta, E., Coviello, A., Spagnolini, U., Magarini, M.: Classification of sensory neural signals through deep learning methods. In: IEEE EUROCON 2023-20th International Conference on Smart Technologies, pp. 313–318. IEEE (2023)
25. Williams, I., et al.: SenseBack - an implantable system for bidirectional neural interfacing. IEEE Trans. Biomed. Circuits Syst. **14**(5), 1079–1087 (2020). https://doi.org/10.1109/TBCAS.2020.3022839

Design Options for Aggregators for In-Body Networks

Johan Engstrand[1]([🖂])[ID], Madhushanka Padmal[1][ID], Bappaditya Mandal[1][ID],
Pramod Rangaiah[1][ID], Mauricio D. Pérez[1][ID], Maria Mani[2][ID],
Robin Augustine[1][ID], and Thiemo Voigt[1][ID]

[1] Department of Electrical Engineering, Uppsala University, Uppsala, Sweden
johan.engstrand@angstrom.uu.se
[2] Department of Surgical Sciences, Uppsala University, Uppsala, Sweden

Abstract. The prevalence of medical implants grows significantly and with it comes a need to network these devices inside the human body. Such an in-body wireless network needs a gateway that provides a connection between the in-body network and the external world. We call this gateway the *aggregator*. Focusing on radio frequency (RF) communication through fat tissue as our intra-body communication paradigm, we explore multiple design options for the aggregator with engineering, security, and medical considerations in mind. We discuss a partially implanted on-skin design and a non-invasive on-skin design for the aggregator. The partially implanted design avoids the losses that human skin present to microwave signals, but requires the patient to go through an invasive procedure. The on-skin aggregator design is easier to realize, but the communication range inside the body is shorter. An implanted wirelessly powered repeater node enables longer communication distances inside the body but requires surgery for the implant. Our discussions show that there is no design that is best in all scenarios and that the aggregator type should be selected for the application at hand. This work also covers signal leakage mitigation and jamming, which are two strategies that the aggregator can implement in order to preserve the privacy of the in-body communication channel.

Keywords: in-body communication · gateway · privacy-preserving

1 Introduction

Already in 2005, 25 million US citizens had medical devices implanted in their bodies for life-critical functions, most often pacemakers [10]. We believe that this number will steadily increase as new application areas for implanted medical devices such as drug delivery systems, intracranial pressure monitoring

---

Supported by SSF, the Swedish Foundation for Strategic Research.

M. Mizmizi et al. (Eds.): BodyNets 2024, LNICST 524, pp. 64–74, 2024.
https://doi.org/10.1007/978-3-031-72524-1_6

devices and artificial kidneys are emerging. Furthermore, with a growing elderly population, more and more people will have multiple diseases with medical conditions that can benefit from implanted devices. As such, it will make sense to network these devices, for example, for in-body control loops where a sensor-actuator pair is physically separated inside the body or to communicate with devices that are deeply embedded into the body so that it is hard to couple out their signals.

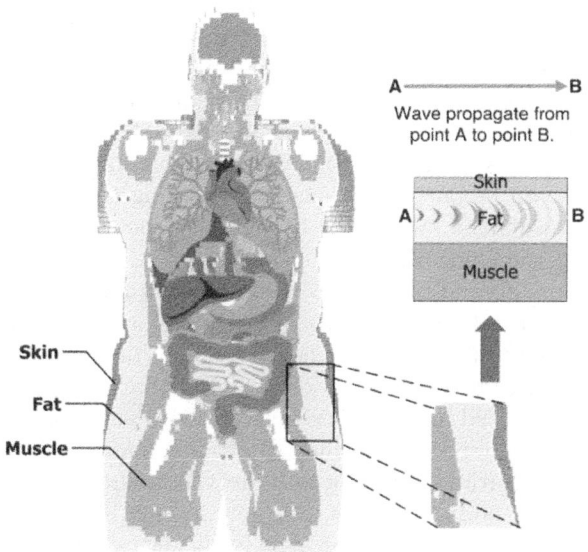

Fig. 1. The fat tissue can be used for communication within the human body. Fat is typically situated between skin and muscle that acts as a waveguide. Reproduced with permission from Badariah Asan, N., Hassan, E., Velander, J., Redzwan Mohd Shah, S., Noreland, D. et al., Sensors, 18(9): 2752; published by MDPI, 2018 [3].

We have earlier shown that the human body's fat tissue is a viable communication channel for radio frequency (RF)-based communication [5]. Fat tissues retain less water and have a lower dielectric constant than muscle and skin. Therefore, radio waves travel better through fat tissues than muscle and skin, and the latter two act as a waveguide for the RF transmissions in the fat tissue as shown in Fig. 1. One major advantage of this approach is that it can support higher data rates [5,21] than current in-body communication methods such as capacitive and galvanic coupling. Therefore we expect to use this type of communication also to support data-intensive applications such as electronic arms and brain-to-machine interfaces.

We call the gateway between the in-body network and the external world the *aggregator*. The aggregator forwards data from the in-body network to the external world, for example, sensor data and implants' status information. The

Table 1. Dielectric properties of human skin, fat and muscle at a frequency of 2.45 GHz [13].

Tissue	ε_r (real part)	Loss tangent	Penetration depth (m)
Skin (dry)	38.0	0.283	0.022
Fat	5.28	0.145	0.115
Muscle	52.7	0.242	0.022

aggregator also relays data from the external world to the in-body network, for example, control commands and code updates. The aggregator may also support other functions such as privacy-enhancing techniques to reduce the information leakage of in-body measurements and hence protect the patients' privacy.

This paper discusses multiple design options for an aggregator for Fat-IBC: First, aggregators can be partially implanted meaning that there is an antenna that penetrates the skin to launch the signals into the subcutaneous fat tissue, i.e., the fat under the skin. Such systems are known from commercial glucose monitoring systems. Second, aggregators can be wearable on the body. In such systems, the aggregator is completely outside and launches its signal through the skin into the fat tissue. Finally, the aggregator may be wearable as in the second case, but with an implanted in-body repeater that has no physical contact with skin but is implanted in the fat tissue. We detail and discuss these multiple options from several perspectives including efficiency and powering, security as well as medical implications. Our focus is on the communication between the aggregator and the in-body networks. Communication between the aggregators and the Internet, for example, a smart edge for healthcare has been studied previously [1, 19, 22, 26]. Finally, we discuss other important tasks of the aggregator that include the ability to defend against battery-draining attacks and protection of the patients' privacy.

The paper continues as follows: In Sect. 2 we describe the concept of fat intra-body communication and in Sect. 3 to Sect. 5 we present different aggregator designs. Section 6 discusses several approaches for privacy-preservation that the aggregators contribute to. Before concluding the paper, we discuss related work in Sect. 7.

2 Fat Intra-body Communication

Human muscle and skin contain around 73–78% and 60–76% water, respectively, while subcutaneous fat tissue has a water content in the range of 5–10% [16]. This leads to a significant disparity in relative permittivity (ε_r) and loss tangent ($\tan \delta$) between the tissues at frequencies such as 2.45 GHz, as shown in Table 1. Fat inherently dissipates less electromagnetic energy than muscle and skin due to its lower loss tangent and relative permittivity, as denoted by a larger penetration depth [16]. Altogether, this forms a structure akin to a three-layered dielectric waveguide, in which the middle layer has significantly lower relative permittivity than the outer layers.

Asan et al. designed a specialised waveguide probe that together with a phantom replicates an implanted Fat-IBC scenario [3]. The waveguide probe is made with an antenna designed using a numerical optimization technique known as *topology optimization* that is mounted inside a larger waveguide structure that one can place against the fat layer of the three-layered planar phantom. We have later used the same probe to transmit at speeds over 90 Mbit/s in a 300 mm phantom at 2.45 GHz with off-the-shelf WiFi (IEEE 802.11n) hardware [21]. An earlier work demonstrated sub-megabit per second data rates at lower transmission powers at 2.0 GHz in a 100 mm phantom using a different probe design [5]. The fat channel is characterized also at 5.8 GHz [4]. The propagation path loss in a three-layer phantom is around 1 dB/cm [3,21], while it is around 2 dB/cm for ex-vivo porcine tissue [3].

The fat channel can be used not only for communication but also for sensing. For example, it can be used for tumour relapse monitoring since obstacles in the fat channel change the communication properties, in particular the signal strength at which packets are received [12,15].

3   Partially Implanted On-Skin Aggregator

This section describes an aggregator that is partially implanted, i.e., it is placed on the skin but has an antenna that penetrates the skin.

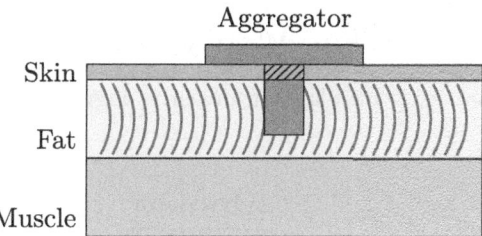

Fig. 2. An on-skin aggregator that is partially implanted into the fat tissue.

Description. Figure 2 illustrates a partially implanted aggregator for Fat-IBC. While the aggregator itself is located onto the skin, it has an antenna that penetrates the skin. This antenna launches signals from the aggregator into the fat channel and receives signals from the fat channel. Such half-implanted systems are used in commercial glucose monitoring systems.

Medical Aspects. This design requires careful consideration of bio-compatibility and infection control due to the risks posed by skin puncture. Infection risks can be mitigated by employing bio-compatible materials and antimicrobial coatings, as well as designing the antenna to minimize skin irritation and facilitate easy cleaning.

Performance. The antenna can be well-matched to the fat tissue, thus avoiding large losses when launching a signal into the fat. The design can cover larger distances within the fat tissue. Earlier works show successful data transmission in phantoms between two implanted nodes separated by up to 30 cm using IEEE 802.11n for high data rates [20,21], and IEEE 802.15.4 for low data rates, with transmission output power levels as low as –55 dBm for the latter case [20].

Power. Power is less of a concern for this type of aggregator. As the aggregator is outside the body, batteries can be replaced or charged externally.

Location. The on-skin aggregator can also be placed at locations where there is less subcutaneous fat. These locations include the upper arm (a typical location for insulin pumps), which usually has less subcutaneous fat than the abdomen or the thigh.

Security Considerations. To ensure secure data transmission, the aggregator should employ robust encryption protocols and secure key management systems to safeguard against unauthorized access and preserve data integrity.

Practical Considerations. This aggregator requires an antenna that penetrates the skin. This setup can be achieved under local anesthetics (to prevent pain) in an outpatient setting, i.e., the patient does not need to stay at a hospital. Once it is set up, the patient cannot move the aggregator to another location. The fact that this aggregator cannot be easily removed may be seen as an advantage if it monitors a life-threatening condition.

4   Non-invasive On-Skin Aggregator

This section describes a wearable, non-invasive aggregator that is put on the skin.

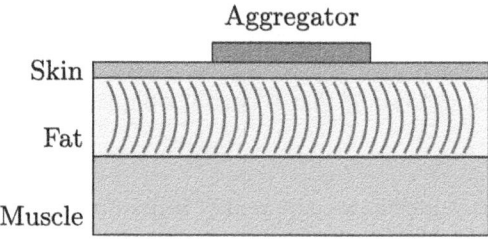

Fig. 3. A non-invasive on-skin aggregator.

Description. This type of aggregator is a wearable device located on the outside of the body that transmits and receives signals through the skin, as shown in Fig. 3. Skin has around 28 dB of loss [20,25], so the antenna should be well-matched to the skin and have a highly directional radiation pattern in order to strongly couple to the fat channel.

Medical Aspects. Opting for a wearable aggregator positioned on the body presents a non-invasive approach, reducing infection risks associated with implanted devices. There could still be irritation or damage to the skin that occurs as a result of friction caused by the aggregator on the skin. There is also less need for surgery (and the associated manpower) which is beneficial for the healthcare systems that are overloaded in many countries.

Performance. This design couples to the fat channel through the skin. A previous work shows successful communication in a phantom between one implanted and one on-skin node placed 30 cm apart [21].

Power. This method ensures that power supply concerns remain external, as batteries can be replaced or charged without affecting the patient. This does, however, raise concerns regarding in-body sensors that may require higher power levels for effective communication. This type of aggregator will receive a weaker signal from the fat channel due to power losses in the skin.

Location. The wearable aggregator is mostly suited for locations with a significant amount of fat in order to be efficient. Suitable locations include the abdomen, i.e., the belly, and the thighs.

Security Considerations. While the other types of aggregator described in the previous and the next section launch the signals directly into the fat channel, the signals here also travel through the air. Therefore, many attacks on wireless low-power communication also apply when this type of aggregator is used [23].

Practical Considerations. Relying on wearable technology for in-body network aggregators comes with its own set of challenges. One major concern is the risk of non-compliance; if a patient forgets to wear the device, it can compromise the effectiveness of the monitoring system. Additionally, there is the issue of comfort. If wearables are not designed with ergonomics in mind, they could be uncomfortable to wear, leading to patients using them inconsistently. Such sporadic use could result in irregular data collection, which is not ideal. So, while having these aggregators as external wearables has its advantages, it is crucial that they are well-designed. They must not only be functional but also easy and comfortable to use, in order to ensure that patients keep wearing them regularly.

5   Wearable Aggregator with an Implanted In-Body Repeater

This section describes a wearable, non-invasive aggregator like in Sect. 4, with the addition of an implanted repeater node.

Description. This system utilizes an implanted node separate from the (wearable) aggregator, which eliminates the need to have an opening in the skin, as seen in Fig. 4. The implanted node functions as a repeater that retransmits signals in order to extend the transmission distance in the fat. Strategic placement of one or multiple repeaters may significantly extend the range of the in-body communication.

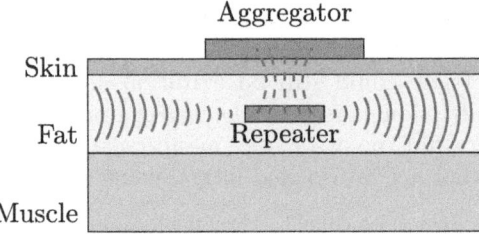

Fig. 4. A wearable aggregator with a wirelessly powered implanted repeater node.

Medical Aspects. This design significantly reduces the risk of infection compared to the methods where the aggregator penetrates the skin. Nevertheless, the repeater must be implanted, which requires surgery.

Performance. A repeater facilitates considerably longer communication distances inside the body, which is advantageous for in-body communication between various internal sensors. It takes weak signals from devices implanted in the body, like sensors or health monitors, and gives them a boost. This way, the signals can travel further through the tissues of the body. By amplifying these signals, the repeater ensures that crucial health information gets where it needs to go, whether that is to another device in the body or to an external monitor. The repeater node could use a miniaturized version of the antenna inside the probe described in Sect. 2.

Power. According to Khan et al., there are various wireless power transfer (WPT) techniques for biomedical implantable devices previously reported in the literature, each one with specific opportunities and challenges [14]. Among these, non-radiative inductive coupling and non-radiative magnetic resonance coupling represent more mature technologies and may be used to power a wireless repeater. Important to note is that for the case of Fat-IBC, where the energy is intended to be transmitted through the fat, the wireless link from the external aggregator and the repeater need only to overcome the skin layer, which could be done while maintaining good enough power transfer efficiency with available WPT techniques at minimum tissue energy absorption.

Location. The wearable aggregator is mostly suited for locations with a significant amount of fat in order to be efficient. Suitable location include the abdomen, i.e., the belly. The thickness of the repeater also affects the location.

Security Considerations. This type of aggregator requires secure communication also between the aggregator and the implanted repeater. As the implanted repeater has limited resources, it cannot afford heavy-weight encryption schemes. One approach to secure the communication is a shield as proposed by Gollakota et al. [8]. Such a shield works by jamming others' messages, something we also discuss in Sect. 6 but in the slightly different context of privacy-preservation.

Practical Considerations. This type of aggregator has largely the same practical considerations as the non-invasive on-skin aggregator in terms of ergonomics and patient compliance. The WPT circuitry may affect the size and shape of this aggregator and it will need a battery with larger capacity in order to power the repeater.

6   Privacy-Preserving Aspects

The skin provides around 28 dB of attenuation to signals that escape the fat channel to the outside world [20, 25]. This strong attenuation implies that the skin on its own provides a level of defense against eavesdropping.

There are a number of available strategies for restricting signal leakage and preserving data privacy. For example, lowering the transmit power of in-body nodes can prevent eavesdroppers outside the body from receiving data packets [20]. Adaptive power control on the in-body nodes can therefore help limit the range of the communication and minimize the risk of unintended signal leakage.

Another privacy-preserving strategy is to generate jamming signals at the aggregator. As the jamming signal increases in strength, external eavesdroppers should experience a progressive failure to decode transmitted packets. For effective jamming, we must fulfill two conditions; at the attacker, the signal strength from the jamming aggregator must surpass that of the in-fat sender; and at the in-fat receiver, the signal strength from the sender must exceed that of the jamming aggregator [25]. For two nodes implanted 10 cm apart in a breast, with an aggregator placed 50 cm away on the thigh and an attacker also 50 cm away from the in-fat sender, the jamming signal from the aggregator appears 10 times stronger than signals from the in-fat sender to the attacker if it is positioned 5 cm above the skin and 250 times stronger when it is 20 cm above the skin [25].

For reasons of privacy, patients may completely want to hide the fact that they have any implants in their body. Such the communication has to be covert [6, 11]. This is typically achieved by one or more friendly jammers. The situation becomes complex when multiple eavesdroppers collude in a coordinated way against two in-fat nodes that try to hide the fact that they are communicating with each other. Increasing the number of eavesdroppers reduces the covertness of the in-fat communication, but a jammer can effectively neutralize the advantages gained by the adversary in such a situation [2].

We assume that a jammer would use the same type of radio that is used for in-body communication. This could be an IEEE 802.15.4 (also called ZigBee) standard-compliant radio, Bluetooth or BLE, as well as a WiFi radio. The partially implanted on-skin aggregator (see Sect. 3) has an antenna that radiates into the fat channel. If the aggregator should act as a jammer also, a second antenna would be required. The same is true for the wearable aggregator with the implanted repeater node described in Sect. 5. The non-invasive on-skin aggregator (see Sect. 4) could use the already existing radio for jamming also, unless it has to jam at the same time as it needs to transmit or receive. The latter scenario might be quite common, for example, when it needs to protect its own transmissions from a neighbouring implant.

7   Related Work

Existing work involves two types of approaches, namely ultrasonic-based and radio-based communication links between the gateway and in-body sensors and nodes.

In papers on ultrasonic-based approaches, Gomez et al. [9] and Kuestner et al. [18] discuss in-body nanosensors and nanobots with free-flowing capabilities enabling remote health monitoring systems. They establish a connection with an on-body gateway located outside the body using an ultrasonic communication uplink based on the placement of the nanosensors. Ultrasonic-based aggregator implementations have a relatively low data rate in the range of kbit/s [9]. They also consider on-body aggregators where the gateway is present outside the body, similar to our on-skin aggregator.

The second approach with a radio-based communication link explores the possibility of establishing a connection between in-body sensors with on-body devices. Usman et al. propose a four-tier architecture for remote health monitoring system, in which the second tier is the connection between in-body sensors and on-body gateways [24]. They place the on-body gateway on the skin, with a radio link connecting the in-body sensors, a scenario reminiscent of our non-invasive aggregator. They analyse security requirements and challenges in such a systematic setup where a patient wears a small radio transmitter on wrist.

Domingo et al. investigate where to position an on-body gateway with respect to in-body sensors placed at different parts of the human body [7]. Their findings propose a model to estimate the optimal gateway positions to minimize the energy consumption of body sensor networks and also to minimize heating effects on human tissues.

We have earlier devised a secure middlebox that defends against remote denial-of-sleep attacks [17]. This approach performs packet filtering in a trusted execution environment to prevent unwanted packets from reaching the implants. Since this approach is based on a trusted execution environment, it tolerates compromise of the middlebox's software, including its operating system. This approach can be implemented on all types of aggregators described in the previous sections.

8   Conclusions

We have explored design options for secure aggregators in fat-intrabody communication (Fat-IBC) networks, which is essential for advancing in-body networks. We have investigated and contrasted various aggregator designs, including partially implanted on-skin, non-invasive on-skin, and wearable aggregators with implanted in-body repeaters, each with unique advantages, medical considerations, and practical implications.

Ultimately, the optimal aggregator design is application-dependent. The non-invasive on-skin aggregator offers a significant advantage by being completely external. This design minimizes medical risks, such as infections, since it does not require any skin penetration or invasive procedures. It can also be integrated into existing wearable technology, making it both convenient and accessible for continuous health monitoring. Its external placement allows for easy mainte- nance, battery replacement, and upgrades, which enhances its practicality for long-term use. The partially implanted aggregator, on the other hand, will receive in-fat communication with higher signal strength but cannot be realized without surgery. The same applies to the aggregator with an implanted repeater, which comes with additional engineering challenges but also strengthens the network. An implanted aggregator could be preferable over a non-implanted aggregator if it monitors a life-threatening condition, as it cannot be removed.

This work also explores privacy preservation techniques such as signal leak- age mitigation and jamming. The aggregator can use adaptive power control to limit the signal range and minimize the risk of unintended leakage. Addition- ally, it can employ jamming techniques, generating signals that interfere with and obscure data transmission from unauthorized external eavesdroppers. This approach ensures that patient data transmitted through the in-body network remains secure and private, safeguarding against potential cybersecurity threats.

References

1. Alabdulatif, A., Khalil, I., Yi, X., Guizani, M.: Secure edge of things for smart healthcare surveillance framework. IEEE Access **7**, 31010–31021 (2019)
2. Arghavani, A., Dey, S., Ahlén, A.: Covert outage minimization in the presence of multiple wardens. IEEE Trans. Signal Process. **71**, 686–700 (2023). https://doi. org/10.1109/TSP.2023.3248869
3. Asan, N., et al.: Characterization of the fat channel for intra-body communication at r-band frequencies. Sensors **18**(9) (2018)
4. Asan, N.B., et al.: Fat-intrabody communication at 5.8 GHz: verification of dynamic body movement effects using computer simulation and experiments. IEEE Access **9**, 48429–48445 (2021). https://doi.org/10.1109/ACCESS.2021.3068400
5. Asan, N.B., et al.: Data packet transmission through fat tissue for wireless intra- body networks. IEEE J. Electromagnetics RF Microwaves Med. Biol. **1**(2) (2017)
6. Chen, X., et al.: Covert communications: a comprehensive survey. IEEE Commun. Surv. Tutor. (2023)
7. Domingo, M.C.: Sensor and gateway location optimization in body sensor net- works. Wirel. Netw. **20**(8), 2337–2347 (2014)
8. Gollakota, S., Hassanieh, H., Ransford, B., Katabi, D., Fu, K.: They can hear your heartbeats: non-invasive security for implantable medical devices. In: Proceedings of the ACM SIGCOMM 2011 Conference, pp. 2–13 (2011)
9. Gómez, J.T., Kuestner, A., Stratmann, L., Dressler, F.: Modeling ultrasonic chan- nels with mobility for gateway to in-body nanocommunication. In: 2022 IEEE Global Communications Conference, GLOBECOM 2022, pp. 4535–4540. IEEE (2022)
10. Halperin, D., Heydt-Benjamin, T.S., Fu, K., Kohno, T., Maisel, W.H.: Security and privacy for implantable medical devices. IEEE Pervasive Comput. **7**(1) (2008)
11. He, B., Yan, S., Zhou, X., Lau, V.K.: On covert communication with noise uncer- tainty. IEEE Commun. Lett. **21**(4), 941–944 (2017)

12. Hylamia, S., et al.: Privacy-preserving continuous tumour relapse monitoring using in-body radio signals. In: IEEE Workshop on the Internet of Safe Things (SafeThings) (2020)
13. IFAC-CNR, Florence (Italy): Dielectric Properties of Body Tissues (2021). http://niremf.ifac.cnr.it/tissprop/htmlclie/htmlclie.php
14. Iqbal, A., Sura, P.R., Al-Hasan, M., Mabrouk, I.B., Denidni, T.A.: Wireless power transfer system for deep-implanted biomedical devices. Sci. Rep. **12**(1), 13689 (2022)
15. Joseph, L., et al.: Non-invasive transmission based tumor detection using anthropomorphic breast phantom at 2.45 GHz. In: 2020 14th European Conference on Antennas and Propagation (EuCAP) (2020)
16. Komarov, V., Wang, S., Tang, J.: Permittivity and measurements. In: Chang, K. (ed.) Encyclopedia of RF and Microwave Engineering. Wiley, New York (2015)
17. Krentz, K.F., Voigt, T.: Reducing trust assumptions with OSCORE, RISC-V, and layer 2 one-time passwords. In: International Symposium on Foundations and Practice of Security, pp. 389–405. Springer (2022)
18. Kuestner, A., Stratmann, L., Wendt, R., Fischer, S., Dressler, F.: A simulation framework for connecting in-body nano communication with out-of-body devices. In: Proceedings of the 7th ACM International Conference on Nanoscale Computing and Communication, NanoCom 2020. Association for Computing Machinery, New York (2020). https://doi.org/10.1145/3411295.3411308
19. Mohapatra, S., Rekha, K.S.: Sensor-cloud: a hybrid framework for remote patient monitoring. Int. J. Comput. Appl. **55**(2), 7–11 (2012)
20. Padmal, M., Engstrand, J., Augustine, R., Voigt, T.: Signal leakage in fat tissue-based in-body communication: preserving implant data privacy. In: Proceedings of the Int'l ACM Conference on Modeling Analysis and Simulation of Wireless and Mobile Systems, MSWiM 2023, pp. 225–232. Association for Computing Machinery (2023). https://doi.org/10.1145/3616388.3617535
21. Rangaiah, P.K.B., Engstrand, J., Johansson, T., Perez, M.D., Augustine, R.: 92Mb/s fat-intrabody communication (Fat-IBC) with low-cost WLAN hardware. IEEE Trans. Biomed. Eng. 1–9 (2023). https://doi.org/10.1109/TBME.2023.3292405. https://ieeexplore.ieee.org/document/10178014
22. Salahuddin, M.A., Al-Fuqaha, A., Guizani, M., Shuaib, K., Sallabi, F.: Softwarization of Internet of Things infrastructure for secure and smart healthcare. arXiv preprint arXiv:1805.11011 (2018)
23. Saleem, S., Ullah, S., Yoo, H.S.: On the security issues in wireless body area networks. Int. J. Digit. Content Technol. Appl. **3**(3), 178–184 (2009)
24. Usman, M., Asghar, M.R., Ansari, I.S., Qaraqe, M.: Security in wireless body area networks: from in-body to off-body communications. IEEE Access **6**, 58064–58074 (2018)
25. Voigt, T., et al.: Jamming to support privacy-preserving continuous tumour relapse monitoring using in-body radio signals. In: Proceedings of the 1st International Workshop on Physical-Layer Augmented Security for Sensor Systems, PLAS 2020, pp. 1–2. Association for Computing Machinery, New York (2020). https://doi.org/10.1145/3417311.3430709
26. Yang, S., Gerla, M.: Personal gateway in mobile health monitoring. In: 2011 IEEE International Conference on Pervasive Computing and Communications Workshops (PERCOM Workshops), pp. 636–641. IEEE (2011)

Visible Light Communications for Implantable Medical Devices

Stefano Caputo[1]([✉]) [iD], Giacomo Borghini[1] [iD], Sara Jayousi[2],
and Lorenzo Mucchi[1] [iD]

[1] Department of Information Engineering, University of Florence, Florence, Italy
{stefano.caputo,giacomo.borghini,lorenzo.mucchi}@unifi.it
[2] Polo Universitario Città di Prato, Prato, Italy
sara.jayousi@pin.unifi.it

Abstract. Implantable medical devices (IMDs) have revolutionized modern healthcare, offering real-time monitoring and therapeutic interventions. However, conventional radio-frequency (RF) technology limits IMD communication due to interference, power consumption, and bandwidth constraints. This paper introduces an innovative solution using optical wireless communication (OWC) for IMDs. OWC transmits data via visible or infrared light, surpassing RF limitations. Recent research explores Visible Light Communication (VLC) for in-body and out-body communication, as it penetrates human tissues effectively. We aim to demonstrate VLC's feasibility and benefits for subcutaneous IMDs in temperature and glycemia measurements using MATLAB simulations. Our contributions encompass: a) a unique VLC approach for Near-Field Communication (NFC); b) an innovative characterization of the in-to-out body communication channel, considering scattering effects; and c) a comparison between single LED and multiple LEDs (MIMO) approaches for IMDs. This paper underscores VLC's transformative potential for IMDs, promising more efficient and reliable IMD-to-external system communication, ultimately enhancing patient outcomes and advancing healthcare.

Keywords: Visible Light Communication · Implantable Medical Device · Channel Characterization · Near-Field Communication · MIMO

1 Introduction

In recent decades, there has been rapid progress in the development of implantable medical device (IMD) technology, driven by advancements in various scientific and engineering fields such as nanomaterials, biotechnology, and microelectronics [1]. The global IMD market, which was estimated at US$ 118.2 Billion in 2022, is projected to grow substantially, reaching a revised size of US$ 188.7 Billion by 2030, with a compound annual growth rate (CAGR) of 6% during the period from 2022 to 2030 [2].

© ICST Institute for Computer Sciences, Social Informatics and Telecommunications Engineering 2024
Published by Springer Nature Switzerland AG 2024. All Rights Reserved
M. Mizmizi et al. (Eds.): BodyNets 2024, LNICST 524, pp. 75–87, 2024.
https://doi.org/10.1007/978-3-031-72524-1_7

The changing post-COVID-19 business landscape has highlighted the importance of tele-monitoring individuals' health status, with a focus on leveraging 6th generation (6G) information and communication technology (ICT) systems. In this context, a crucial element is the automatic acquisition of data from individuals' bodies. In-body sensors encompass nano-devices, implants, or molecules serving as biological communication systems, while on-body sensors refer to wearable devices designed for measuring bio-parameters such as blood pressure, pulse oximetry, and electrocardiogram (ECG) data acquisition [3].

The field of IMDs has primarily been explored in the medical domain: numerous papers emphasize the significance of IMDs for monitoring and treating patients. This demand has given rise to an innovative technological branch focused on creating sensors, actuators, and devices suitable for implantable applications.

Historically, conventional IMDs have relied on radio frequency (RF) technology. Only recently ICT field begun to delve into IMD domain, in order to come up with new and more efficient solutions.

Traditional IMDs operate within the RF band, which is often saturated in terms of bandwidth (BW) [4]. These devices typically use transmission power in the range of several tens of milliwatts [5]. Consequently, they face challenges in achieving the high data rates required to emulate human organs effectively [6,7]. Moreover, conventional IMDs are susceptible to interference from other sources operating within the same RF band, leading to significant performance degradation.

To cope with these challenges, a novel approach involving optical wireless communications (OWC) has been considered for very short communication ranges [8]. OWC technology inherently provides enhanced security compared to RF technologies, offering a highly secure link for in- to out-body communications [9]. This is a key element in IMD applications due to the highly personal and health-related nature of the transmitted data [10].

Recent literature has explored the use of OWC for both in- to out-body communications, with studies characterizing tissue penetration of optical electromagnetic waves [11–13]. In particular, the usage of VLC (Visible Light Communications) is supported. VLCs are a subset of OWCs, and make use of the visible portion of the light spectrum, ranging from 400 to 800 THz.

Figure 1 highlights the advantages of using VLC for communication within human tissue, with particular emphasis on the low absorption coefficient of red light (Fig. 1b).

This work addresses these main questions regarding the use of VLC in IMD applications:

- Why is there a growing interest in using VLC for IMD applications?
- What advantages does VLC offer for communication within human tissue?
- How does VLC address the in-to-out body communications associated with IMD applications?
- Can the transmission from inside to outside the body be improved by using multiple LEDs and MIMO schemes?

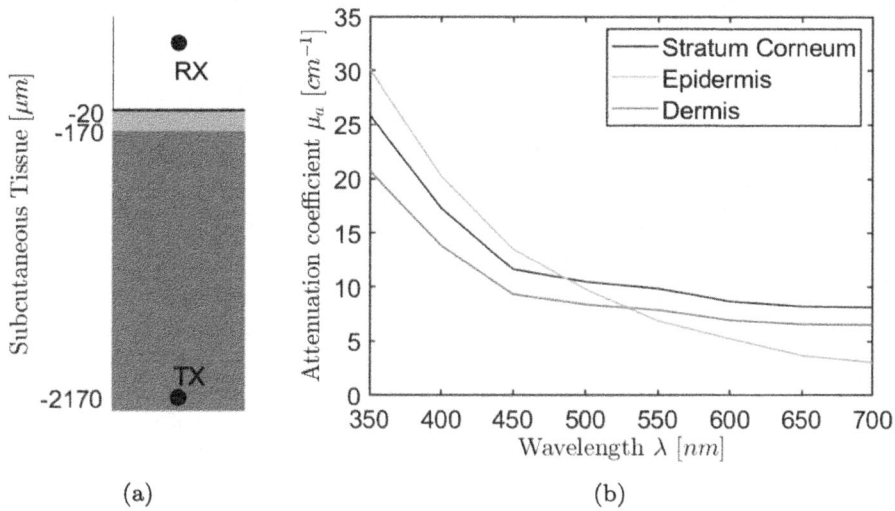

Fig. 1. Human skin absorption for wavelength at different skin layers: 1. Stratum Corneum; 2. Epidermis; 3. Dermis.

To answer these questions, it is essential to consider the following insights. First, the growing interest in VLC for IMD applications stems from their capacity to offer highly safe and efficient communication within the human body, effectively overcoming the limitations associated with conventional RF technologies. Second, VLC shows low absorption coefficient, which enables optical signals to penetrate human tissue effectively, making it an ideal choice for in-to-out body communications. Lastly, VLC addresses the critical security concerns associated with IMD applications by ensuring enhanced data privacy and protection. Given the sensitivity and personal nature of data transmitted within the body, VLC emerges as the preferred solution over RF technologies.

In this study, a MATLAB simulation has been implemented to demonstrate the feasibility and advantages of OWC, specifically VLC, for in-to-out body communications of implantable subcutaneous devices. These devices are commonly used for measurements such as temperature and glycemia, as depicted in Fig. 1a. This paper provides a model of light propagation thorugh the skin layers (in-body channel) as well as a model of light propagation from the outside skin on (out-body channel). The communication source (LED) is under the skin, while the receiver (photodetector) is outside the body. Both single LED single photodetector (SISO) and multiple LEDs multiple photodetectors (MIMO) communication is considered. The performance of SISO and MIMO LED-based VLC systems is characterized by means of the bit error rate (BER) as a function of the distance and angle of the receiver from the skin.

This research contributes to the growing body of knowledge in the field of implantable medical devices and optical wireless communications.

The key contributions of this paper include:

– A feasible approach to Near-Field Communication (NFC) for VLC systems
within IMD scenarios;
– A characterization of the communication channel for VLC systems in IMD
scenarios. Notably, this encompasses a novel approach to accounting for scattering effects in in-body channel characterization and an assessment of how
scattering impacts the out-body channel;
– An exploration of the potential application of MIMO techniques in IMD scenarios to manage and control the receiver region.

The rest of the paper is structured as follows: Sect. 2 provides a comprehensive explanation of the implemented MATLAB model, encompassing its mathematical foundations and treatment. Section 3 presents the outcomes and findings
derived from the conducted simulations, offering an insightful examination of the
obtained results. Finally, concluding remarks and a summary of this study key
takeaways is reported in Sect. 4.

2   System Model

In the case of NFC, it is not feasible to approximate the light spot on the skin as
a point emission source because the distance between the receiver and the skin is
comparable to the dimensions of the spot. Hence, to address this issue, a 50 mm
square section of skin was subdivided into smaller square areas measuring 0.1 mm
each. Each of these small skin areas was individually analyzed as a micro-LED
(μ-LED) with its pattern and its intensity of emission.

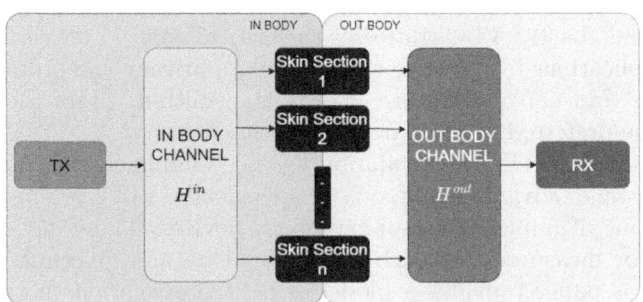

Fig. 2. VLC System Model

The VLC system was analyzed in terms of four components for each
route from transmitter to receiver: two corresponding to the telecommunication
devices, i.e. the transmitter (implanted LEDs) and the receiver (photodiode),
and two associated with the optical channel, i.e. one for characterizing light diffusion inside the body and one for external diffusion. The system model used for
simulation is shown in Fig. 2.

2.1 In-Body Channel Model

The evaluation of the in-body channel's characteristics was derived from a review of the literature, as discussed in [14]. This review includes considerations of both light power absorption (as depicted in Fig. 1b) and scattering. Absorption and scattering collectively contribute to the formation of a light spot on the skin.

To define the impact of absorption and scattering, Stochastic Monte Carlo (MC) modeling is the most used solution in the literature. In fact, over the past decade, several MC algorithms for simulating the propagation of optical radiation in biological media have been developed for diverse applications [14,15].

The simulation is based on modelling a large number of possible trajectories of the light from the source to the skin surface. Intensity path loss has been modeled using the Beer-Lambert law, which is represented as:

$$I_i = I_{i-1}e^{-\mu_a l} \tag{1}$$

where I_i is the light intensity during the i-th step of simulation, μ_a is the attenuation coefficient and l is the distance covered by the photon.

The scattering event is simulated by generating a random propagation angle denoted as θ, which determines the new direction of the photon. This angle follows a Henyey-Greenstein scattering phase function [16]:

$$p(\theta) = \frac{1}{4\pi} \frac{1 - a_f^2}{(1 + a_f^2 - 2a_f \cos\theta)^{3/2}} \tag{2}$$

Here, the parameter a_f represents the anisotropy factor, which is essentially the average cosine of the scattering angle θ. The value of g falls in the range $[-1, 1]$: when a_f is less than 0, it indicates back-forward scattering; when a_f equals 0, it means isotropic (Rayleigh) scattering, and when a_f is greater than 1, it denotes forward scattering (Mie scattering).

The simulation has been depicted in two dimensions because the LED's emission is axisymmetric. Consequently, the transfer function ($\boldsymbol{H}^{in}$) has been established in relation to the distance between a skin section and the symmetry axis ($\boldsymbol{d} = [d_1, \cdots, d_N]$ with N is the number of skin section). In this simulation, the LED's emission has been presumed to exhibit uniformity concerning the angle, then the transfer function has been defined as:

$$\boldsymbol{H}^{in} = I_0 \boldsymbol{f}(\boldsymbol{d}) \tag{3}$$

where I_0 is the uniform intensity of transmitter and $\boldsymbol{f}(\boldsymbol{d})$ is the path loss that depends on light absorption and scattering (see Fig. 3).

2.2 Out-Body Channel Model

Moreover, the MC simulation is used to define the emission pattern $\boldsymbol{g}(\boldsymbol{\alpha}, \boldsymbol{\beta})$ of each small skin area that depends on the angle formed between the symmetry axis of transmission and the line joining the transmitter to the respective small emission area (α) and the angle formed between the perpendicular to the skin surface and the line joining the respective small emission area to the receiver (β). The photodiode's area, utilized as the receiver, has been intentionally kept small since it's designed for short-range communications. Consequently, the distance involved is not on the same scale as the photodiode's surface area, enabling an approximation as a point receiver.

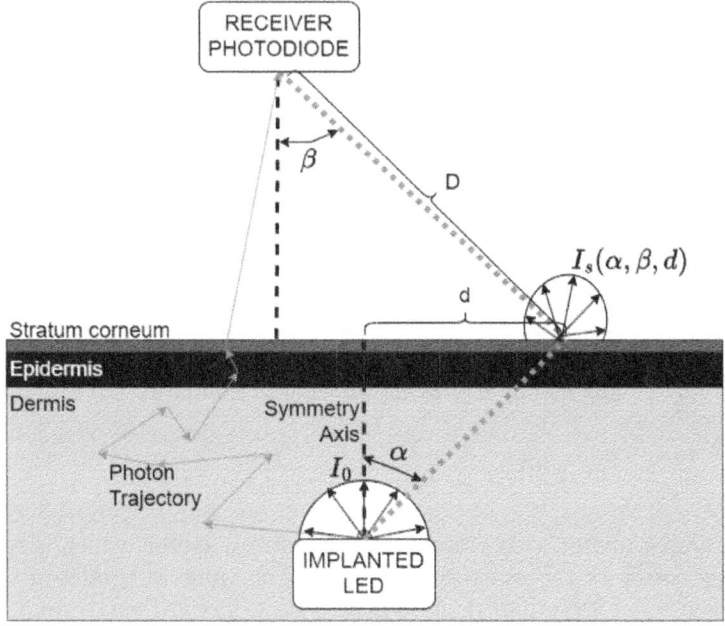

Fig. 3. Simulated Model

The photodetector has been positioned in a grid arrangement oriented perpendicular to the skin. This grid is centered at the center of the light spot, with the x-axis aligned parallel to the skin and z-axis aligned perpendicular to the skin. Along the x-axis, the grid points align with the segmented areas of the 50mm skin region, while along the z-axis ranges from 5mm to 50 mm, increasing in 5mm intervals.

For each receiver position, the out-body channel path loss (H^{out}) between specific receiver position and each small emission areas has been calculated as follows:

$$H^{out} = \frac{g(\alpha, \beta) \cos \beta}{D^2} \qquad (4)$$

where D represents the distance from a given receiver position to each of the individual small emission areas (see Fig. 3), the cosine of β depends on the characteristic of the geometric characteristics of the system.

2.3 VLC System Model: Single LED

The prevalent modulation scheme employed in VLC applications is Amplitude Sub-carrier BPSK as suggested in standard IEEE 802.15.7 [17], chosen to maintain the LED's primary function of providing constant light signaling for human eye. For this reason, the data transmitted $s_{tx}(t)$ can assume value of 1 or -1 in baseband. We assume here a binary phase shift keying (BPSK) modulation.

The received data $s_{rx}(t)$ in baseband was characterized for the follow equation, because the amplitude sub-carrier frequency is in the led modulation band, i.e., the out-body channel is characterized only on path loss component:

$$
s_{rx}(t) = \left(\underbrace{\sum \boldsymbol{H}^{in} * \boldsymbol{H}^{out}}_{H_{tot}} \right) s_{tx}(t) + n(t)
\tag{5}
$$

where $n(t)$ is the complex noise of Additive White Gaussian Noise (AWGN) for VLC link in amplitude sub-carrier frequency used in modulation scheme. The operator ($*$) is a multiplication corresponding elements between two array and $\sum$ is a sum of all element of the array. The characterization of out-body communication channel for NFC application was defined as $H_{tot} = \sum \boldsymbol{H}^{in} * \boldsymbol{H}^{out}$ (see Eq. (5)).

The data receiver in baseband was demodulated with the sign of real part of signal in BPSK modulation.

2.4 VLC System Model: MIMO

The MIMO used for simulation is a 2×2, i.e., the system is composed by two transmitting implanted LEDs and two photodiodes as receiver out of the body.

The mathematical treatment for MIMO application is similar to the single LED emission described above. Also in this case, as reference portion skin of 50 mm square section was subdivided into smaller square areas measuring 0.1 mm each and analyzed as a μ-LED matrix. The geometrical differences between a two system model are the position of led and photodiode in reference portion of skin and in position of receiver respectively. In the previous case, the position of led is in the center of reference portion skin, while in MIMO system model the middle point between two led is positioning in the middle of 50 mm square section of skin, i.e. the two leds are located at $d_{led}/2$ from the center reference portion skin along x-axis one to the right and the other to the left respect of the center (see Fig. 4).

The same applies for position photodiode, in the previous case the position of photodiode coincided with the position of receiver, while the two photodiodes are located at $d_{ph}/2$ from receiver position along x-axis as leds position (see Fig. 4).

For each transmitter, the transfer functions of in-body channel ($\boldsymbol{H}_1^{in}$ and $\boldsymbol{H}_2^{in}$) has been calculated, similar to the single LED case (as shown in Eq. (3)). The transfer functions for the out-body channel, as per formulation (4), are

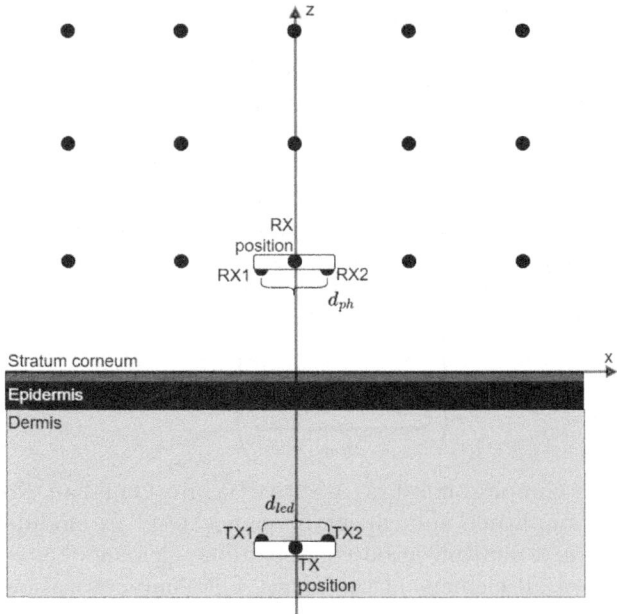

Fig. 4. MIMO System Model

contingent on the angles α and β, and consequently, they rely on the positioning of both the transmitter and receiver. For each receiver position, four distinct transfer functions denoted as $\boldsymbol{H}_{i,j}^{out}$ (with $i, j = 1$ or 2) have been defined, where i and j represent the specific LED and photodiode that transmitting and receiving data, respectively.

The two LEDs transmit distinct data streams ($s1_{tx}(t)$ and $s2_{tx}(t)$). The data received from the two photodiodes ($s1_{rx}(t)$ and $s2_{rx}(t)$) at each grid position in the baseband has been characterized using linear equations, as follows:

$$
\underbrace{\begin{bmatrix} s1_{rx}(t) \\ s2_{rx}(t) \end{bmatrix}}_{\boldsymbol{s}_{rx}(t)} = \underbrace{\begin{bmatrix} \sum \boldsymbol{H}_1^{in} * \boldsymbol{H}_{1,1}^{out} & \sum \boldsymbol{H}_2^{in} * \boldsymbol{H}_{2,1}^{out} \\ \sum \boldsymbol{H}_1^{in} * \boldsymbol{H}_{1,2}^{out} & \sum \boldsymbol{H}_2^{in} * \boldsymbol{H}_{2,2}^{out} \end{bmatrix}}_{\boldsymbol{H}_{tot}} \underbrace{\begin{bmatrix} s1_{tx}(t) \\ s2_{tx}(t) \end{bmatrix}}_{\boldsymbol{s}_{tx}(t)} + \underbrace{\begin{bmatrix} n1(t) \\ n2(t) \end{bmatrix}}_{\boldsymbol{N}(t)} \tag{6}
$$

where $\boldsymbol{N}(t)$ is a vector of two noises ($n1(t)$ and $n2(t)$) to characterize two different additive Gaussian noise channels.

To demodulate the two different data in the simulation, the inverted function of Eq. (6) has been calculated as:

$$
\boldsymbol{s}_{tx}^*(t) = \boldsymbol{H}_{tot}^{-1} \, \boldsymbol{s}_{rx}(t) \tag{7}
$$

where $\boldsymbol{s}_{tx}^*(t)$ are the estimation of transmitted signals. Once the two transmitted signals have been separated, the received data in the baseband is demodulated using the sign of the real part of the signal in the BPSK modulation.

3   Results

This section has been divided in two parts: initially, through MC simulation, the functions $f(d)$ and $g(\alpha, \beta)$ were computed (as outlined in Subsect. 3.1). Subsequently, these computed functions were utilized to simulate a potential transmission scenario between a single LED and a single photodiode, as well as for MIMO,2×2 transmission setups. The communication simulations were employed to calculate the Bit Error Rate (BER), which served as an assessment metric for the performance of the two prospective communication systems (as discussed in Subsect. 3.2). The skin coefficients used in the simulation were taken from literature [18], and it has been summarized in Table 1.

Table 1. Skin Parameters used in the MC simulation

Skin Parameter	Stratum Corneum	Epidermis	Dermis
Absorption coefficient (μ_a) [cm^{-1}]	8.15	3.07	6.52
Anisotropy Factor (a_f)	0.942	0.804	0.715
Layer Thickness [μm]	20	150	2000

3.1   Channel Characterization

Through MC simulation, the light intensity and direction have been established, as illustrated in Fig. 5. Notably, the summation of light beam intensities emanating from the skin surface, in relation to the distance from the LED's symmetry axis, is depicted in Fig. 5a. These data points have been effectively approximated with a Gaussian distribution, as indicated by the red line in Fig. 5a. This distribution is used to define Transfer Function $\boldsymbol{H}^{in}$.

For each skin section used to the defined $\boldsymbol{H}^{in}$, the summation of light beam intensity in angle clusters has been used to define the pattern of emission of single skin section, $g(\alpha, \beta)$. The average of the distribution of light intensity in angle cluster highlights the refraction effect of the light. In fact, in Fig. 5b the data has been fitted with a linear function with a different angular coefficient compared to α that characterized a single skin section. This angular coefficient defined similar to refractive index, n_{refr}.

The results obtained have been utilized to scale the emission pattern of a single skin section, incorporating all simulation data in the evaluation of the emission pattern caused by scattering.

The data has been modeled using a Gaussian distribution, as demonstrated in Fig. 5c. Figure 5d presents the emission pattern of a single skin section. The peak of the Gaussian distribution is equal to 1 since it's scaled against $\boldsymbol{H}^{in}$, and it is centered at an angle of 0 rad, which is achieved by translating the angle by $n_{\text{refr}}\alpha$.

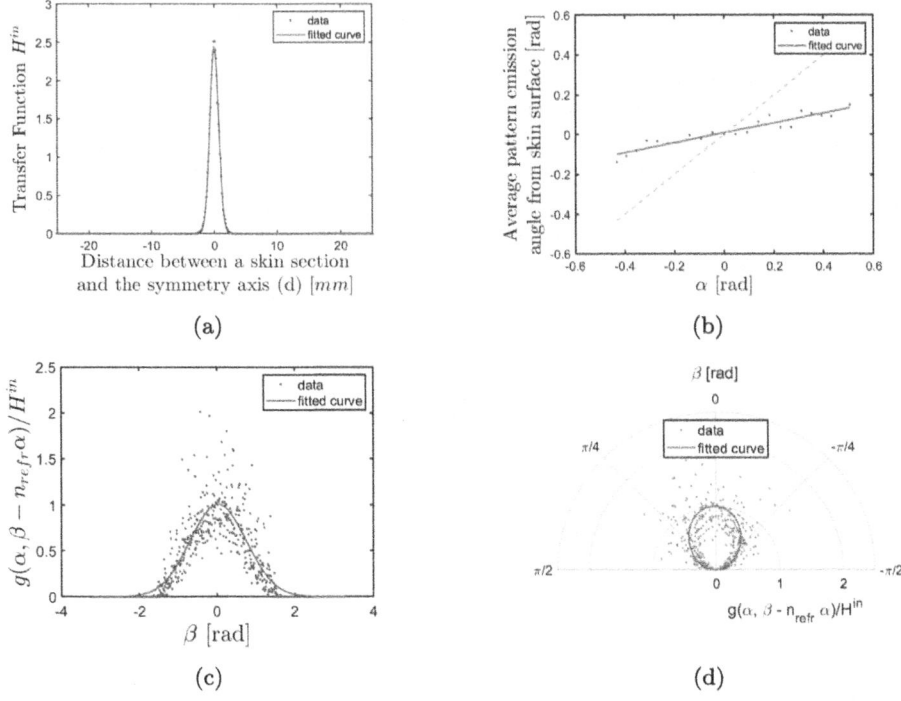

Fig. 5. Transfer Function of In-body Channel: in (a) the distribution of light intensity along the skin surface; in (b) the refraction effect. Pattern emission of skin scaled to intensity and average direction: (c) Cartesian plot (d) Polar plot.

3.2 System Performance: Bit Error Rate

In this section the BER is reported as a function of the position of the transmitters (LEDs) and receivers (photodiodes). The signal to noise ratio (SNR) at the receiver is dependent only on the path loss as depicted in (5). In particular, the received power depends on the in-body and out-body path loss as depicted in (3) and (4), respectively. The path loss depends on the position of the receiver, given the location of the transmitter, as depicted in Fig. 3.

The performance of the simulated implanted VLC system is assessed by analyzing the BER. A total of 1×10^5 symbols with Manchester coding were transmitted from the transmitter to the receiver.

In the case of single LED communication, the BER remains below 1×10^{-5} up to a distance of 35 mm, as illustrated in Fig. 6a.

In the MIMO case, the alignment between LEDs and photodiodes becomes more critical. In this simulation, both transmitters and receivers are positioned along the same axis, which represents the optimal configuration. Moreover, the system is not axisymmetric, in contrast to the previous case. Consequently, the position of the receiver along the x-axis (as shown in Fig. 6b) differs from its position along the y-axis (as depicted in Fig. 6c). In both cases, the BER remains below 1×10^{-5} up to a distance of 30 mm. However, the width of the maximum BER region is narrower compared to the previous case when the position of the receiver is in the plane (xz) including the segment joining the two transmitters/receivers (as shown in Fig. 6b), while the maximum BER region is comparable to the previous case when the position of the receiver is in the plane (yz) orthogonal to the segment joining the two transmitters/receivers (as shown in Fig. 6c).

It is worth noting that the maximum BER limit is 30 mm for the MIMO case, while it is 35 mm for the single LED case. This is due to the self-interference of the LEDs in the MIMO case.

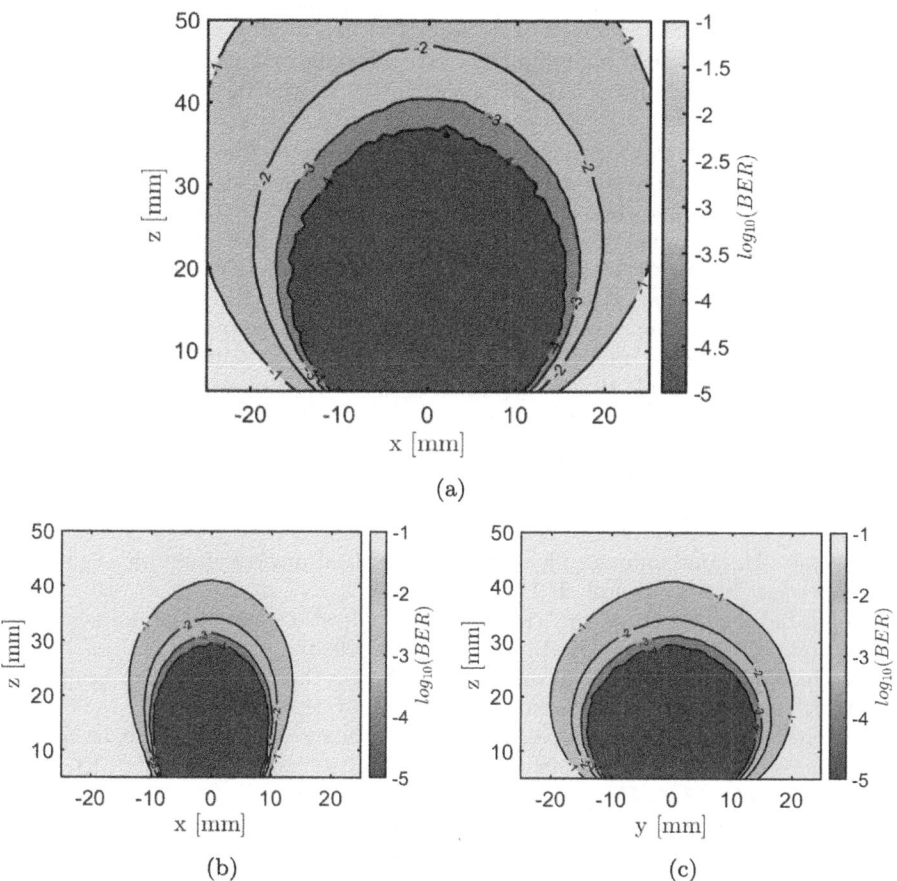

Fig. 6. Bit error rate (BER) over the vertical plane for the single LED (a) and multi-LED (b)–(c) systems.

4 Conclusion

This paper has presented a comprehensive study on the use of optical wireless communication (OWC), in particular visible light communication (VLC), for implantable medical devices (IMDs). The paper has explored the potential application of single LED and multiple LEDs multiple-input multiple-output (MIMO) techniques in IMD scenarios to manage and control the receiver region. Through MATLAB simulations, we demonstrated the feasibility and advantages of using VLC for subcutaneous IMDs used in temperature and glycemia measurements. We also evaluated the impact of the receiver's movement on the bit error rate (BER) of the VLC system and identified the optimal receiver placement for VLC systems in IMD scenarios. Finally, we proposed a novel approach for OWC-based communication in IMDs, which can potentially improve the reliability and efficiency of IMDs. These contributions can pave the way for the development of more advanced and effective OWC-based IMDs in the future.

Acknowledgments. This work was supported in part by the Italian Ministry of Foreign Affairs and International Cooperation, grant number US23GR04 (CUP: D43C23000350001). This work was also partially supported by the European Union under the Italian National Recovery and Resilience Plan (NRRP) of NextGenerationEU, partnership on "Telecommunications of the Future" (PE00000001 - program "RESTART"), by the European Telecommunication Standard Institute (ETSI), Smart Body Area Networks (SmartBAN) Technical Committee, by the European Union's Horizon 2020 programme under grants No. 872752 and No. 101017331, and by Fondazione Cassa di Risparmio di Firenze (project: SmartHUB on Medical & Social ICT for Territorial Assistance).

References

1. Joung, Y.-H.: Development of implantable medical devices: from an engineering perspective. Int. Neurourol. J. **17**(3), 98 (2013)
2. Global Industry Analysts Inc.: Implantable medical devices global market. Technical report, Global Strategic Business Report (2023)
3. Mucchi, L., et al.: How 6G technology can change the future wireless healthcare. In: 2020 2nd 6G Wireless Summit (6G SUMMIT). IEEE (2020)
4. Chi, N., Haas, H., Kavehrad, M., Little, T.D., Huang, X.-L.: Visible light communications: demand factors, benefits and opportunities [guest editorial]. IEEE Wirel. Commun. **22**, 5–7 (2015)
5. Agarwal, K., Jegadeesan, R., Guo, Y.-X., Thakor, N.V.: Wireless power transfer strategies for implantable bioelectronics. IEEE Rev. Biomed. Eng. **10**, 136–161 (2017)
6. Kim, H.-J., Hirayama, H., Kim, S., Han, K.J., Zhang, R., Choi, J.-W.: Review of near-field wireless power and communication for biomedical applications. IEEE Access **5**, 21264–21285 (2017)
7. Thompson, A.C., Wade, S.A., Pawsey, N.C., Stoddart, P.R.: Infrared neural stimulation: influence of stimulation site spacing and repetition rates on heating. IEEE Trans. Biomed. Eng. **60**, 3534–3541 (2013)

8. Latva-aho, M., Leppänen, K., et al.: Key drivers and research challenges for 6G ubiquitous wireless intelligence (2019)

9. Katz, M., Ahmed, I.: Opportunities and challenges for visible light communications in 6G. In: 2020 2nd 6G Wireless Summit (6G SUMMIT). IEEE (2020)

10. Caputo, S., Borghini, G., Jayousi, S., Rashid, A., Mucchi, L.: Visible light communications for healthcare applications: opportunities and challenges. In: 2023 IEEE 17th International Symposium on Medical Information and Communication Technology (ISMICT). IEEE (2023)

11. Sohn, I., Jang, Y.H., Lee, S.H.: Ultra-low-power implantable medical devices: optical wireless communication approach. IEEE Commun. Mag. **58**, 77–83 (2020)

12. Ahmed, I., Halder, S., Bykov, A., Popov, A., Meglinski, I.V., Katz, M.: In-body communications exploiting light: a proof-of-concept study using ex vivo tissue samples. IEEE Access **8**, 190378–190389 (2020)

13. Minotto, A., et al.: Visible light communication with efficient far-red/near-infrared polymer light-emitting diodes. Light Sci. Appl. **9** (2020)

14. Tuchin, V.V.: Light scattering study of tissues. Phys. Usp. **40**, 495–515 (1997)

15. Meglinski, I.V., Matcher, S.J.: Quantitative assessment of skin layers absorption and skin reflectance spectra simulation in the visible and near-infrared spectral regions. Physiol. Meas. **23**, 741–753 (2002)

16. Henyey, L.C., Greenstein, J.L.: Diffuse radiation in the galaxy. Astrophys. J. **93**, 70 (1941)

17. IEEE standard for local and metropolitan area networks–part 15.7: Short-range optical wireless communications

18. Bashkatov, A.N., Genina, E.A., Tuchin, V.V.: Optical properties of skin, subcutaneous, and muscle tissues: a review. J. Innov. Opt. Health Sci. **04**, 9–38 (2011)

Spectral Features-Based Machine Learning Approach to Detect SARS-COV-2 Infection Using Cough Sound

Shadab Azam Siddique[1][✉], Sudhir Kumar[2], Prabhat Kumar Upadhyay[3], Fardad Vakilipoor[4], and Davide Scazzoli[4]

[1] Department of Electronics and Communication Engineering, Supaul College of Engineering, Supaul, Supaul, India
shadab086@gmail.com

[2] Department of Electrical Engineering, Indian institute of Technology, Patna, Patna, India
sudhir@iitp.ac.in

[3] Department of Electrical Engineering, Indian Institute of Technology, Indore, Indore, India
pkupadhyay@iiti.ac.in

[4] Department of Electronics, Information and Bioengineering, Politecnico di Milano, Milan, Italy
{fardad.vakilipoor,davide.scazzoli}@polimi.it

Abstract. In this paper, a spectral features based automated techniques for the classification of Severe Acute Respiratory Syndrome coronavirus using cough audio sound is presented. The proposed technique has following major stages: pre-processing, feature extraction, feature representation, and classifications. COUGHVID dataset is used for this study which comprises cough audio data of both Corona Virus disease 19 (COVID-19) positive and healthy subjects. Different audio features such as Mel Frequency Cepstral Coefficients and Zero Crossing Rate were extracted and represented using different methods. We found that frame-level labeling and feature representation is providing the best accuracy. The feature vector was taken as input to the classifier with 5-fold cross-validation. Support Vector Machine, Random Forest, K Nearest Neighbor, and Light Gradient Boosting Method model are tested in this paper to classify the COVID-19 positive and healthy subjects achieving an accuracy of 88.52%, 88.91%, 98.34%, and 81.95%, respectively.

Keywords: COVID19 · KNN · SVM · RF · LGBM

1 Introduction

Since the outbreak of Corona Virus disease 19 (COVID-19), there have been more than 605 million people infected and 6.5 million lives have been lost globally due

© ICST Institute for Computer Sciences, Social Informatics and Telecommunications Engineering 2024
Published by Springer Nature Switzerland AG 2024. All Rights Reserved
M. Mizmizi et al. (Eds.): BodyNets 2024, LNICST 524, pp. 88–101, 2024.
https://doi.org/10.1007/978-3-031-72524-1_8

to COVID-19 (SARS-COV-2) virus till September, 2022 [1]. Rapid increase in the cases and tremendous load on healthcare system a fast diagnosis tool can help to slow down or stop the spread of disease in the area. Fast diagnosis techniques are essential for early disease detection in low-income counties with limited testing facilities. Usually, when patients experience symptoms, they either contact their physician or seek out medical professionals in clinical settings, where test can be done using various COVID-19 screening tools such as rapid antibody tests, antigens, and RT-PCR [2]. Diagnostic decisions are made based on input provided by the patient and their test reports. These approaches are relatively expensive, limiting their ability to test the public on a large scale.

A predominant symptom of respiratory disease is coughing and this is widely used by physician as one of the parameter for diagnosis and analysing the progress of treatment [3]. This motivates and allow the researchers to investigate pulmonary health using cough sounds. Asthma, COVID-19, pertussis, and tuberculosis are most common respiratory disease [4]. Machine Learning (ML) or Deep Learning (DL) algorithm can be used to diagnose respiratory disease by processing respiratory data such as speech, coughing, sneezing and breathing. COVID-19 was caused by the SARS-COV-2, which affects the respiratory system [3,5]. Several medical laboratory tests which are available to diagnose COVID-19, these includes molecular test, sputum test, antigen, plolymerase chain reaction, and rapid diagnostic test [2], X-ray [6,7] and Computed Tomography (CT) scan [8]. All of these diagnostic methods are expensive in the context of developing countries and require trained specialists and in some cases, laboratory facilities.

In this context, a simple, affordable, rapid, non-invasive, and machine aided remote diagnosis COVID-19 testing tool would be required. In modern technology systems, researchers are at rapid pace to develop signal processing, machine learning, or deep learning based, an automated low powered mobile device to replace primary screening by healthcare practitioners to reduce the risk of disease transmission. For the present work, a ML based classifier is used for automatic detection and classification of cough sound. This can be done by using the auditory features extracted from the cough audio data. Mel Frequency Cepstral Coefficients (MFCCs) and their variants have been extensively used in speech recognition task [2,9–15]. To increase the system performance, other features such as spectral, cepstral, and periodicity features are also paired with those of MFCCs [2,9,11–14]. In forgoing sections, related works, methodology, results and discussions, conclusion, and future work of the proposed model will be discussed.

2   Related Works

Diagnosing COVID-19 from cough audio has become the thrust area of research to artificial intelligence community. In [9], respiratory sounds were used to extract handcrafted features of 477 dimensions and Visual Geometry Group Network (VGGNet) based features of 256 dimensions. These features are concatenated to get a total features of 733 dimensions. Gradient Boosting (GB)

Table 1. Summary of related work

Ref	Dataset	Features	Classifier	Performance
[2]	Coughvid, Coswara	NMF Spectrogram, MFCCs, MFCCs Stats	SVM, KNN, XGBoost	Accuracy 73.3%
[9]	Own developed dataset	SC, ZCR, duration, period, onset, tempo, RMS energy, MFCCs, and their variants	SVM, GB Tree, LR, VGGNet	AUC-ROC 80%
[10]	Virufy	MFCCs	SVM	Accuracy 95.86%
[11]	DiCOVA, COUGHVID	Spetrogram	VGG13	AUC-ROC 78.3%
[12]	Coughvid	ZCR, RMS, PSD, MFCCs	Stack ensemble model	Accuracy 79.86%
[16]	Coughvid	MFCC and Mel Spectrogram Images	DNN	Best AUC-ROC 91%
[13]	Coughvid	MFCCs	CNN	AUC-ROC 94%
[14]	Coughvid, Coswara	MFCCs	Ensemble DNN	AUC-ROC 77.1%
[15]	Cambridge	Log frequency power spectrogram	DNN (VGGNet)	AUC-ROC 74%

Ref: References, NMF: Non-Negative Matrix Factorisation, SC: Spectral centroid, SB: Spectral Bandwidth, XGBoost: Extreme Gradient Boost, CNN: Convolution Neural Network, DNN: Deep Neural Network.

Trees, Logistic Regression (LR), and Support Vector Machine (SVM) are used as a classification model to get the best performance as Area Under Curve of Receiver Operating Characteristics (AUC-ROC) of 80%.

In [10], the classification accuracy of 95.86% were reported with MFCCs feature on radial basis kernel function based SVM. In [11], spetrogram images were extracted from cough audio data. They used deep network architecture VGG13 to get an average AUC-ROC of 78.3%. In [12], the author extracted ZCR, Root Mean Square (RMS), Power Spectral Density (PSD), and MFCCs features. The performance of ten different ML algorithms were reported and compared. They have proposed stacked ensemble of ML models that yields the best performance, with an accuracy of 79.86%. Some of the related works are summarized in Table 1. Authors in [2,12–14,16] used the COUGHVID dataset and proposed different DL and ML approach for the classification of cough audio data. In [6,7], chest X-ray images have been used for the prediction of COVID-19. In [8], authors extracted features from X-ray and CT images using various DL models to detect and assess the severity of COVID-19 effect on lungs. These methods [6–8] required a clinical visit, well-trained technician, and medical practitioner for data acquisition. Current research focuses on the development of an improved COVID-19 system based on cough audio sound. Several cough based COVID-19 classification methods have been discussed in Table 1. There is still scope for improvement in terms of feature representation, detection accuracy, and computational complexity. In this article we have proposed a pre-processing of raw cough audio data, segmentation of pre-processed data, feature extraction, labelling of feature in a frame wise manner, then we have used different shallow ML classifier to get the best performance. Due to the use of shallow ML classifier it can be implemented in a low cost micro-controller based device for commercial applications.

3 Methodology

This section describes the proposed methodology, which consists of dataset, data augmentation, pre-processing, feature extraction, feature representation, and ML classifiers. For the classification, the audio recordings of COUGHVID dataset were first passed through a pre-processing module. Next our pre-processed dataset is splitted into training and test sets with the ratio of 80:20. Now, to extend the training set and solve the class imbalance problem, two data augmentation methods were applied. ML based model is used to produce binary classification and the results were obtained based on MFCCs features and spectral feature ZCR. Five fold cross-validation method is used to validate the model. To assess the classification performance of the proposed model we have computed accuracy, precision, sensitivity, specificity, AUC-ROC and, F1 score evaluation metrics.

3.1 Dataset

In this article, COUGHVID [3] dataset is used, which is publicly available crowd-sourcing dataset. This dataset has been gathered through a web application developed by researchers from the Embedded Systems Laboratory (ESL), Swiss Federal Institute of Technology Lausanne (EPFL). COUGHVID contains more than 20,000 cough audio recordings along with each of them has one metadata comprises of their self-reported information such as gender, age, respiratory condition, geographic location, COVID-19 status (healthy, symptomatic, COVID-19, none), etc. Out of 20,000 cough audio recording only 1,050 of them claimed to have been exposed to COVID-19. A total of around 1,000 cough audio recordings were annotated by pulmonologist, the annotated attributes include audible nasal congestion, audible dyspnea, audible stridor, audible choking, audible wheezing, quality, and type of cough.

In addition, this dataset required data cleaning as some participants did not report their self-reported information while uploading their cough sounds. Apart from cough sound the dataset also contains complete silent audio files and non-cough sound. A cough detection ML model is applied to predict whether the sound file is really a cough recording. This is included in the metadata called as cough detected and their entry is a float number from 0 to 1 that indicates the probability of cough detection. The data cleaning is done with cough detected value 0.7 to get an audio recording contains only cough records. After filtering of dataset we have 5,386 recordings in our cleaned dataset, each labelled with one class either positive or negative. The raw cough audio data is available as a .JSON format that has been converted to a .wav format for further processing.

3.2   Pre-processing

The audio present in the COUGHVID dataset were recorded on voluntary basis by different users in different environments. Hence the audio quality varied significantly within the dataset [5]. Spectrogram of one cough signal is investigated in Fig. 1. Also it is evident from the literature that for cough audio, significant amount of information is present within the 10 kHz bandwidth [17]. From the perusal of Fig. 1, it is observed that significant information is within 8 kHz bandwidth. Therefore, to remove unwanted signal components not related to human speech, all the audio signals are passed through a 10 kHz low-pass filter. The cough audio recording is resampled at sampling rate of 22,050 Hz. To remove the outliers and adjusting the amplitude levels within a minimum and maximum range the normalization is required. All the cough audio $y_j(t)$, is normalised using (1), where j is j^{th} cough audio sample.

$$y_j(t) = 0.9 \times \frac{y_j(t)}{|max(y_j(t))|} \quad .$$

(1)

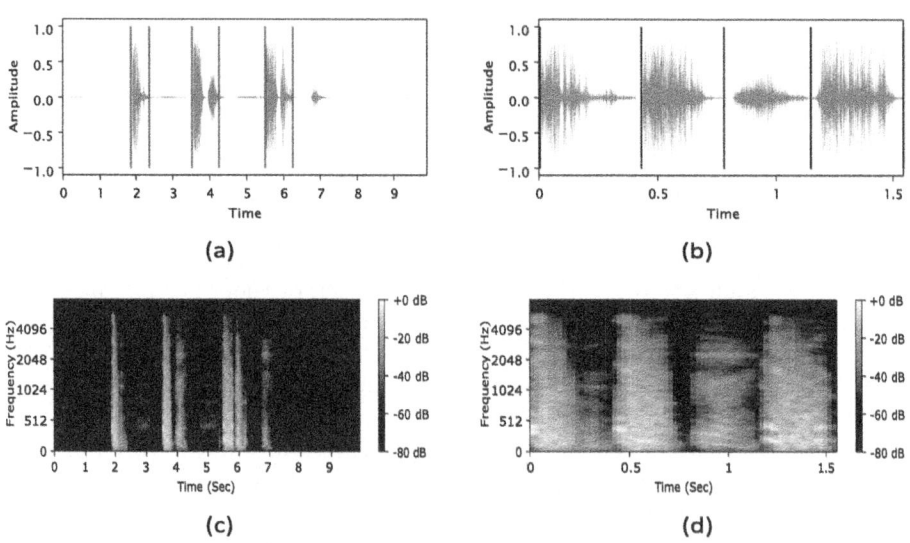

Fig. 1. (a) Raw cough audio data (b) spectrogram of raw cough audio data (c) processed cough audio data (d) spectrogram of processed cough audio data

It is evident from Fig. 1 that the first and last segment of audio signals are prone to silence, which can be removed by trimming the silence using a short term energy based silence detection algorithm. The background noise levels and silence in the cough audio files badly affect the overall performance of speech recognition systems [18,19]. Each audio files were segmented and split on silence where we set a threshold of 10 dB and minimum silence length of 50 ms. We divided each non-silent piece of segmented audio files into chunks if their amplitude was higher than the threshold and their length was longer than the minimum silence length. Now, all the chunks is passed through trim effects where we set a threshold of 10 dB, below this reference we consider as silence and trim that part. These values were determined manually and interactively. Finally, all the audio chunks were stacked and we get a silence and noise free audio signal (cf. Fig. 1).

3.3 Data Augmentation

In ML, the problem of small and unbalanced dataset is the biggest challenge. The better results can be obtained when data is fed in balanced groups, so equalizing data can help us to train a good model [13]. We have applied two data augmentation techniques to the COVID-19 positive labelled audio samples. First, the pitch of the recording is randomly shifted, secondly, white noise is added. We have increased COVID-19 positive labelled audio recordings from 420 to 1,260. From the other class we have randomly selected 1,260 audio recordings. This results in a balanced dataset of 2,520 audio recordings. To ensure the validity of our network performance and to avoid the repeated occurrence of the same original audio files in different splits, the dataset was split into training and test set prior to the data augmentation.

3.4 Feature Extraction

After data augmentation and pre-processing of the COUGHVID dataset, a total of 2,520 pre-processed cough audio data is filtered in which 1,260 observations of COVID-19 positive and randomly chosen 1,260 observations of healthy subjects each of same length. We have used MFCCs features which are extracted from pre-processed audio signal. MFCCs have been used successfully as a feature for audio signal analysis, especially as a feature for automatic speech recognition. They have been successfully used to distinguish between dry and wet coughs and to identify tuberculosis, asthma and COVID-19-associated cough [20–22]. From the literature it has been established that MFCCs features are most significant for audio signals, therefore MFCCs features along with ZCR are selected to train our ML classifier. We have used librosa package [23] where default sampling rate is 22,050 Hz, frame length of 2,048 samples $\cong 93ms$, hop length of 512 samples $\cong 23ms$, Hann window type and frame rate 44 frames/Sec (cf. Fig. 2). Frame rate can be found with the ratio of sampling rate to the hop length. We have extracted the first 40 MFCCs features hence we got the 2 dimensional vector of size $m \times n$, where all m frames of a particular sample are labelled same as sample label. Conversion from linear frequency domain to Mel-frequency domain can be seen in (2) [24].

$$f_{mel} = 2595 \log_{10}(1 + \frac{f}{700}) \tag{2}$$

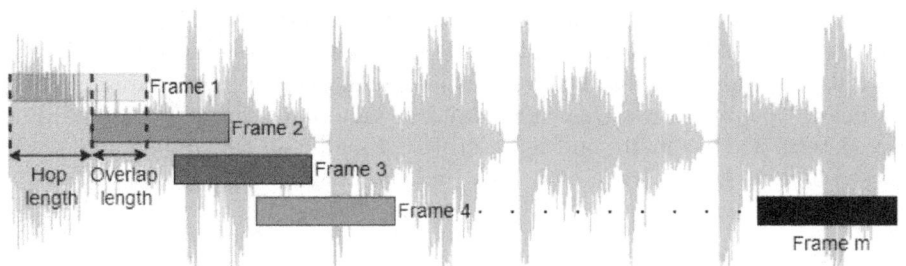

Frame length = hop length + ovelap length

Fig. 2. Segmentation of pre-processed cough audio data.

Algorithm for computing MFCCs feature and labelling frame wise:
Pre-emphasis of the audio signal $s(n)$: flatten the signal spectrally and uses high pass filter that will put an emphasis to increase the amplitude of high frequency signals.

$$p(n) = s(n) - \alpha s(n-1) \qquad (3)$$

where $0.9 < \alpha < 1$. Segmentation of the signal $p(n)$ into i number of smaller time frames (length $= m$ points)

$$p(n) = p_1, p_2, p_3, p_4, \ldots\ldots, p_i \qquad (4)$$

Apply Hanning window $w(n)$ to each frame.

$$f(n) = p(n) \times w(n) \qquad (5)$$

Now, the Fast Fourier Transform is applied on $f_i(n)$ in order to obtain the magnitude spectrum signal for each frame.

$$X(k) = \sum_{n=0}^{N-1} f(n) e^{\frac{i2\pi nk}{N}} \qquad (6)$$

For mel frequency wrapping J number of filters are used and for each filter i^{th} mel spectrum X_i is computed.

$$X_i = \log\left(\sum_{n=0}^{N-1} |X(k)|H_i(k)\right) \qquad (7)$$

where $i = 1, 2, 3, \ldots\ldots, J$ and $H_i(k)$ is the ith triangular filter.
Using discrete cosine transform m number of cepstrum coefficients are calculated

$$Y_n = \sum_{i=0}^{J} X_i cos(n(i - 0.5)\pi/J) \qquad (8)$$

where $n = 1, 2, 3, \ldots., N$ (no. of coefficient required).

MFCC feature vector of $m \times n$ used for feature representation. ZCR are calculated for $s(n)$ and concatenated with MFCC feature. Final feature vector is $m \times (n + 1)$.

$$\hat{Z}(n) = \frac{1}{2l_{p_i}} \sum_{n=0}^{N-1} |sgn(s_i(n)) - sgn(s_i(n - 1))| \tag{9}$$

where l_{p_i} is the length of p_i and $sgn(x(n)) = \begin{cases} 1 & x(n) \geqslant 0 \\ -1 & x(n) < 0 \end{cases}$

The $m \times (n + 1)$ feature vector is represented using different feature representation method described below.

For feature representation few techniques were explored. In the first method, two dimensional feature vector $m \times (n + 1)$ were reshaped to one dimensional feature vector $1 \times m(n + 1)$ to get the most significant features. In the second method, the mean of these $(n + 1)$ columns are computed to get a 1 dimensional feature vector $1 \times (n + 1)$. For third method, all the m rows of features are labelled the same as the input signal $s(n)$, which is a frame level feature (Fig. 3 depicts the method 3.

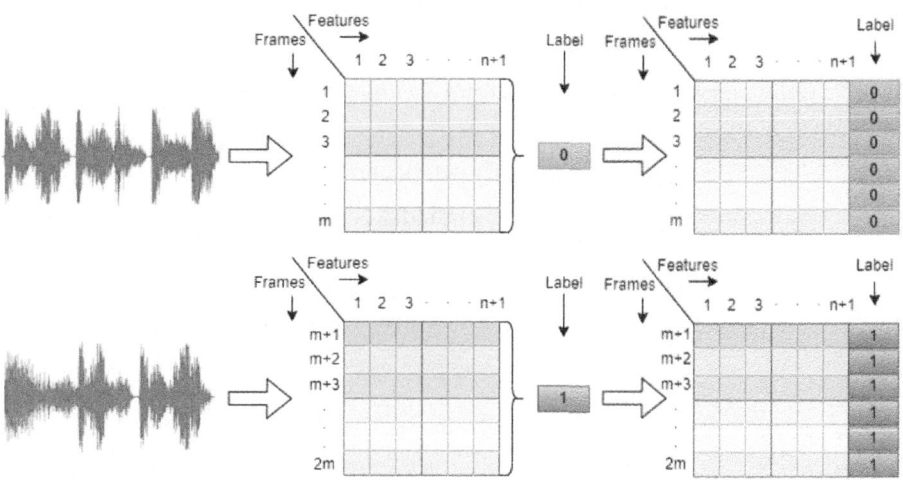

Fig. 3. Frame level feature extraction and labelling.

3.5 Machine Learning Classifier

Machine learning classifier is used to for the classification of the cough data to identify the COVID-19 patients. We have performed a comprehensive analysis by applying various machine learning classification techniques including SVM, K-Nearest Neighbour (KNN), Random Forest (RF), Linear Discriminant Analysis

(LDA), Extreme Gradient Boosting Machine (XGBM), Light Gradient Boosting Machine (LGBM) and Neural Network (NN), on the features obtained by applying the different method mentioned above. Out of these ML classifier SVM, KNN, RF, and LGBM outperform among all the classifiers. 80% data are used to train the model and the best model is exported. The model is then tested at 20% data from the entire dataset. The hyper-parameters for these models were chosen empirically to achieve the best performance. For SVM, a radial basis kernel function was used, the value of k for KNN was set to 5, and the n-estimators parameter for RF was 400 which specifies the number of trees in the forest.

4   Results and Discussions

The proposed model is evaluated with in-depth analysis using the COUGHVID [3] dataset to detect the COVID-19 in cough sounds along with the corresponding test results. The main focus of our research is to propose a novel machine learning-based system that will lead to adequate COVID-19 diagnostic capabilities.

The classifier versus test accuracy for all the proposed feature representation method discussed in Sect. 3.4 are presented in Table 2. It is evident from Table 2, that method 3 outperformed the first two methods.

Table 2. Comparison of different classifier's accuracy for different feature representation method.

Classifier	Method-1	Method-2	Method-3
SVM	85.51%	85.51%	**88.52%**
KNN	74.20%	82.34%	**98.34%**
RF	88.09%	88.88%	**88.91%**
LGBM	85.51%	**85.91%**	81.95%

4.1   Performance Evaluation

The model performance is evaluated in terms of accuracy (AC), precision (PR), sensitivity (SE), specificity (SP), and F1 score metrics and are presented as follows.

$$AC = \frac{TP + TN}{TP + TN + FP + FN} \tag{10}$$

$$PR = \frac{TP}{TP + FP} \tag{11}$$

$$SE = \frac{TP}{TP + FN} \tag{12}$$

$$SP = \frac{TP}{TN + FP} \tag{13}$$

$$F1 - Score = 2 \times \frac{PR \times SE}{PR + SE} \tag{14}$$

For method 3 described in the above section, the confusion matrix of the proposed models is presented in Table 3. The performance parameters were calculated from Table 3 and presented in Table 4. For different methods used in this article, we evaluated the curve of the Receiver Operating Characteristic (ROC) graphed to estimate the Area Under Curve (AUC) parameter. It is evident from Fig. 4 that method 3 outperformed method 1 and method 2. Using method 3 the AUC-ROC is 98.5%, 96%, 94.8%, and 89.5% for KNN, RF, SVM, and LGBM classifier respectively.

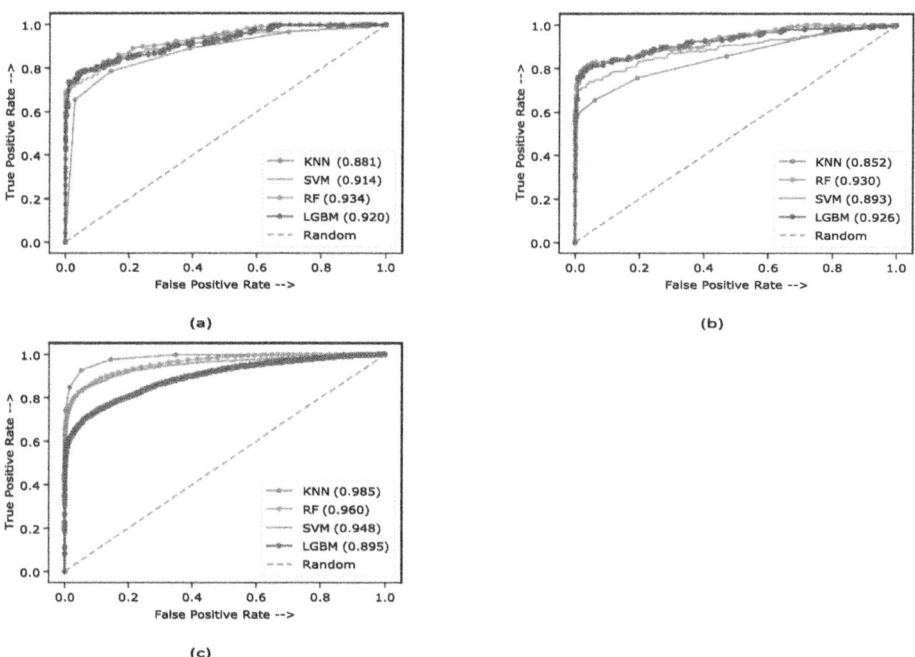

Fig. 4. AUC-ROC plot of different classifier for (a) method 1 (b) method 2 (c) method 3.

Table 3. Confusion matrix of the proposed methods.

		Predicted Class	
		Negative	**Positive**
Actual Class	**Negative**	TN (True Negative)	FP (False Positive)
	Positive	FN (False Negative)	TP (True Positive)

(a) Confusion matrix

		Negative	Positive
Actual Class	**Negative**	97.61%	2.39%
	Positive	18.24%	81.76%

(b) Confusion matrix for SVM

		Negative	Positive
Actual Class	**Negative**	98.06%	1.94%
	Positive	1.38%	98.62%

(c) Confusion matrix for KNN

		Negative	Positive
Actual Class	**Negative**	84.34%	15.66%
	Positive	33.02%	66.98%

(d) Confusion matrix for RF

		Negative	Positive
Actual Class	**Negative**	93.59%	6.41%
	Positive	29.60%	70.40%

(e) Confusion matrix for LGBM

Table 4. Performance comparison of different models.

Classifier	Accuracy	Precision	Sensitivity	Specificity	F1-Score
SVM	89.48%	96.98%	81.76%	97.46%	88.72%
RF	87.91%	97.14%	78.20%	97.70%	86.65%
KNN	98.39%	98.11%	98.67%	98.10%	98.39%
LGBM	82.00%	91.66%	70.4%	93.59%	79.63%

From Table 4 it can be concluded that KNN performs best among all the classifier.

4.2 Comparative Discussion

Comparison of proposed model with the other available technology are compared in the Table 5. Spectral features such as MFCCs and ZCR were extracted from COUGHVID dataset and used as an input to different classifiers [2,10,12], the maximum accuracy of 95.86% were achieved with MFCCs feature and SVM classifier. A novel approach for feature representation is used in this article and here KNN classifier shows an average accuracy of 98.39% with MFCCs and ZCR feature extracted from pre-processed cough audio data.

Table 5. Performance comparison with existing models.

Reference	Feature	Classifier	Accuracy
[10]	MFCCs	SVM	95.86%
[12]	MFCCs, ZCR, RMS, PSD	Stack Ensemble Model	79.86%
[2]	MFCCs, MFCCs Stats, NMF Spectrogram	SVM, KNN, XGBoost	73.3%
Proposed work*	MFCCs, ZCR	SVM	89.48%
		RF	87.91%
		LGBM	85.91%
		KNN	98.39%

5 Conclusion

In this article, we have used cough recordings from COUGHVID dataset to perform pre-processing, feature extraction, feature representation, and modelling techniques for a COVID-19 classification system. The cleanliness of the dataset such as normalization of data, low pass filtering, and silence removal has a significant impact on the performance of classification. The dataset has been shown to perform better with clean sound recordings. To handle the imbalance dataset data augmentation technique is used. Audio sample level extracted MFCCs features vectors are stacked, where each row represents frame level MFCCs feature, these row are labelled with the same label as the audio sample. It can be concluded that frame level labelled MFCCs feature improve the classification performance. We have evaluated different ML model for the detection of COVID-19 from cough audio signal. As compared to all the classifier KNN tend to produce better performance with test accuracy of 98.39%, specificity of 98.10%, sensitivity of 98.67%, F1 score of 98.39% and AUC-ROC of 98.50%. Testing for COVID-19 using cough samples could benefit clinical diagnostic systems as well as regular monitoring of infected patients at low cost. This study could be a step towards better COVID-19 pre-screening.

6   Future Work

In the present work, we have introduced a non-invasive automatic cough detection method based on machine learning that can accurately distinguish between COVID-19 positive subjects and healthy subjects. Additionally, we will create a smartphone application-driven tool to identify COVID-19, also a digital signal processing and microcontroller-based device can be created to detect COVID-19, where by inputting a cough sound using an on-board microphone, the device will be able to provide the status of disease.

Acknowledgement. This work was supported in part by the Vishleshan I-hub Foundation, Technology Innovation Hub (TIH), Indian Institute of Technology Patna (IIT Patna), India under project titled "Auditory Scene Analysis in Audio Signal Processing using Deep Learning Methods" and part by Italian Ministry of Foreign Affairs and International Cooperation, grant number US23GR04 (CUP: D43C23000350001).

References

1. Lebourgeois, S., et al.: Differential activation of human neutrophils by SARS-CoV-2 variants of concern. Front. Immunol. **13**, 1010140 (2022)
2. Rahman, D.A., Lestari, D.P.: COVID-19 classification using cough sounds. In: 2021 8th International Conference on Advanced Informatics: Concepts, Theory and Applications (ICAICTA), pp. 1–6. IEEE (2021)
3. Orlandic, L., Teijeiro, T., Atienza, D.: The COUGHVID crowdsourcing dataset, a corpus for the study of large-scale cough analysis algorithms. Sci. Data **8**(1), 1–10 (2021)
4. Imran, A., et al.: AI4COVID-19: AI enabled preliminary diagnosis for COVID-19 from cough samples via an app. Inform. Med. Unlocked **20**, 100378 (2020)
5. Sharma, A., Tiwari, S., Deb, M.K., Marty, J.L.: Severe acute respiratory syndrome coronavirus-2 (SARS-CoV-2): a global pandemic and treatment strategies. Int. J. Antimicrobial Agents **56**(2), 106054 (2020)
6. Tabik, S., et al.: COVIDGR dataset and COVID-SDNet methodology for predicting COVID-19 based on chest X-ray images. IEEE J. Biomed. Health Inform. **24**(12), 3595–3605 (2020)

7. Tang, S., et al.: EDL-COVID: ensemble deep learning for COVID-19 case detection from chest X-ray images. IEEE Trans. Ind. Inf. **17**(9), 6539–6549 (2021)
8. Kassania, S.H., Kassanib, P.H., Wesolowskic, M.J., Schneidera, K.A., Detersa, R.: Automatic detection of coronavirus disease (COVID-19) in X-ray and CT images: a machine learning based approach. Biocybern. Biomed. Eng. **41**(3), 867–879 (2021)
9. Brown, C., et al.: Exploring automatic diagnosis of COVID-19 from crowdsourced respiratory sound data. arXiv preprint arXiv:2006.05919 (2020)
10. Manshouri, N.M.: Identifying COVID-19 by using spectral analysis of cough recordings: a distinctive classification study. Cogn. Neurodyn. **16**(1), 239–253 (2022)
11. Rao, S., Narayanaswamy, V., Esposito, M., Thiagarajan, J., Spanias, A.: Deep learning with hyper-parameter tuning for COVID-19 cough detection. In: 2021 12th International Conference on Information, Intelligence, Systems & Applications (IISA), pp. 1–5. IEEE (2021)
12. Gupta, R., Krishna, T.A., Adeeb, M.: Cough sound based COVID-19 detection with stacked ensemble model. In: 2022 4th International Conference on Smart Systems and Inventive Technology (ICSSIT), pp. 1391–1395. IEEE (2022)
13. Sabet, M., Ramezani, A., Ghasemi, S.M.: COVID-19 detection in cough audio dataset using deep learning model. In: 2022 8th International Conference on Control, Instrumentation and Automation (ICCIA), pp. 1–5. IEEE (2022)
14. Chaudhari, G., et al.: Virufy: global applicability of crowdsourced and clinical datasets for AI detection of COVID-19 from cough. arXiv preprint arXiv:2011.13320 (2020)
15. Xia, T., et al.: COVID-19 sounds: a large-scale audio dataset for digital respiratory screening. In: Thirty-Fifth Conference on Neural Information Processing Systems Datasets and Benchmarks Track (Round 2) (2021)
16. Fakhry, A., Jiang, X., Xiao, J., Chaudhari, G., Han, A., Khanzada, A.: Virufy: a multi-branch deep learning network for automated detection of COVID-19. arXiv preprint arXiv:2103.01806 (2021)
17. Ai, O.C., Hariharan, M., Yaacob, S., Chee, L.S.: Classification of speech dysfluencies with MFCC and LPCC features. Expert Syst. Appl. **39**(2), 2157–2165 (2012)
18. Le Prell, C.G., Clavier, O.H.: Effects of noise on speech recognition: challenges for communication by service members. Hearing Res. **349**, 76–89 (2017)
19. Dash, T.K., Solanki, S.S., Panda, G.: Improved phase aware speech enhancement using bio-inspired and ANN techniques. Analog Integrated Circuits Signal Process. **102**(3), 465–477 (2020)
20. Botha, G.H.R., et al.: Detection of tuberculosis by automatic cough sound analysis. Physiol. Measur. **39**(4), 045005 (2018)
21. Pahar, M., Smith, L.S.: Coding and decoding speech using a biologically inspired coding system. In: 2020 IEEE Symposium Series on Computational Intelligence (SSCI), pp. 3025–3032. IEEE (2020)
22. Han, W., Chan, C.-F., Choy, C.-S., Pun, K.-P.: An efficient MFCC extraction method in speech recognition. In: 2006 IEEE International Symposium on Circuits and Systems (ISCAS), pp. 4–pp. IEEE (2006)
23. McFee, B., et al.: Librosa: audio and music signal analysis in Python. In: Proceedings of the 14th Python in Science Conference, vol. 8, pp. 18–25. Citeseer (2015)
24. Hossan, Md.A., Memon, S., Gregory, M.A.: A novel approach for MFCC feature extraction. In: 2010 4th International Conference on Signal Processing and Communication Systems, pp. 1–5. IEEE (2010)

Smart Healthcare Applications

Smart Healthcare System for Detection of Diabetic Retinopathy Using Transfer Learning

Pooja Ranjan[1], Shubham Kumar[1], Mustafa Sameer[1], Sanchita Ghosh[2],
Davide Scazzoli[3], and Bharat Gupta[1]([✉])

[1] Department of Electronics and Communication Engineering, National Institute of Technology
Patna, Patna, Bihar, India
{poojar.pg20.ec,shubhamk.ug18.ec,mustafa.ec17,bharat}@nitp.ac.in
[2] Department of Information Technology, Institute of Engineering and Management, Kolkata,
West Bengal, India
sanchita.ghosh@iemcal.com
[3] Department of Electronics, Information and Bioengineering, Politecnico di Milano, Milan,
Italy
davide.scazzoli@polimi.it

Abstract. The Diabetic Retinopathy (DR) causes significant vision loss, especially among the working-age population. Manual diagnosis by Ophthalmologists
is slow due to a shortage of skilled clinicians. An automated system for early DR
detection is needed. Deep Learning (DL) shows promise in medical image analysis but requires ample training images, challenging in the DR domain. Transfer
Learning (TL) addresses this data scarcity issue, combining TL with CNNs for DR
detection. This study proposes a smart healthcare model using EfficientNetV1 and
V2 CNNs with TL on IDRiD dataset for DR detection. EfficientNetV1 (B0-B7)
performance is compared, evaluating sensitivity, specificity, and accuracy. Effi-
cientNetV2's performance on the same dataset is also assessed. EfficientNetV2
being a smaller model size achieved 80.09% sensitivity, establish it as a state-of-
the-art model that excels in both training efficiency and parameter efficiency compared to its predecessors, a novel model for DR detection and classification. The
study showcases advancements in early DR diagnosis, promising broader accessi-
bility. Future efforts will focus on enhancing model performance and deploying it
in smart healthcare settings. The proposed smart healthcare model holds significant
promise for DR diagnosis and treatment.

Keywords: Diabetic Retinopathy · Transfer Learning · IDRiD ·
EfficientNetV1 · EfficientNetV2

© ICST Institute for Computer Sciences, Social Informatics and Telecommunications Engineering 2024
Published by Springer Nature Switzerland AG 2024. All Rights Reserved
M. Mizmizi et al. (Eds.): BodyNets 2024, LNICST 524, pp. 105–126, 2024.
https://doi.org/10.1007/978-3-031-72524-1_9

1 Introduction

Diabetes is becoming a serious global disease which is primarily caused by the pancreas' inability to produce enough insulin [1]. Diabetes has been recognized as a medical condition for thousands of years, with evidence of its existence dating back to ancient civilizations.

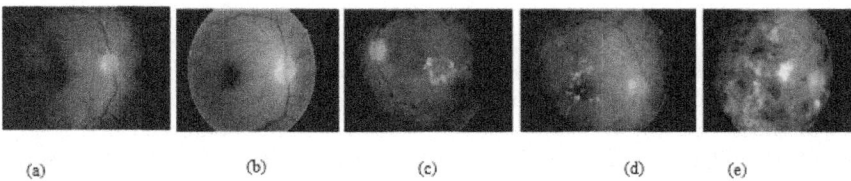

(a)   (b)   (c)   (d)   (e)

Fig. 1. Random Samples of Diabetic Retinopathy of various Levels. (a) Level 0, (b) Level 1, (c) Level 2, (d) Level 3, and e) Level 4.

However, the understanding and awareness of diabetic retinopathy as a specific complication of diabetes likely developed in the 20th century with advancements in medical research and technology. Thereafter, dramatic rise of DR cases from 108 million in 1980 to 422 million in 2014 has been observed and further a rise of 700 million has been predicted by 2045. Diabetes has evolved into a fatal disease that has claimed the lives of 1.5 million people worldwide in 2019 [1, 2]. It has been found to cause serious problems to the retina, heart, nerves, and lower limb [3]. DR is one of the most prevalent significant diabetes-related diseases [4]. This is the most common blindness causing disease in which the blood vessels of the retina are damaged [5]. Preservation of fluids or expansion of the macula is a distinguishing aspect of the two, which can occur at any stage of DR. People with diabetic Mellitus are more likely to experience a variety of short- and long-term difficulties as a result of macular abnormalities, which can result in life-threatening vision loss [6]. Adults (> 18 years of age) with diabetes accounted for 8.5% of the population in 2014, nearly doubling the 4.7% in 1980 [7]. DR is responsible for at least 2.6% of blindness worldwide.

These worldwide reports indicate the percentage of a person's usual life that has been impacted. Diabetes patients who have been sick with the condition for a long time are more likely to have DR. Hence regular retinal screening should be done for early detection of DR which can help avoid blindness, but review of retinal images requires a lot of efforts and labor which makes it a difficult undertaking [8]. As a result, a reliable detection technique is required to aid healthcare professionals in the analysis of DR [9].

The deciding factor of diabetic retinopathy is visual lesions on retinal images which are named as microaneurysms (MA), hemorrhages (HM), and soft and hard exudates (EX) are examples of these lesions [10]. MA comes first in the severity hierarchy of DR and is identified as a little red spherical spots on the retina. The weakening in the retinal vascular wall is one of the major contributing factors of DR. Other symptoms include Hemorrhages (HM) which are red lesions seen on the retina (rear of the eye) as irregular marginal bigger patches while hard exudates and soft exudates are the brightest lesions that appear on the outer layer of the retina [11]. Depending on the occurrence of these lesions, there are five level of DR. According to Wilkinson et al. [12] level 0 is normal with no signs of DR, level 1 indicates the presence of mild DR, level 2 indicates moderate DR, level 3 indicates severe DR, and level 4 indicates new vascular proliferation, with risk of blindness. The different levels of DR are shown in Fig. 1.

Deep learning (DL) approach has proved to be an advantageous method in image classification and several other applications [13, 14].Deep learning is a subdivision of machine learning structured on artificial neural networks utilized for extraction of progressively higher level features from data [15]. Non-dependence on handcrafted features makes deep learning methodologies a better technique as compared to traditional machine learning methods. Furthermore, DL methods scale significantly better than classical ML methods in dealing with larger amount of data [16]. However, the absence of properly labelled data for evaluating the models makes it difficult to build a deep learning algorithm and thus consumes large amount of time in building the required model [17]. These are some reasons behind massive shifting towards TL. Unlike deep learning, TL is another machine learning technique where components of a trained model are reused on a desired new network with a different but comparable problem [18]. In general, the task of feature extraction is done based on previously trained models' layers having some weight instead of changing the weights of the model's layers during training with new data for the current task. This technique significantly reduces the time required for feature engineering and training. Moreover, TL can be applied on lesser available datasets which makes it more suitable for use. This can also be used in predicting the behavior of model on assigned tasks while training process. The previously trained model helps in reducing the training time and generalization error after its application on newer model [19]. TL is quite effective, particularly in situations when huge amounts of data are unavailable and minimal computing costs are required [20–22]. There have been several proposed methods to automate the image classification process to make the diagnosis process accurate. CNN architectures are one of the most widely used approaches for image classification [23–27] which justifies the evidence of various methods of classification of DR using CNN, either through deep learning or by incorporating unique architectures.

1.1 Related Work

This section discusses about the existing work of DR classifications using pre-trained CNN architectures and TL technique in terms of different dataset selected, employed architectures and performance measures. TL is capable of transferring learned knowledge to new task with different datasets and gives comparatively faster and accurate results. Hence, this approach inspired many authors to study TL on different datasets and different domain. Gulshan et al. [28] were the first to use deep learning to diagnose referable and non-referable diabetic retinopathy, the two classes of DR using CNN inception-V3. The model was trained on a huge private dataset called EyePACS-1, which contains approximately 120,000 fundus images. They obtained sensitivity as 97.5% and specificity as 93.4% on the dataset. M. T. Esfahan et al. [29] employed ResNet34 for classification of DR images into two classes namely normal or DR image. They used Kaggle dataset and applied image processing technique including Gaussian filter, weighted addition and image normalization for improvement of the quality of images. They obtained an accuracy of 85% and a sensitivity of 86%. Masood et al. [30] applied the InceptionV3 model for classification of DR into five classes using the Kaggle dataset. Total 4000 images were chosen and trimmed to 500 pixels for their classification task. The authors measured the model's performance using accuracy, which came in at 48.8%. Wang et al. [31] tested the usage of TL for detecting DR by comparing three different pre-trained CNNs namely InceptionNetV3, AlexNet and VGG16 on the Kaggle datasets. They classified their result into five classes of DR. InceptionNetV3 achieved the highest average accuracy (ACC) of 63.23% among three. T. Li et al. [32] used the GoogLeNet, DenseNet-121, ResNet-18, SE-BN-Inception and VGG-16 accessible pre-trained networks on DDR datasets for conducting his experiments. There are 13,673 fundus images in their dataset. They performed cropping and resampling of images while preprocessing in order to balance the classes. With an accuracy of 82.84%, the SE-BN-Inception network was found to be most precise. However, the authors' technique failed in finding visual spots in images. Xu et al. [33] investigated the DenseNet on a private collection of dataset comprising of 10,000 images and graded into five levels. The author experimented using fine-tuning technique and observed the behavior in both of the condition of fine-tuning. For balancing and resizing of dataset among different classes, the authors utilized image augmentation and obtained collection of 20,000 images labeled into five balanced classes. For training from scratch, the authors utilized a stochastic gradient descent (SGD) optimizer with an LR of 0.1 and an LR of 0.01 for fine-tuning the network. The authors claimed that TL improved the model's accuracy. Wan et al. [34] examined a variety of pre-trained models namely AlexNet, ResNet, GoogleNet and VGGNet that had been fine-tuned using the Kaggle EyePACS dataset with five classes. Among them, VGGNet architecture showed best results outperforming other more sophisticated architectures with accuracy of 95.68%, specificity of 97.43%, sensitivity of 86.47%, and an AUC of 0.979. M.Khalifa et al. [35] compared different TL models namely SqueezeNet, AlexNet, GoogleNet, ResNet18 VGG16, and VGG19 over APTOS 2019 datasets for detection of five classes of DR. They used augmentation techniques to avoid the overfitting problem and increased the image size of the dataset to four times that of the original dataset. The AlexNet model found to achieve the highest testing accuracy of 97.9%, precision, and F1 score percentage among all other models. Murcia et al. [36] tested two different architectures namely the ResNet-18 and ResNet-50 along with other previously trained models including SqueezeNet, AlexNet, VGGnet-16 and VGGnet-19, and an additional residual network, ZhangNet on the Messidor dataset. The author used data augmentation in terms of random horizontal flipping, evaluation parameters such as sensitivity, specificity, global correct rate (CR), ROC and AUC while training of all models. They concluded ResNet-based models outperformed all other models in both of multiclass and binary grading problems with a very good sensitivity and accuracy. Choi et al. [37] tested the performance of pre-trained model such as VGG 19 and AlexNet architecture on STARE dataset for the classification of multi-categorical retinal disease by using TL. They compared the architecture by applying different classifiers like SVM, RF and found the highest accuracy of about 90.1% by using VGG 19 architecture with RF classifier. Le et al. [38] used the inherited feature of retraining of layers for further use of TL for automated OCTA classification. They investigated VGG 16 architecture and obtained pre-trained weights from the ImageNet dataset. The author used data augmentation via horizontal and vertical flips, random rotation on the datasets during each iteration. They performed this experiment on datasets composed of 24 eyes from 17 patients affected with diabetes having no DR, 75 eyes from 60 patients suffering from DR, and 32 healthy eyes with 20 control subjects40.

Chetoui et al. [39] investigated the recent CNN architecture EfficientNet-B7 for detecting DR on publicly available dataset EyePACS and APTOS 2019.The dataset includes 82,547 fundus images from the EYEPACS in which more than 55,000 used for training, 18851 for validation and tested with more than 8000 image data. APTOS 2019 dataset images were used for testing purpose. They preprocessed the image and cropped it to 224 × 224 pixels and fixed the learning rate of 0.003 after employing SGD algorithm were applied. The author obtained a sensitivity of 0.917, a specificity of 0.989 and an AUC of 0.984 on EyePACS test set while sensitivity of 0.914, specificity of 0.972 and AUC of 0.966 over APTOS 2019 datasets for detecting RDR. On the other hand, they achieved highest scores on EyePACS test set with an AUC of 0.994, a sensitivity of 0.981 and a specificity of 0.9374 while AUC of 0.998, Sensitivity of 0.981 and specificity of 0.925 over APTOS 2019 for detection of Vision-Threatening DR. Laurensia et al. [40] tested the performance of EfficientNet and XGboost to extract image features and for classification of images. They used APTOS 2019 datasets on more than 3000 images which were filtered using Gaussian filter and resized to 224 × 224 pixels. In order to avoid overfitting problem, they used GlobalAveragePooling2D. This work achieved accuracy of 80% for binary classification. Lazuardi et al. [41] employed two of the EfficientNet family namely EfficientNet-B4 and EfficientNet-B5 for automation of the DR severity classification task over Kaggle datasets composed of mixed ratios of various classes. They used Contrast Limited Adaptive Histogram Equalization (CLAHE) and central image cropping preprocessing technique. They employed the quadratic weighted kappa (QWK) score as evaluation metrics and achieved a comparable QWK, F1, and accuracy scores for the two models, i.e. of approximately 0.79, 0.82, and 83.88% respectively. Pham et al. [42] employed modified EfficientNet-B5 on APTOS 2019 retinal image dataset. They used Group normalization instead of batch normalization and used RAdam (Rectified Adam) optimizer as modification. They used an efficient preprocessing strategy as the average local color was eliminated employing technique called Gaussian mask, which improved the QWK score by 0.03 and finally achieving score of 0.90. Zhang et al. [43] studied EfficientNet-B3 over private dataset which was combination of images of EYEPACS and APTOS The author utilized this architecture for features extraction from fundus images simultaneously and diagnose the severity levels of DR through a regression method. The reported result showed that this model achieved quadratic weighted kappa score 0.935 on the considered dataset. They used K-Fold cross validation and Pseudo-Level technique to improve the performance of the pre-trained models. Momeni Pour et al. [44] proposed a novel diabetic screening model for the classification of DR. The authors preprocessed the image using CLAHE resulting in uniform equalization of intensities and improvement in image quality. They employed efficientnet-B5 model in the proposed work. The authors tested the model once on both of the two datasets, Messidor-2 and IDRiD combined, while evaluating the result. The AUC is boosted from 0.936 to 0.945, achieving one of the highest among other recent works. They also analyzed the performance of the model by training on a combination of datasets, Messidor-2 and Messidor and testing on the IDRiD dataset. The AUC recorded for this was 0.932. Sugeno et al. [45] employed a CNN architecture for detection of DR based on pre-trained model named EfficientNet-B3 over training dataset of APTOS 2019 after mixing it with unnatural noise. From the dataset, the blur and duplicate images were removed after applying numerical threshold method. The edges of masked images helped in further expansion of fundus region of processed images to a diameter of 416 pixels. They evaluated this model on DIARETDB1 database and calculated specificity and sensitivity values > ~0.98. Karki et al. [46] studied the combination of EfficientNet family members for severity level multi- classification. Ensemble of EfficientNet B1, B2, B3 and B5 were used to obtain the model. For training, different combinations of datasets including EyePACS plus APTOS were used. However, the APTOS test datasets came out to be best among the two attaining 0.924377 quadratic kappa score. Anitha et al. [47] have compared one of the members of EfficientNet family that is EfficientNet B5 with other existing models such as VGG16 and ResNet50 in terms of accuracy. The authors chose APTOS dataset for five class categorization of DR. Among the chosen models for research, EfficientNet B5 were 7 times better than ResNet50 while 21 times better than VGG16 in its performance.

1.2 Challenges and Issues

There have been several studies done in classification using machine learning, DL and TL techniques. Most of the studies discussed above used conventional machine learning techniques which start with feature extraction at the beginning after moving ahead for classification purpose. On the other hand, some of the studies used DL techniques which required a lot of data for training purpose. Finding authentic and suitable dataset is one of the biggest problems now-a-days. Moreover, both ML and DL techniques takes a lot of time in training which makes them unsuitable for frequent use for creating a model. These short-comings of these two methods lead to the shifting towards another popular technique TL. This method proves its suitability when we have smaller labelled datasets and we are bound to create a model for such datasets. Under TL, there are various pre-trained CNN architectures that are the choice of researchers while investigating such classification tasks. There are several studies based on these CNN architectures where the authors use depth or width scaling of the models to increase their performance. Another popular method is to increase or decrease the image resolution of the models as per the requirement. Even if scaling in two or three dimensions at the same time is conceivable, human tweaking is still necessary, resulting in sub-optimal precision and efficiency. The three dimensions must be balanced, which can be accomplished by using a fixed aspect ratio in each dimension. EfficientNet is one architecture that can execute such scaling equally in all dimensions using a coefficient compound which we will discuss in later chapters. Most of the studies used till now have used complex CNN architectures which take a lot of training time and consequently require significant system power. Moreover, the bigger architecture are slower due to computational complexity involved. These were several short-comings that we observed while literature review and took a recently proposed CNN model for classification and detection of DR. This model is 8.4x smaller and found 6.1x faster while training over ImageNet dataset that consists of about 14 million of non-medical datasets. Further, the robustness and performance of the used CNN architecture can be seen in the result section. This paper is organized as follows: Sect. 2 presents the description of datasets while Sect. 3 briefly explains methodology used. Section 4 shows the result and performance of the proposed work. Section 5 presents conclusion and discussion of the paper.

2 Datasets

In this work, the models has been trained and tested on the human fundus images from IDRiD (INDIAN DIABETIC RETINOPATHY IMAGE DATASET) dataset [48]. Indian DR Image Dataset is the world's first database of DR images. This dataset comprises of annotated pixels of typical DR lesions and normal retinal components. Thus the information provided by this dataset helps in creating and testing of image analysis algorithms for DR early detection. The dataset contains 516 images with different images of DR and DME. The CSV file contains grading information for all of the photographs. The International Clinical Diabetic Retinopathy Scale was used to split the diabetic retinal images into groups. The images were acquired at 50-degree FOV centering near to the macula ranging from 4288×2848 pixels. The distribution of the five classes of DR images present in the IDRiD dataset is shown in Fig. 2.

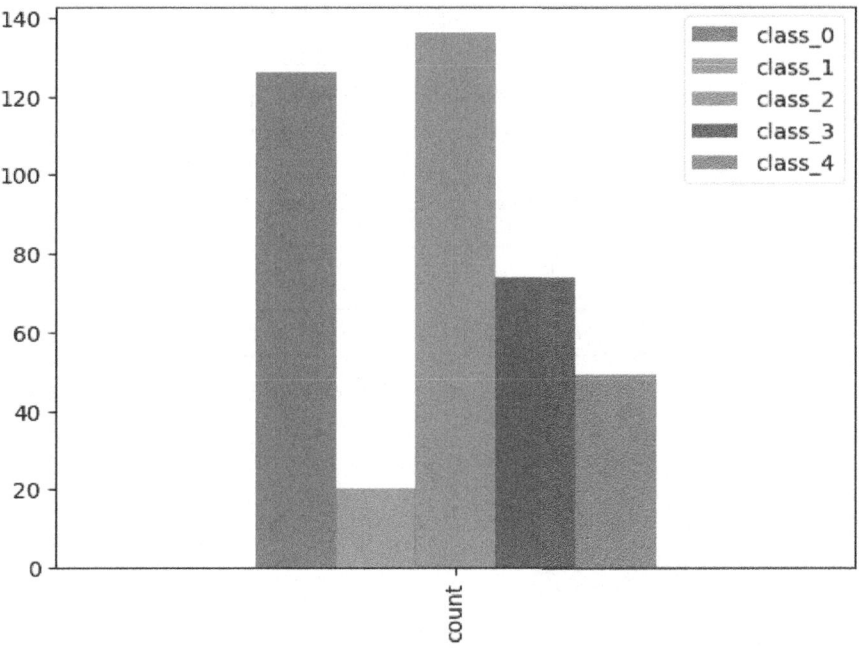

Fig. 2. Distribution of IDRiD Fundus Retinal Image Dataset

3 Methodology

3.1 Proposed Model

The proposed model is based on TL techniques. In this model, a recently proposed CNN architecture named EfficientNet has been used over publicly available human fundus retinal images from IDRiD. One of the most important specialties of this EfficientNet model is compound scaling feature. In this feature, simultaneous scaling of network width, depth and image resolution takes place which avoids the previously discussed problems. Moreover, this Convolutional network is smaller in size and faster in nature as compared to previously available models. Flow chart of the proposed model is shown in Fig. 3.

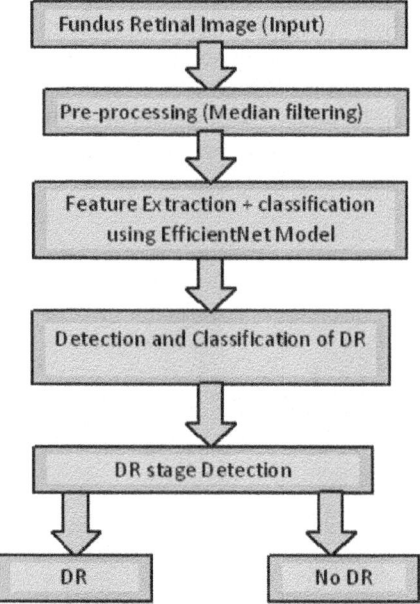

Fig. 3. Flow chart of Proposed Model.

3.2 Pre-processing Technique

Pre-processing techniques are one of preliminary stage for preparation of input images involving activities such as removing the edge errors, opacity and misalignment of camera images for obtaining the best quality input images. The errors in input images have an impact on visual contrast, lighting, and color. As a result, fundus image preparation is a necessary step [49]. Contrast Enhancement and De-noising techniques, median filtering, Gaussian filtering, histogram equalization (HE), and partial differential equation filters, and so on are all examples of pre-processing techniques.

Many studies recommend scaling images to a set resolution to make them network-ready. The images which were obtained after cropping images were used to remove the image's excess portions, followed by data normalization to normalise the images into a comparable distribution. In some works, only the green channel of images was retrieved, whereas in others, such as, the images were turned to gray scale.

In this work, median filtering was employed to improve the image quality in terms of its edges smoothening and removing noise from it. This filtering technique has been selected on the basis of a study conducted in [50] where author has implemented and compared several filtering and smoothening techniques.

Median filtering is a noise elimination filtering technique which is extensively used in digital image processing for its ability to preserve edges while reducing noise under specific conditions. It has many advantages such as smoothening, removal of noises and preserves edges and highlights blood vessel.

3.3 Model Description

In this work, EfficientNet family starting from baseline architecture B0 to EfficientNet B7 was used to extract the features from the fundus images. EfficientNet is a CNN architecture which is the outcome of limitation of dimensional scaling of network. In the previous version of CNN, network were scaled of either width, depth or resolution which led researcher to fill the gap of finding a most efficient scaling method to scale the network and achieve better performance. This idea led to the development of an efficient scaling method named compound scaling method wherein all dimensions of network width, depth and resolution are uniformly scaled using a compound coefficient $\emptyset$ that is fixed scaling coefficients.

The algorithms of EfficientNetV1 [51] is powerful enough to compute 2^N times more computational resources. Moreover, the parameters such as the depth of the network can be increased by α^N, width can be increased by β^N, and image size can be increased by γ^N to achieve this. Here α; β; γ are constant coefficients determined by a small grid search on the original small model. The formulae of designing of EfficientNet using a compound coefficient uniformly scaling network width, depth, and resolution are as follows:

This technique applied to help in achieving higher accuracy than existing models while reducing overall FLOPS and model size dramatically.

There were two steps given to scale up baseline EfficientNet-B0 by compound scaling method:-

$$
\left.\begin{array}{l}
Depth\, d = \alpha^{\emptyset} \\
Width\, w = \beta^{\emptyset} \\
Resolution\, r = \gamma^{\emptyset} \\
s.t.\, \alpha \cdot \beta^2 \cdot \gamma^2 \approx 2
\end{array}\right\} \tag{1}
$$

STEP 1: Fixing $\emptyset = 1$ and running over a small grid search of α, β, γ, with assumption of twice as many resources are available. After that choose the best values for EfficientNet-B0 that is $\alpha = 1:2$; $\beta = 1:1$; $\gamma = 1:15$, under constraint of $\alpha \cdot \beta2 \cdot \gamma2 \approx 2$.

STEP 2: Fixing α; β; γ as constants and scaling up baseline network with different φ using Eq. 1, to obtain EfficientNet-B1 to B7.

These mathematical computation forms the base behind the EfficientNet family models. The baseline architecture that is EfficientNetB0 is shown in the Table 1.

Table 1. EfficientNetB0 baseline architecture.

Stage	Operator	Resolution	Channels	Layers
1	Conv 3×3	224×224	32	1
2	MBConv1, k3 $\times$ 3	112×112	16	1
3	MBConv6, k3 $\times$ 3	112×112	24	2
4	MBConv6, k5 $\times$ 5	56×56	40	2
5	MBConv6, k3 $\times$ 3	28×28	80	3
6	MBConv6, k5 $\times$ 5	14×14	112	3
7	MBConv6, k5 $\times$ 5	14×14	192	4
8	MBConv6, k3 $\times$ 3	7×7	320	1
9	Conv 1×1 & Pooling & FC	7×7	1280	1

However, recent developments have been made by Google in the EfficientNetV1 and named that family of CNN as EfficientNetV2. EfficientNetV2 [52] is a successor of EfficientNetV1 which overcame the limitations of the former model. In the EfficientNetV1 model, memory usage was greater due to its larger image size. Since the total memory is fixed on GPU and TPU, the researchers trained the model in smaller batch size slowing down the training time. Other shortcomings were found in depthwise convolutions which was slow in early layers. The reason behind this slowness is fewer parameters and FLOPS (floating point operations per second) as compared to regular convolutions. The architecture of EfficientNetV2 uses fused MBCONV which replaces the depthwise convolutional block of EfficientNetV1 with regular convolutional block. In this way, it improves the training speed and reduces the excess load from parameters. Since EfficientNet is known for its unique uniform scaling method of stages however, these stages could not contribute to the training speed and parameter efficiency. These limitations of EfficientNetV1 were met by its newer versions named EfficientNetV2. In this version, training-aware Neural Architecture Search (NAS) and scaling is combined for optimization of training speed and parameter efficiency. It also supported progressive learning adaptively adjusting with regularization and image size.

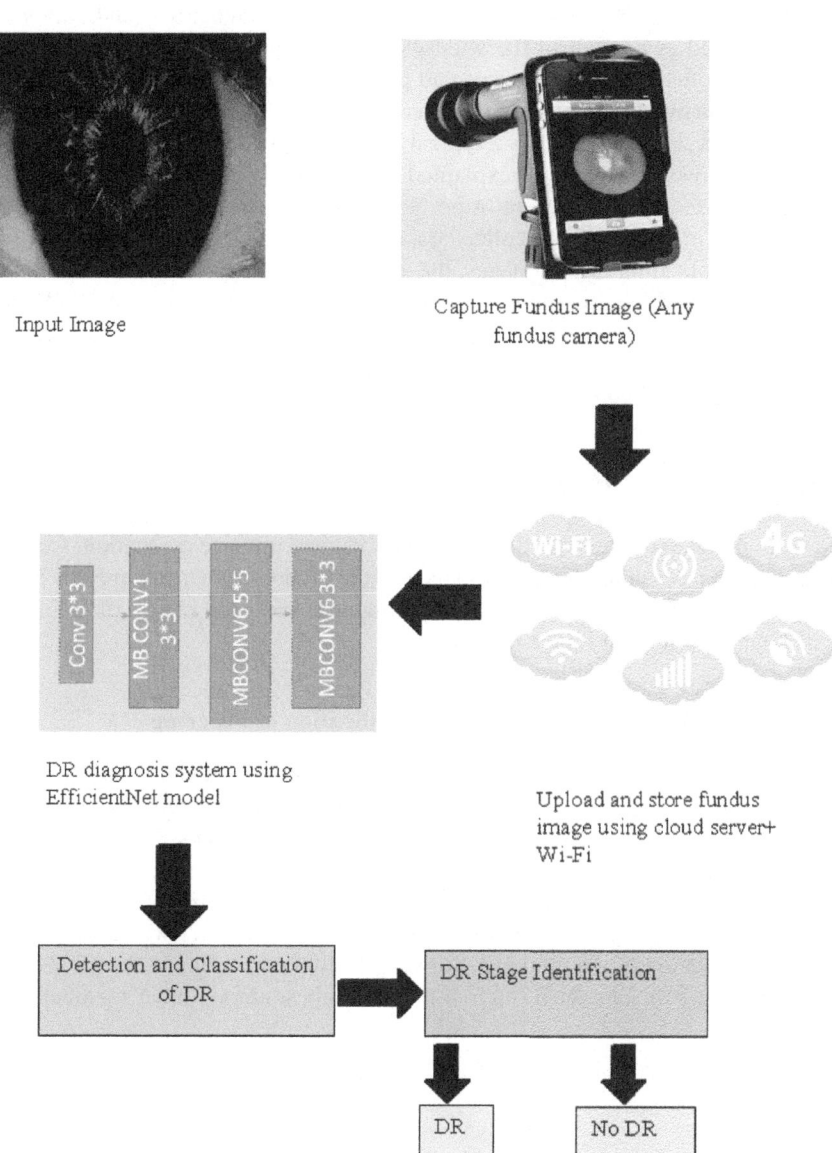

Fig. 4. Suggested Smart healthcare model for detection of DR

3.4   Exploration of Smart Healthcare System

Smart healthcare has expanded beyond electronic and mobile health in recent times. These systems transform data from mobile and sensory devices into personalised healthcare data. Integration of deep learning technologies with healthcare systems has wide possibility in medical field. Clinicians' health monitoring, diagnosis, and data gathering have increased as a result of the widespread use of portable smart health devices, allowing them to make early diagnoses and provide prompt treatment. However, there is a threat to security of patient's data that has been collected through several means of sharing platforms. Figure 4 depicts a typical smart healthcare for detection of diabetic retinopathy. The workflow can be explained as first the data has to be collected from either of specialized fundus camera or portable camera or lens integrated with mobile application. The images samples collected can be uploaded to cloud storage for better analysis. After uploading of the images, the architectural model based on suitable EfficientNet algorithm which is compatible with mobile has been used to detect and classify diabetic retinopathy in this work. This would help patient understand the severity level of their disease and further can decide to consult experienced clinicians. Moreover, this would assist ophthalmologist in accurate diagnosis.

4   Experiment and Results

In this section, the experiment is discussed with its performance evaluation. Confusion matrix was used to evaluate the performance of the models. Other parameters like sensitivity and specificity were calculated from obtained confusion matrix of the model to study its behavior on input image dataset.

4.1   EfficientNetV1 Performance Before Application of Filtering

We have studied the behavior of the EfficientNetV1 (B0-B7) model on IDRiD dataset. The model employed a fully connected CNN with 512 hidden units, ReLU activation and a final softmax layer. The model was trained for 10 epochs and tested on same specified dataset. After obtaining the training and testing accuracy, confusion matrix for each of the members of the model were obtained and performance parameters like sensitivity and specificity were calculated for each of the model which are shown in Fig. 5. The calculation of the models before application of filtering is shown in Table 2. The sensitivity of EfficientNet B7 is found to be highest among other members with a value of 0.83.

Table 2. Performance metrics calculation (in %) before filtering.

Models	Training accuracy	Testing Accuracy	Sensitivity	Specificity
EfficientNet B0	96.3	82.2	82.5	66.6
EfficientNet B1	97.5	76	73.4	81.2
EfficientNet B2	96	76	69.2	90.3
EfficientNet B3	96.4	72.9	83	58
EfficientNet B4	98.3	75	79.6	65.6
EfficientNet B5	97.0	73.9	65.0	72.7
EfficientNet B6	97.4	75.5	73	77
EfficientNet B7	90.62	75	83.1	64.5

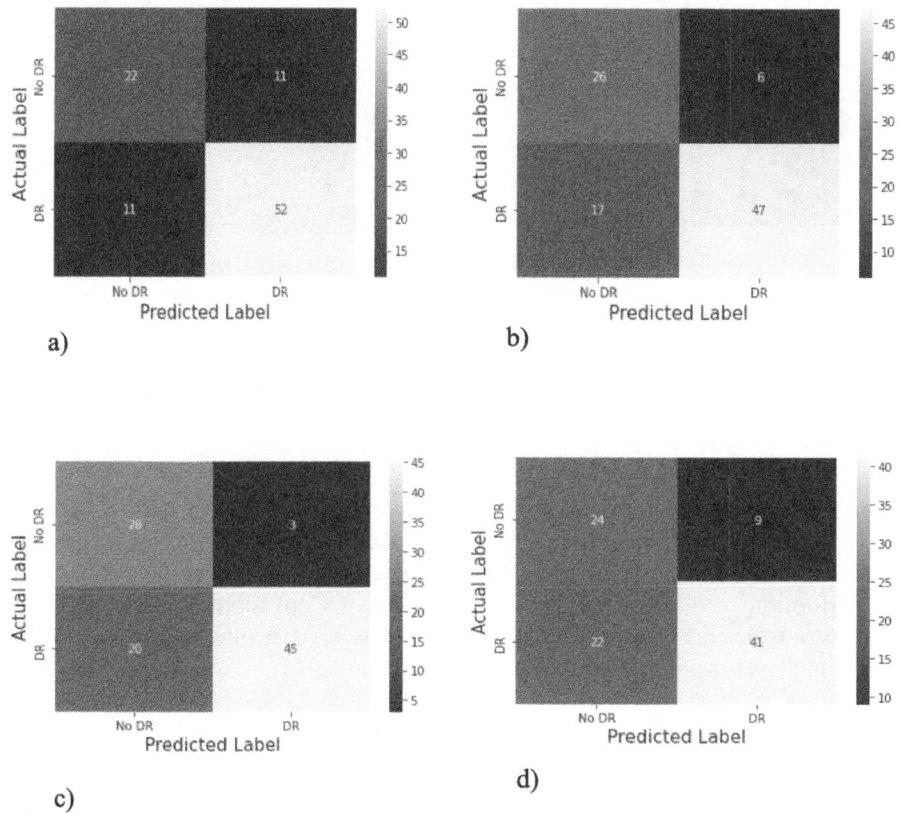

Fig. 5. Confusion matrix for each of the members of EfficientNetV1 models before filtering (a) EfficientNetB0, (b) EfficientNetB1, (c) EfficientNetB2, (d) EfficientNetB3, (e) EfficientNetB4, (f) EfficientNetB5, (g) EfficientnetB6, (h) EfficientNetB7.

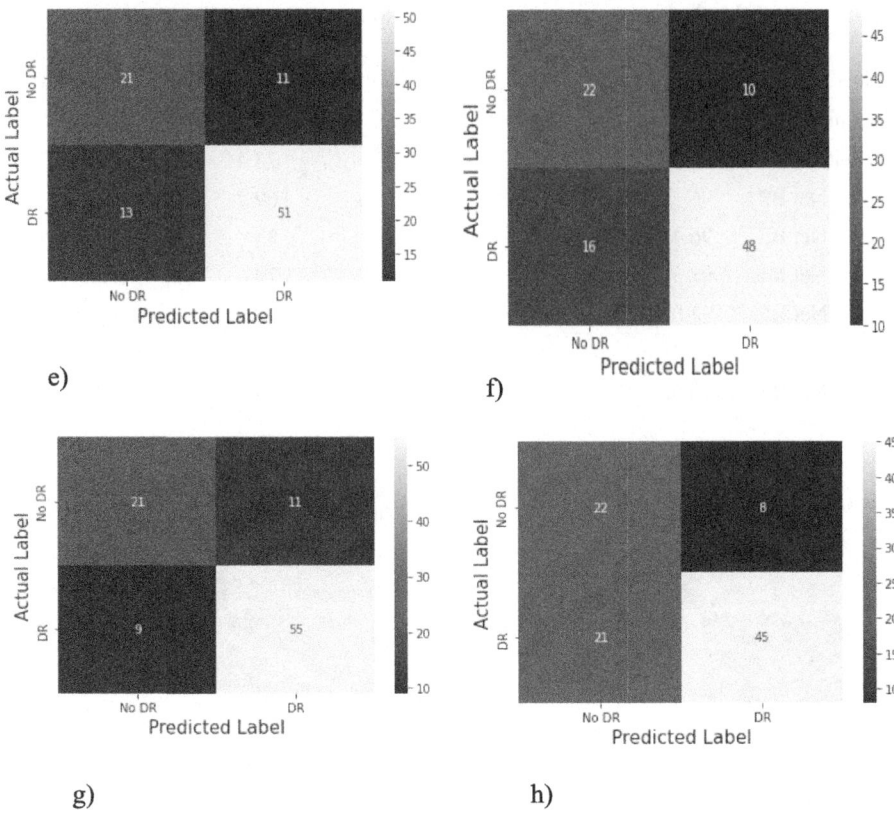

e)   f)

g)   h)

Fig. 5. (*continued*)

4.2 EfficientNet V1 Performance After Application of Filtering

Further, to study the performance of the models on more enhanced version of retinal images, filtering was used. From different available filters, median filtering was used which showed a dramatic increase in the performance of the models. The calculations after performing median filtering are shown in Table 3. Confusion matrix of each of the members of EfficientNetV1 models are shown in Fig. 6. After filtering, EfficientNet B0 attained highest sensitivity of 92.18% among other members.

Table 3. Performance metrics calculation (in %) after filtering.

Models	Training accuracy	Testing Accuracy	Sensitivity	Specificity
EfficientNet B0	98.07	78.12	92.18	43.75
EfficientNet B1	94.79	80.20	84.61	74.9
EfficientNet B2	94.94	76	81.25	62.5
EfficientNet B3	92.06	78.12	87.5	62.5
EfficientNet B4	97.62	81.25	84.61	67.74
EfficientNet B5	96.73	73.95	75	68.75
EfficientNet B6	93.9	81.25	78.12	71.87
EfficientNet B7	90.62	75	83.07	64.5

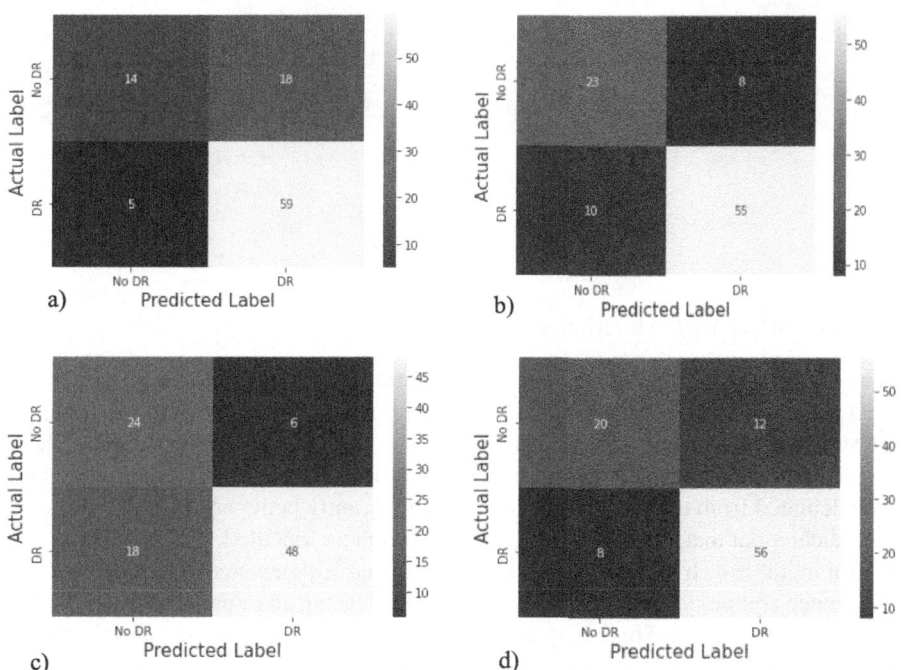

Fig. 6. Confusion matrix for each of the members of EfficientNetV1 models after filtering (a) EfficientNetB0, (b) EfficientNetB1, (c) EfficientNetB2, (d) EfficientNetB3, (e) EfficientNetB4, (f) EfficientNetB5, (g) EfficientnetB6, (h) EfficientNetB7.

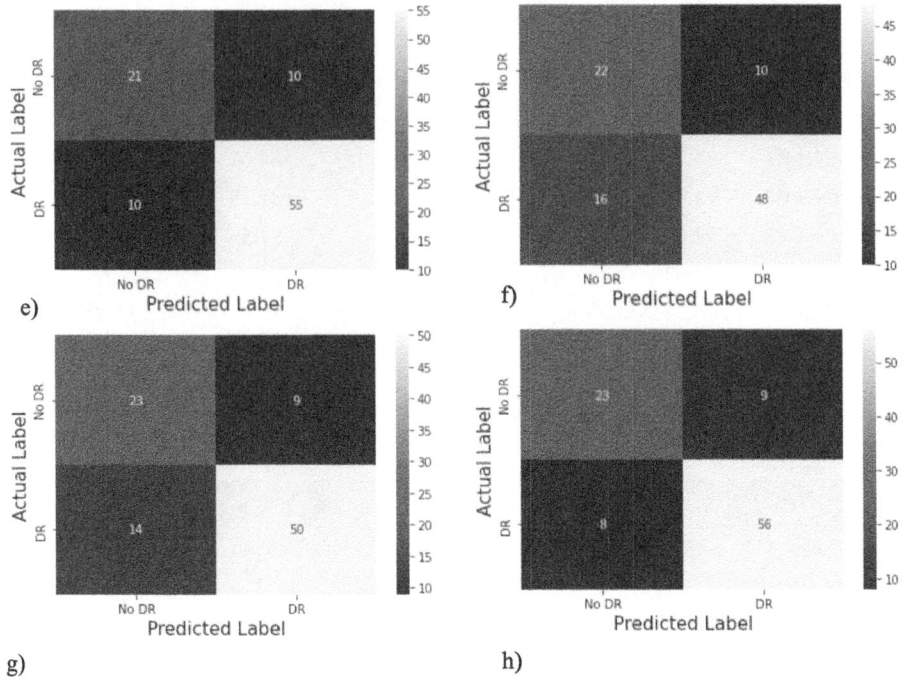

Fig. 6. (*continued*)

4.3   EfficientNet V2 Performance

In the search of best model which can be compatible with mobile application, we used newest version of EfficientNet model that is EfficientNetV2. Similar approach of training and testing were employed for this architecture as well. Confusion matrix which is shown in Fig. 7 were obtained for its performance evaluation and its sensitivity and specificity were calculated from the matrix which came significantly better according to the sensitive medical input that we applied to it. The performance calculation of EfficientNet V2 is shown in Table 4. It can be seen from the table that EfficientNetV2 exhibits superior performance compared to its previous version, showcasing an impressive 80.09% sensitivity on the task at hand. This exceptional sensitivity achieved within lesser training time makes it a novel and highly effective classification model for detecting and classifying DR lesions.

4.4   Comparison of Studied Models

In this section, the discussion is focused on the training timing of different versions of the EfficientNet model. The latest version, EfficientNet V2, has demonstrated a remarkable reduction in training time compared to its predecessors, making it highly efficient in terms of training efficiency and computational complexity.

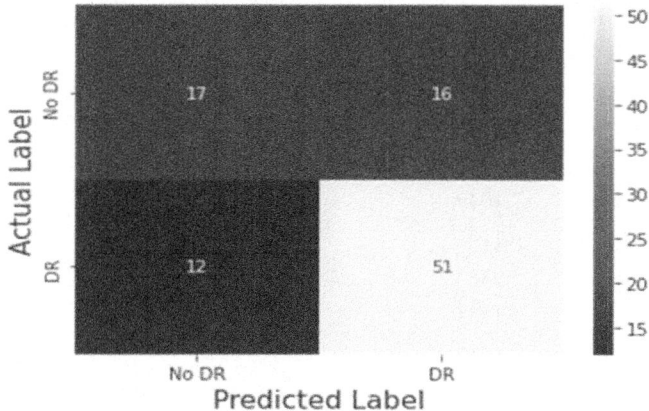

Fig. 7. Confusion matrix of EfficientNetV2

Table 4. Performance metrics calculation (in %) without filtering

Models	Training accuracy	Testing Accuracy	Sensitivity	Specificity
EfficientNet V2	98.1	71.8	80.9	51.5

The study conducted on EfficientNet V2 highlights its superiority over previous versions in terms of parameter efficiency [52]. Not only does the model achieve impressive results with reduced training time, but it also requires fewer parameters to achieve comparable performance.

The table presented in the research paper demonstrates how EfficientNet V2 outperforms its earlier iterations, showcasing its enhanced efficiency in model training. This advancement is crucial as it significantly reduces the computational resources required, making it more feasible to deploy on various platforms and devices with limited resources (Table 5).

4.5 Comparison of Obtained Result with Existing Models

In this section, the comparison of proposed model with other similar pre-trained models employing CNN has been done and shown in Table 6. The table shows the newest version of CNN based EfficientNet model has better performance than existing models. Some existing models might show better sensitivity but they are very big in size and some other models could not compete with newest version of EfficientNet models in terms of its performance and size. The sensitivity of the model towards the detection of disease is notable that is 80.9% and proves its suitability for clinical practice and mobile applications.

Table 5. Comparison of Training time of studied models

Model Name	Total Training Time (in sec)	Parameters
EfficientNet B0	750	43 M
EfficientNet B1	817	
EfficientNet B2	1049	
EfficientNet B3	1197	
EfficientNet B4	936	
EfficientNet B5	1133	
EfficientNet B6	1277	
EfficientNet B7	1460	
EfficientNet V2	680	24 M

Table 6. Comparison of proposed work with existing work

Study	Year	Architecture	Number of Classes	Dataset	Performance Measures	Results
Gulshan et al.	2016	InceptionV3	2 classes	Private	Sensitivity	97.5%
Masood et al.	2017	InceptionV3	5 classes	Kaggle	Accuracy	48.8%
Wang et al.	2018	AlexNet VGG16 InceptionV3	5 classes	Kaggle (166)	Accuracy	37.43% 50.03% 63.23%
Karki et al.	2021	Ensemble of EfficientNet B1,B2, B3 and B5	5 classes	APTOS	Quadratic kappa score	0.924377
Anitha et al.	2022	VGG16, ResNet50 EfficientNetB5	5 classes	APTOS	Accuracy	76.47% 90.2% 97.2%
Proposed Work	2022	EfficientNetV2	2 classes	IDRiD	Sensitivity	80.9%

5   Conclusion

This study identifies prospective technical breakthroughs in the healthcare and medical fields, particularly in the early diagnosis of a variety of ailments. Every life-threatening disease such as cancer, DR, and many others health problems, can be recovered if it is identified in its early stages. Furthermore, automated models made for detection and diagnosis purpose saves a lot of time and is cost-effective in nature, serving a wide range of populations and geographies, and can be used by any practitioner once they are familiar with the model's processing and output. We created a deep CNN based on the EfficientNet (B0-B7) CNN model that was recently constructed. Further we developed another CNN model based on EfficientNetV2 and observed the improvement in the performance of the model on the same dataset. The model was trained and tested on IDRiD dataset for the detection and binary classification of DR based on severity level. On comparing the performance of discussed models, EfficientNetV2 has been found to be best with 80.9% sensitivity value which shows its high possibility in implementation in smart healthcare systems. Hence, it can be concluded that the proposed work is indeed a good model for two category classification for earlier detection and diagnosis of DR. Moreover, the research findings clearly establish EfficientNet V2 as a state-of-the-art model that excels in both training efficiency and parameter efficiency compared to its predecessors. This progress has significant implications for the practical implementation of deep learning models, as it allows for faster training and deployment in resource-constrained environments.

Authors Contribution.   All authors made substantial contributions to all of the following:

1. The conception and design of the study: Pooja Ranjan, Mustafa Sameer, Bharat Gupta.

2. Software implementation and interpretation of results: Pooja Ranjan, Shubham Kumar, Mustafa Sameer.

3. Drafting the article or revising it critically for important intellectual content: Pooja Ranjan, Shubham Kumar, Mustafa Sameer, Sanchita Ghosh, Bharat Gupta.

4. Final approval of the version to be submitted: approved by all authors.

Funding.   All authors have no sources of funding to report.

Data Availability Statement.   The dataset is publicly available on the link: https://ieee-dataport.org/open-access/indian-diabetic-retinopathy-image-dataset-idrid.

Declarations.

Ethical Approval.   Not Applicable.

Conflict of Interest.   The authors declare no conflict of interest.

References

1. Diabetes. https://www.who.int/news-room/fact-sheets/detail/diabetes
2. Sarwar, N., Gao, P., Seshasai, S.R.K., et al.: Diabetes mellitus, fasting blood glucose concentration, and risk of vascular disease: a collaborative meta-analysis of 102 prospective studies. Lancet (Lond. Engl.) **375**(9733), 2215–2222 (2010). https://doi.org/10.1016/S0140-6736(10)60484-9
3. Alyoubi, W.L., Shalash, W.M., Abulkhair, M.F.: Diabetic retinopathy detection through deep learning techniques: a review. Inform. Med. Unlocked **20**, 100377 (2020)
4. Faust, O., Acharya, U.R., Ng, E.Y.K., et al.: Algorithms for the automated detection of diabetic retinopathy using digital fundus images: a review. J. Med. Syst. **36**(1), 145–157 (2012). https://doi.org/10.1007/s10916-010-9454-7

5. Acharya, U.R., Chua, C.K., Ng, E.Y.K., et al.: Application of higher order spectra for the identification of diabetes retinopathy stages. J. Med. Syst. **32**(6), 481–488 (2008). https://doi.org/10.1007/s10916-008-9154-8

6. Kandel, I., Castelli, M.: Transfer learning with convolutional neural networks for diabetic retinopathy image classification. A review. Appl. Sci. **10**(6) (2020). https://doi.org/10.3390/app10062021

7. Eszes, D.J., Szabó, D.J., Russell, G., et al.: Diabetic retinopathy screening in patients with diabetes using a handheld fundus camera: the experience from the South-Eastern region in Hungary. J. Diabetes Res. **2021**, 6646645 (2021). https://doi.org/10.1155/2021/6646645. Sokolovska J. (ed.)

8. Abramoff, M.D., Niemeijer, M., Russell, S.R.: Automated detection of diabetic retinopathy: barriers to translation into clinical practice. Expert Rev. Med. Devices **7**(2), 287–296 (2010). https://doi.org/10.1586/erd.09.76

9. Tsiknakis, N., Theodoropoulos, D., Manikis, G., et al.: Deep learning for diabetic retinopathy detection and classification based on fundus images: a review. Comput. Biol. Med. **135**, 104599 (2021). https://doi.org/10.1016/j.compbiomed.2021.104599

10. Grading diabetic retinopathy from stereoscopic color fundus photographs–an extension of the modified Airlie House classification. ETDRS report number 10. Early Treatment Diabetic Retinopathy Study Research Group. Ophthalmology **98**(5 Suppl.), 786–806 (1991)

11. Alyoubi, W.L., Abulkhair, M.F., Shalash, W.M.: Diabetic retinopathy fundus image classification and lesions localization system using deep learning. Sensors **21**(11) (2021). https://doi.org/10.3390/s21113704

12. Wilkinson, C.P., Ferris, F.L., III., Klein, R.E., et al.: Proposed international clinical diabetic retinopathy and diabetic macular edema disease severity scales. Ophthalmology **110**(9), 1677–1682 (2003)

13. Alzubaidi, L., Zhang, J., Humaidi, A.J., et al.: Review of deep learning: concepts, CNN architectures, challenges, applications, future directions. J. Big Data **8**(1), 53 (2021). https://doi.org/10.1186/s40537-021-00444-8

14. Xie, S., Girshick, R., Dollár, P., et al.: Aggregated residual transformations for deep neural networks (2017). https://doi.org/10.48550/arXiv.1611.05431

15. Mahony, N., Murphy, T., Panduru, K., et al.: Adaptive process control and sensor fusion for process analytical technology. In: 2016 27th Irish Signals and Systems Conference (ISSC), pp. 1–6 (2016)

16. Deng, L.: Three classes of deep learning architectures and their applications: a tutorial survey. APSIPA Trans. Signal Inf. Process. 57–58 (2012)

17. Najafabadi, M.M., Villanustre, F., Khoshgoftaar, T.M., et al.: Deep learning applications and challenges in big data analytics. J. Big Data **2**(1), 1 (2015). https://doi.org/10.1186/s40537-014-0007-7

18. Zhou, Y., Wang, B., Cui, S., et al.: A benchmark for studying diabetic retinopathy: segmentation, grading, and transferability (2020)

19. Simonyan, K., Zisserman, A.: Very deep convolutional networks for large-scale image recognition (2015)

20. Pan, S.J., Yang, Q.: A survey on transfer learning. IEEE Trans. Knowl. Data Eng. **22**(10), 1345–1359 (2010)

21. Yosinski, J., Clune, J., Bengio, Y., et al.: How transferable are features in deep neural networks? In: Advances in Neural Information Processing Systems, vol. 27 (2014)

22. Kornblith, S., Shlens, J., Le, Q.V.: Do better imagenet models transfer better? In: Proceedings of the IEEE/CVF Conference on Computer Vision and Pattern Recognition, pp. 2661–2671 (2019)

23. Hershey, S., Chaudhuri, S., Ellis, D.P., et al.: CNN architectures for large-scale audio classification. In: 2017 IEEE International Conference on Acoustics, Speech and Signal Processing (ICASSP), pp. 131–135. IEEE (2017)
24. Abamh, M.M., Krg, M.K.: A combined machine-learning and graph-based framework for the segmentation of retinal surfaces in SD-OCT volumes Biomed. Opt. Express **4**(12), 2712 (2013)
25. Akselrod-Ballin, A., Karlinsky, L., Alpert, S., et al.: A region based convolutional network for tumor detection and classification in breast mammography. In: Deep Learning and Data Labeling for Medical Applications: First International Workshop, LABELS 2016, and Second International Workshop, DLMIA 2016, Held in Conjunction with MICCAI 2016, Athens, Greece, October 21, 2016, Proceedings 2, pp. 197–205. Springer (2016)
26. Ishtiaq, U., Abdul Kareem, S., Abdullah, E.R.M.F., et al.: Diabetic retinopathy detection through artificial intelligent techniques: a review and open issues. Multimed. Tools Appl. **79**, 15209–15252 (2020)
27. Pratt, H., Coenen, F.M., Broadbent, D., Harding, S.P., Zheng, Y.: Convolutional neural networks for diabetic retinopathy. Procedia Comput. Sci. **90**, 200–205 (2016)
28. Gulshan, V., Peng, L., Coram, M., et al.: Development and validation of a deep learning algorithm for detection of diabetic retinopathy in retinal fundus photographs. JAMA **316**(22), 2402–2410 (2016)
29. Esfahani, M.T., Ghaderi, M., Kafiyeh, R.: Classification of diabetic and normal fundus images using new deep learning method. Leonardo Electron. J. Pract. Technol. **17**(32), 233–248 (2018)
30. Masood, S., Luthra, T., Sundriyal, H., et al.: Identification of diabetic retinopathy in eye images using transfer learning. In: 2017 International Conference on Computing, Communication and Automation (ICCCA), pp. 1183–1187 (2017). https://doi.org/10.1109/CCAA.2017.8229977
31. Wang, X., Lu, Y., Wang, Y., et al.: Diabetic retinopathy stage classification using convolutional neural networks. In: 2018 IEEE International Conference on Information Reuse and Integration (IRI), pp. 465–471 (2018)
32. Li, T., Gao, Y., Wang, K., et al.: Diagnostic assessment of deep learning algorithms for diabetic retinopathy screening. Inf. Sci. **501**, 511–522 (2019)
33. Xu, X., Lin, J., Tao, Y., et al.: An improved densenet method based on transfer learning for fundus medical images. In: 2018 7th International Conference on Digital Home (ICDH), pp. 137–140 (2018)
34. Wan, S., Liang, Y., Zhang, Y.: Deep convolutional neural networks for diabetic retinopathy detection by image classification. Comput. Electr. Eng. **72**, 274–282 (2018)
35. Khalifa, N.E., Loey, M., Taha, M., et al.: Deep transfer learning models for medical diabetic retinopathy detection. Acta Informatica Medica **27**, 327 (2019). https://doi.org/10.5455/aim.2019.27.327-332
36. Martinez-Murcia, F.J., Ortiz, A., Ramírez, J., et al.: Deep residual transfer learning for automatic diagnosis and grading of diabetic retinopathy. Neurocomputing **452**, 424–434 (2021). https://doi.org/10.1016/j.neucom.2020.04.148
37. Choi, J.Y., Yoo, T.K., Seo, J.G., et al.: Multi-categorical deep learning neural network to classify retinal images: a pilot study employing small database. PLoS ONE **12**(11), e0187336 (2017)
38. Le, D., Alam, M., Yao, C.K., et al.: Transfer learning for automated OCTA detection of diabetic retinopathy. Transl. Vis. Sci. Technol. **9**(2), 35 (2020). https://doi.org/10.1167/tvst.9.2.35
39. Chetoui, M., Akhloufi, M.A.: Explainable diabetic retinopathy using EfficientNET(). In: Annual International Conference of the IEEE Engineering in Medicine and Biology Society IEEE Engineering in Medicine and Biology Society Annual International Conference, pp. 1966–1969 (2020). https://doi.org/10.1109/EMBC44109.2020.9175664

40. Laurensia, Y., Young, J.C., Suryadibrata, A.: Early detection of diabetic retinopathy cases using pre-trained EfficientNet and XGBoost. Int. J. Adv. Soft Comput. Appl. **12**(3) (2020)
41. Lazuardi, R.N., Abiwinanda, N., Suryawan, T.H., et al.: Automatic diabetic retinopathy classification with EfficientNet. In: 2020 IEEE Region 10 Conference (TENCON), pp. 756–760 (2020). https://doi.org/10.1109/TENCON50793.2020.9293941
42. Pham, H., Tan, R., Cai, Y., et al.: Automated grading in diabetic retinopathy using image processing and modified EfficientNet, pp. 505–515 (2020). https://doi.org/10.1007/978-3-030-63007-2_39
43. Zhang, Z.: Deep-learning-based early detection of diabetic retinopathy on fundus photography using efficientnet. In: Proceedings of the 2020 the 4th International Conference on Innovation in Artificial Intelligence, pp. 70–74 (2020)
44. Pour, A.M., Seyedarabi, H., Jahromi, S.H.A., et al.: Automatic detection and monitoring of diabetic retinopathy using efficient convolutional neural networks and contrast limited adaptive histogram equalization. IEEE Access **8**, 136668–136673 (2020). https://doi.org/10.1109/ACCESS.2020.3005044
45. Sugeno, A., Ishikawa, Y., Ohshima, T., et al.: Simple methods for the lesion detection and severity grading of diabetic retinopathy by image processing and transfer learning. Comput. Biol. Med. **137**, 104795 (2021). https://doi.org/10.1016/j.compbiomed.2021.104795
46. Karki, S.S., Kulkarni, P.: Diabetic retinopathy classification using a combination of efficientnets. In: 2021 International Conference on Emerging Smart Computing and Informatics (ESCI), pp. 68–72 (2021). https://doi.org/10.1109/ESCI50559.2021.9397035
47. Nair, A.T., et al.: Disease grading of diabetic retinopathy using deep learning techniques. In: 2022 6th International Conference on Computing Methodologies and Communication (ICCMC), pp. 1019–1024 (2022). https://doi.org/10.1109/ICCMC53470.2022.9754113
48. Porwal, P., Pachade, S., Kokare, M., et al.: IDRiD: diabetic retinopathy - segmentation and grading challenge. Med. Image Anal. **59**, 101561 (2020). https://doi.org/10.1016/j.media.2019.101561
49. Lu, D., Weng, Q.: A survey of image classification methods and techniques for improving classification performance. Int. J. Remote Sens. **28**(5), 823–870 (2007)
50. Priya Henry, A.G., Jude, A.: Convolutional neural-network-based classification of retinal images with different combinations of filtering techniques. Open Comput. Sci. **11**(1), 480–490 (2021). https://doi.org/10.1515/comp-2020-0177
51. Tan, M., Le, Q.V.: Efficientnet: rethinking model scaling for convolutional neural networks. arXiv 2019. arXiv preprint arXiv:190511946 (2020)
52. Tan, M., Le, Q.: Efficientnetv2: smaller models and faster training. In: International Conference on Machine Learning, pp. 10096–10106. PMLR (2021)

Type 2 Diabetes Mellitus Monitoring Through Non-invasive IoT-Based System

Aamir Hussain[1,2(✉)], Attique ur Rehman[1], Altaf Hussain[1], Qimeng Li[2], Raffaele Gravina[2], and Giancarlo Fortino[2]

[1] Department of Computer Science, Muhammad Nawaz Sharif Agriculture University Multan, Multan, Pakistan
aamir.hussain@mnsuam.edu.pk, ch.attiqurrehman183@gmail.com,
2021-uam-2722@mnsuam.edu.pk
[2] Department of Computer Engineering, Modeling, Electronics and Systems,
University of Calabria, 87036 Rende, CS, Italy
{qimeng.li,giancarlo.fortino}@unical.it, r.gravina@dimes.unical.it

Abstract. Type 2 diabetes (T2d), also known as diabetes mellitus or adult-onset diabetes, is a chronic condition that disrupts the body's insulin regulation, a crucial hormone for controlling blood glucose levels. Glucose, a form of sugar, is the primary energy source for cells in the human bloodstream. Regulating glucose metabolism is vital for the body's proper functioning. The primary challenges in managing T2d include blood sampling, timely analysis, risk of skin infections, and blood-borne diseases. This paper presents the design of an IoT-based, non-invasive system for monitoring blood glucose levels. Our system utilizes medical sensors to gather data, which is then cleaned and transformed using data mining algorithms. Subsequent analysis compares the accuracy and sensitivity of this data with results from pathology labs and glucometers. The system generates specific warning notifications and provides standard medical advice in response to these alerts, aiding T2d patients in painlessly and effortlessly monitoring and controlling their blood sugar levels.

Keywords: Type 2 Diabetes Mellitus · Non-invasive · Wearable Sensor

1 Introduction

Diabetes, particularly Type 2 diabetes (T2d), represents a rapidly escalating global health crisis in the 21st century. Characterized by high blood sugar levels due to insulin resistance or deficiency, T2d can lead to severe health complications, including permanent disability and reduced life expectancy [1]. The escalation of this crisis highlights the growing importance of advanced human-machine systems in healthcare, as discussed in Fortino et al.'s "Handbook of Human-Machine Systems" [23]. These systems offer new avenues for monitoring

© ICST Institute for Computer Sciences, Social Informatics and Telecommunications Engineering 2024
Published by Springer Nature Switzerland AG 2024. All Rights Reserved
M. Mizmizi et al. (Eds.): BodyNets 2024, LNICST 524, pp. 127–137, 2024.
https://doi.org/10.1007/978-3-031-72524-1_10

and managing chronic diseases like diabetes. Lifestyle factors such as obesity, smoking, unhealthy diets, and lack of physical activity have been identified as significant contributors to the rising incidence of T2d [2]. The global prevalence of diabetes, including T2d, is alarmingly high, with about 9.3% of the world's population affected, making it the seventh leading cause of death according to the World Health Organization (WHO) [4].

Recent advancements in wearable body sensor networks have opened new possibilities for continuous health monitoring and disease management [24]. These technologies, as explored in Gravina and Fortino's study, are particularly pertinent in the context of T2d, where consistent monitoring of blood glucose levels is crucial. Additionally, the integration of situation-aware sensor-based wearable computing systems, as reviewed by D'Aniello et al. [25], aligns well with the need for personalized and adaptive health monitoring solutions. These systems could significantly enhance the quality of life for individuals with T2d by providing real-time data and insights into their health status.

The advent of mobile and Internet of Things (IoT) technologies has further introduced innovative approaches to managing T2d. These include mobile applications for self-monitoring and desktop applications facilitating doctor-patient communication. Traditional blood glucose measurement methods, often invasive and uncomfortable, are being challenged by the development of non-invasive sensor technologies [12]. These advancements are crucial in making diabetes care more accessible and less burdensome for patients.

This paper introduces an innovative non-invasive, sensor-based system for monitoring blood glucose levels in individuals with T2d. Our contribution lies in designing and validating a wearable device that employs state-of-the-art sensor technology to offer a pain-free and convenient alternative for diabetes monitoring. By integrating this system with cloud-based data management, we facilitate real-time tracking and analysis of patient data, enhancing the capability for remote monitoring and timely intervention. Our study not only bridges the gap in current diabetes management practices but also paves the way for future research in non-invasive health monitoring technologies.

2   Related Work

Previous research in the field of diabetes management has primarily focused on the compilation of patient datasets, including basic details such as name, age, and gender. However, managing these datasets can be cumbersome, as they often involve fragmented data across various functions such as Information Systems (IS), analysis, and record updating. This includes updating records to include new patients [13] and the use of insulin pumps for diabetes control [14].

A notable study indicated that 62% (n=29) of the research focused exclusively on type 2 diabetes, with the remaining 38% (n=18) addressing total diabetes cases across 47 studies. These studies highlighted the increasing prevalence of diabetes in various age groups up until 2000, after which the trend either stabilized or decreased. This necessitates a systematic approach to review all incidence data, focusing on age and gender patterns [15].

In Pakistan, the prevalence of T2d is particularly alarming, currently standing at 17% and projected to rise to 13.8 million cases by 2030. Cultural and familial factors play significant roles in managing and controlling T2d in the country, underscoring the need for interventions that consider these aspects to promote physical activity and improve diabetes management [6].

The effectiveness of eHealth interventions in enhancing the psychosocial and physical well-being of adults with diabetes has been a major focus of recent studies. Various interventions, such as the iDecide program, Medical Guard Diabetes (MGD) system, and GlucoBeep device, have been employed to improve metabolic control and self-management [16].

Mobile health (mHealth) Randomized Controlled Trials (RCTs) targeting Type 1, Type 2, and pre-diabetes patients have been examined in 25 studies. Research published between 2010 and 2020 was reviewed, indicating that digital health technologies can significantly enhance diabetes management through efficient data exchange between patients and healthcare providers [17].

The development of skin-based wearable devices for health monitoring has also gained traction [10]. These devices focus on various health indicators, leveraging advanced materials and fabrication techniques to enhance sensitivity, durability, and biocompatibility, thereby contributing significantly to healthcare technology.

Research on invasive sensors for T2d has also been documented, highlighting the need for more reliable health and fitness technology [18]. The evolution in technology has shown a positive trend towards developing non-invasive glucose testing methods. Notably, spectroscopy technologies have been promising in studying the wavelengths of light absorbed or emitted by various objects [20].

Current technological advancements indicate that blood glucose levels can be monitored using non-invasive sensors. These sensors, often employing LED signals in the 940nm wavelength range, translate signal intensity and variations to determine glucose levels [21].

Standard health checks for non-communicable diseases typically involve invasive procedures for testing blood sugar, cholesterol, and uric acid, posing challenges for those with phobias of needles or busy schedules [4]. Addressing these shortcomings, our proposed study utilizes a non-invasive MAX30105 IR sensor, selected for its speed and accuracy in data analysis. We have developed an IoT-based non-invasive diabetes monitoring system to record and regularly update patient glucose levels, facilitating effortless monitoring for those requiring continuous observation.

3   Methodology

Type 2 diabetes (T2d) predominantly affects the elderly, often due to insufficient insulin production by the pancreas. Our methodology involves the use of a non-invasive sensor, which minimizes discomfort during analysis.

3.1   Non-invasive Prototype Design and Implementation

We developed a non-invasive prototype that calculates variations in blood circulation using a photodetector emitting light onto the skin surface. A MAX30105 sensor is integrated into this prototype, where patients can scan their finger. The sensor then measures the infrared readings from the patient's finger. The data from the biosensor are transmitted to a Raspberry Pi 4, which processes the correlation coefficient between readings from an invasive glucometer and the non-invasive MAX30105 sensor. The outputs are displayed on a screen as shown in Fig. 1 and are also sent to the cloud for access by authorized personnel, such as caregivers and doctors, for monitoring and advising patients.

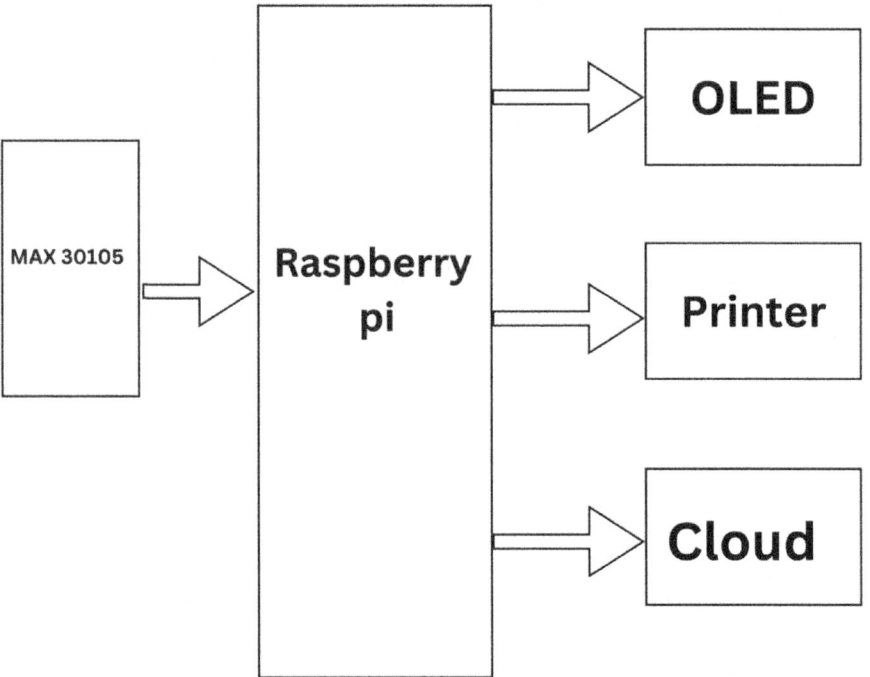

Fig. 1. Block diagram of the proposed system.

3.2   Data Flow Chart

The T2d monitoring system begins with initialization, followed by the biomedical sensor reading data from the patient's finger. After successful data acquisition, the information is forwarded to a microcontroller for processing. The results are then displayed on the screen, can be printed, and are also sent to the cloud. This system flow process is illustrated in Fig. 2.

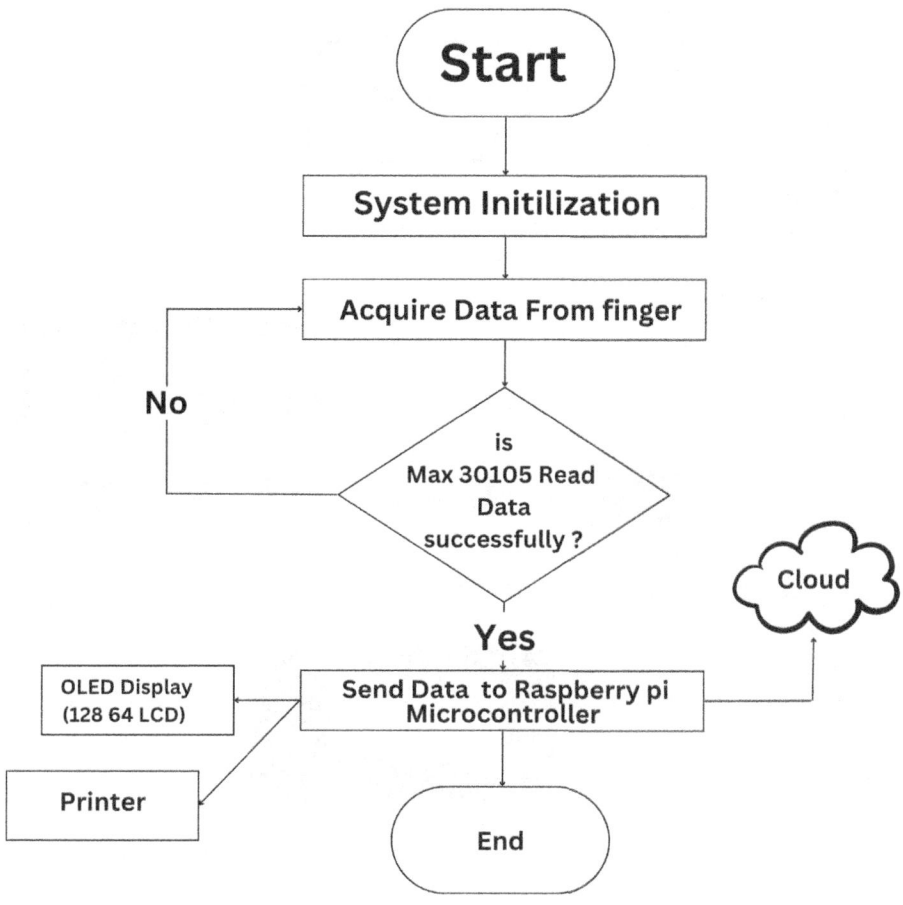

Fig. 2. Data flow diagram.

3.3   System Architecture

The system architecture incorporates a Raspberry Pi 4 microcontroller to receive input data from the MAX 30105 biomedical sensor. Three outputs are used to record and display data, as depicted in Fig. 3:

1. An OLED (LCD12864) screen displays the MAX30105 readings.
2. A crystal printer (QR204) prints the sensor readings for presenting to doctors or for maintaining a physical record.
3. A GSM module attached to the Raspberry Pi 4 forwards data to the cloud.

The raw data collected by the biosensor are converted into meaningful information using processing techniques (referenced from the Arduino website) before being sent to the data processing unit. This processed data can be easily interpreted by doctors and endocrinologists.

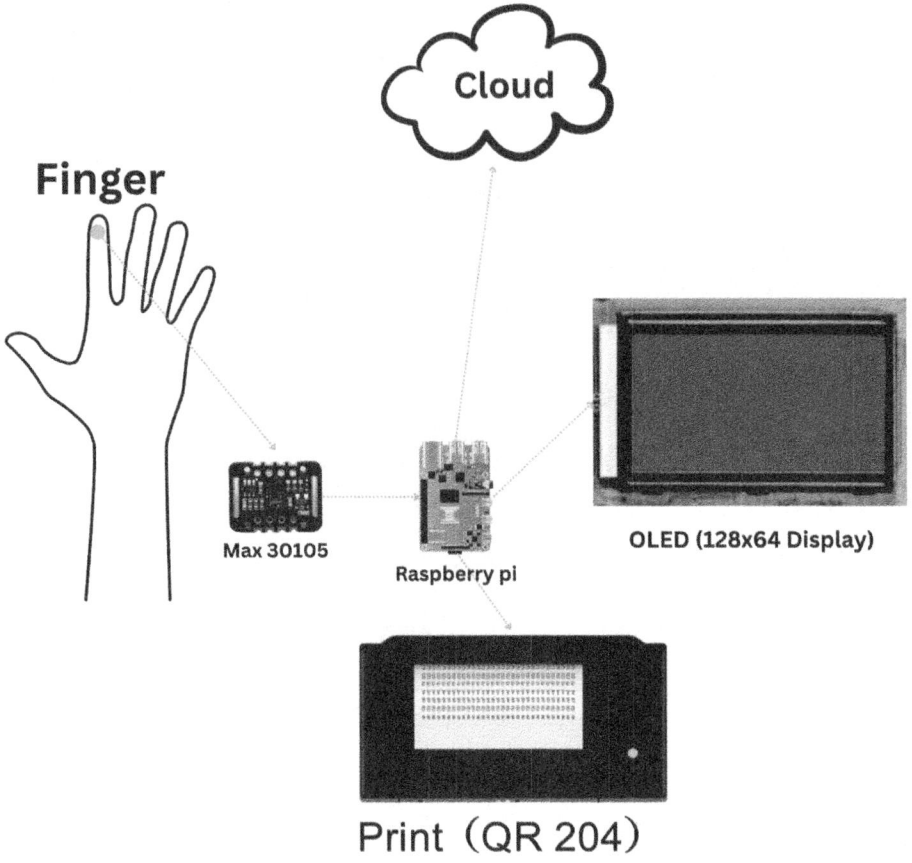

Fig. 3. System Architecture.

4   Data Analysis

This applied research was validated by comparing the results of our proposed system with those obtained using a Certeza glucometer, to assess accuracy. A total of one hundred volunteers were tested using both the proposed system and the glucometer concurrently, as depicted in Fig. 4.

– **Error Calculation of the Non-Invasive System** - The error percentage in the readings of the non-invasive system was determined using the following formula:

$$\text{Error}(\%) = \frac{\text{Proposed System Reading} - \text{Glucometer Reading}}{\text{Glucometer Reading}} \times 100 \quad (1)$$

– **Accuracy Check of the Non-Invasive System** - The accuracy of the system was calculated as:

$$\text{Accuracy} = 100\% - \text{Error}(\%) \quad (2)$$

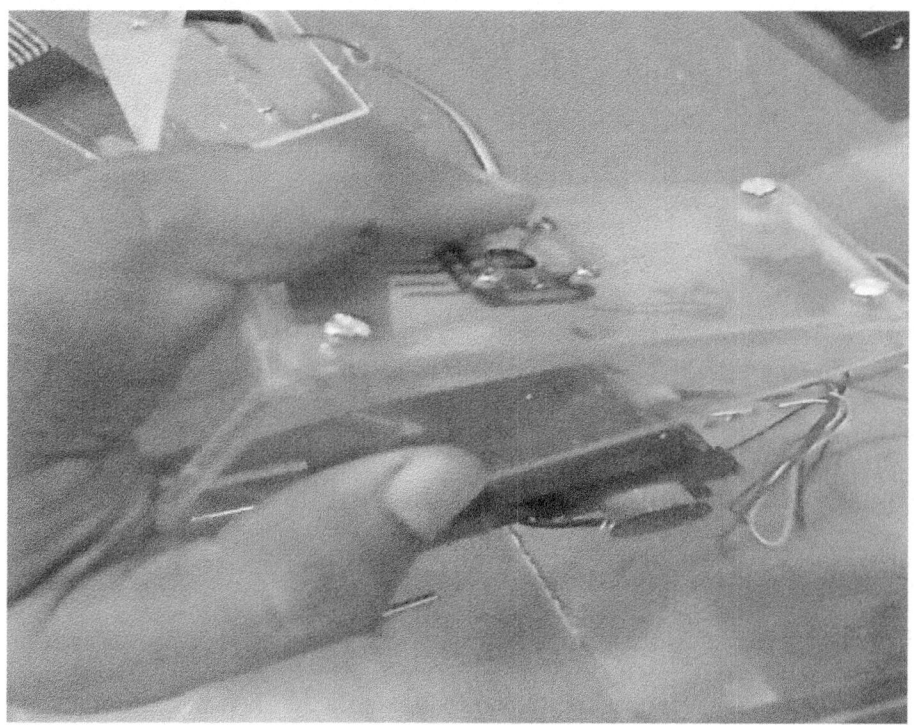

Fig. 4. Glucose monitoring through non-invasive device.

A strong linear relationship was observed between the readings from the proposed system and the glucometer. This relationship was quantified using the Pearson correlation coefficient, which measures the strength of the linear association between two variables, as illustrated in Fig. 5.

Further validation was carried out by including more data to ensure that the observed relationship remained consistent. This approach confirmed that the sample size was adequate for the calculation of the correlation formula. Subsequent to data collection, the readings from the glucometer and the biosensor module were utilized to develop an algorithm for non-invasive blood glucose testing. This algorithm integrates a formula that enables the Max30105 biosensor to assess blood glucose levels accurately.

When the correlation coefficient between two values lies between 0 and 1, it indicates a positive correlation. In our study, the proposed system demonstrated a correlation of 0.97 with the Certeza glucometer readings [22].

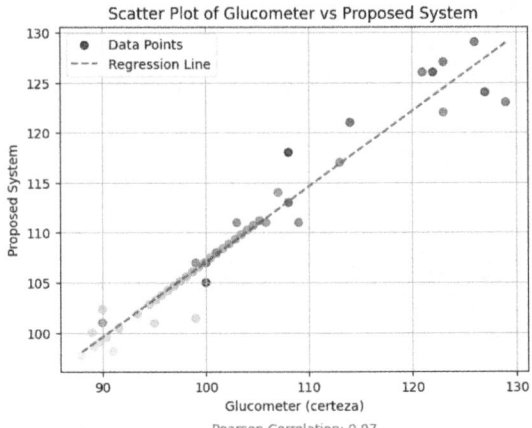

Fig. 5. Experiment data of Proposed system and glucometer.

5 Results and Discussion

The efficacy of the MAX30105 sensor-based system module was evaluated by comparing its results with those obtained from an invasive blood glucose monitoring device. This comparison aimed to establish the correlation between the non-invasive and invasive methods.

5.1 Correlation Analysis

The non-invasive sensor's results are presented in Table 1, where the glucose levels of 20 patients were measured using both the proposed system and the Certeza glucometer. The data suggest a strong correlation between the readings of the proposed non-invasive system and the invasive glucose monitoring device. This comparison is graphically represented in Fig. 6.

5.2 Discussion

The observed strong correlation indicates that the MAX30105 sensor-based non-invasive system can be a reliable alternative to traditional invasive blood glucose monitoring methods. This finding is significant, considering the need for less intrusive and more patient-friendly approaches in diabetes management. The convenience and ease of use offered by the non-invasive system can potentially enhance patient compliance and regular monitoring, thus improving overall diabetes management.

It is crucial to note that while the initial results are promising, further research involving a larger sample size and diverse patient demographics is necessary to validate these findings comprehensively. Additionally, continuous improvement and calibration of the non-invasive system are essential to maintain its accuracy and reliability over time.

Table 1. Patient Results Comparison with Certeza Device.

Patient ID	Gender	Age	Proposed System	Glucometer (Certeza)	Difference	Accruary (%)
10101	M	40	118	108	10	90.74
10102	M	42	105	100	5	95.00
10103	M	32	107	100	7	93.00
10104	M	36	126	122	4	96.72
10105	M	53	124	127	3	97.64
10106	M	48	113	108	5	95.37
10107	M	35	121	114	7	93.86
10108	M	32	129	126	3	97.62
10109	M	41	127	123	4	96.75
10110	F	46	133	129	4	96.90
10111	F	48	126	121	5	95.87
10112	M	44	125	123	2	98.37
10113	M	43	111	109	2	98.17
10114	M	28	108	101	7	93.07
10115	M	29	111	103	8	92.23
10116	M	30	117	113	4	96.46
10117	M	45	107	99	8	91.92
10118	M	51	114	107	7	93.46
10119	M	39	101	90	11	87.78

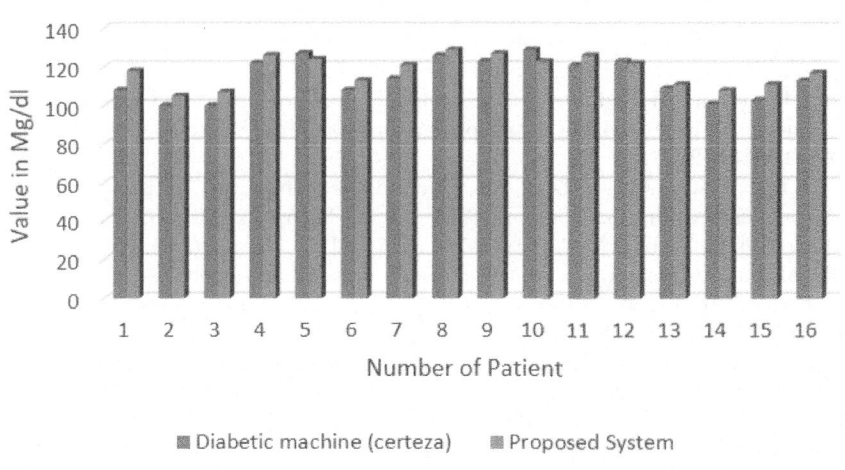

Fig. 6. Results comparison.

6   Conclusion

This study focused on developing a wearable sensor-based system for monitoring diabetes, specifically T2d. Our experimentation with a biomedical sensor device revealed that blood glucose levels can be accurately monitored using the device's non-invasive sensor. Despite the global prevalence of T2d, there is a notable lack of systems capable of non-invasively and accurately monitoring blood glucose levels without the need for needles. Our system successfully addresses this gap by providing a means to regularly monitor the glucose levels of T2d patients, recording data both on the cloud and in print form. Future work will involve exploring other non-invasive sensors, such as those in the MAX optical particle sensors series, to further enhance the accuracy of our system. The development of such non-invasive monitoring tools represents a significant step forward in diabetes care, potentially easing the burden for patients and improving overall management of the condition.

References

1. Heald, A.H., et al.: Estimating life years lost to diabetes: outcomes from analysis of National Diabetes Audit and Office of National Statistics data. Cardiovasc. Endocrinol. Metab. **9**(4), 183 (2020)
2. Connolly, V., Unwin, N., Sherriff, P., Bilous, R., Kelly, W.: Diabetes prevalence and socioeconomic status: a population based study showing increased prevalence of type 2 diabetes mellitus in deprived areas. J. Epidemiol. Community Health **54**(3), 173 (2000)
3. Chan, J.C., et al.: The Lancet Commission on diabetes: using data to transform diabetes care and patient lives. Lancet **396**(10267), 2019–2082 (2020)
4. Fauzi, R.N., et al.: Non-invasive detection system for blood sugar, cholesterol, uric acid, and body temperature using MAX30105 and MLX90614 sensors, pp. 1–7 (2022)
5. Rghioui, A., Lloret, J., Harane, M., Oumnad, A.: A smart glucose monitoring system for diabetic patient. Electronics **9**(4), 678 (2020)
6. Sun, H., et al.: IDF diabetes atlas: global, regional and country-level diabetes prevalence estimates for 2021 and projections for 2045. Diabetes Res. Clin. Pract. **183**, 109119 (2022)
7. Li, A.P.Z., Kariyawasam, D.: 4.10 - type 2 diabetes mellitus. In: Kenakin, T. (ed.) Comprehensive Pharmacology, pp. 225–243. Elsevier, Oxford (2022)
8. Galaviz, K.I., Weber, M.B., Straus, A., Haw, J.S., Narayan, K.M.V., Ali, M.K.: Global diabetes prevention interventions: a systematic review and network meta-analysis of the real-world impact on incidence, weight, and glucose. Diabetes Care **41**(7), 1526–1534 (2018)
9. Shokrekhodaei, M., Quinones, S.: Review of non-invasive glucose sensing techniques: optical, electrical and breath acetone. Sensors **20**(5), 1251 (2020)
10. Jin, H., Abu-Raya, Y.S., Haick, H.: Advanced materials for health monitoring with skin-based wearable devices. Adv. Healthcare Mater. **6**(11), 1700024 (2017)
11. Lehmann, V., et al.: Machine learning for non-invasive sensing of hypoglycemia while driving in people with diabetes. Diab. Obes. Metab. (2023)

12. Ali, M.S., Shoumy, N., Khatun, S., Kamarudin, L., Vijayasarveswari, V.: Non-invasive blood glucose measurement performance analysis through UWB imaging, pp. 513–516 (2016)

13. Hussain, A., Wenbi, R., Xiaosong, Z., Hongyang, W., Da Silva, A.L.: Personal home healthcare system for the cardiac patient of smart city using fuzzy logic. J. Adv. Inf. Technol. **7**(1) (2016)

14. Villena Gonzales, W., Mobashsher, A.T., Abbosh, A.: The progress of glucose monitoring-a review of invasive to minimally and non-invasive techniques, devices and sensors. Sensors **19**(4), 800 (2019)

15. Magliano, D.J., et al.: Trends in incidence of total or type 2 diabetes: systematic review. BMJ **366** (2019)

16. Bassi, G., Mancinelli, E., Dell'Arciprete, G., Rizzi, S., Gabrielli, S., Salcuni, S.: Efficacy of eHealth interventions for adults with diabetes: a systematic review and meta-analysis. Int. J. Environ. Res. Public Health **18**(17), 8982 (2021)

17. Stevens, S., Gallagher, S., Andrews, T., Ashall-Payne, L., Humphreys, L., Leigh, S.: The effectiveness of digital health technologies for patients with diabetes mellitus: a systematic review. Front. Clin. Diab. Healthcare **3** (2022)

18. Reddy, V.S., et al.: Recent advancement in biofluid-based glucose sensors using invasive, minimally invasive, and non-invasive technologies: a review. Nanomaterials **12**(7), 1082 (2022)

19. Song, K.-H., et al.: REP1 inhibits FOXO3-mediated apoptosis to promote cancer cell survival. Cell Death Dis. **8**(1), e2536–e2536 (2018)

20. Guevara, E., Torres-Galván, J.C., Ramírez-Elías, M.G., Luevano-Contreras, C., González, F.J.: Use of Raman spectroscopy to screen diabetes mellitus with machine learning tools. Biomed. Opt. Express **9**(10), 4998–5010 (2018)

21. Narkhede, P., Dhalwar, S., Karthikeyan, B.: NIR based non-invasive blood glucose measurement. Indian J. Sci. Technol. **9**(41), 1–7 (2016)

22. Godfrey, K., Gatare, I., Rushingabigwi, G.: Non-invasive IoT-based embedded device for testing diabetes mellitus type 2 for early detection and prediction, pp. 1–5 (2023)

23. Fortino, G., Kaber, D., Nürnberger, A., Mendonça, D.: Handbook of Human-Machine Systems. Wiley, Hoboken (2023)

24. Gravina, R., Fortino, G.: Wearable body sensor networks: state-of-the-art and research directions. IEEE Sens. J. **21**(11), 12511–12522 (2021). https://doi.org/10.1109/JSEN.2020.3044447

25. D'Aniello, G., Gravina, R., Gaeta, M., Fortino, G.: Situation-aware sensor-based wearable computing systems: a reference architecture-driven review. IEEE Sens. J. **22**(14), 13853–13863 (2022). https://doi.org/10.1109/JSEN.2022.3180902

Automatic Voice Classification of Autistic Subjects

Jessica Vacca[1], Natascia Brondino[2], Fabio Dell'Acqua[3], Anna Vizziello[3], and Pietro Savazzi[3(✉)]

[1] Department of Electrical, Computer, Biomedical Engineering,
University of Pavia, Pavia, Italy
[2] Department of Brain and Behavioral Sciences, University of Pavia, Pavia, Italy
natascia.brondino@unipv.it
[3] Department of Electrical, Computer, Biomedical Engineering, University of Pavia,
& CNIT Consorzio Nazionale Interuniversitario per le Telecomunicazioni, Pavia, Italy
{fabio.dellacqua,anna.vizziello,pietro.savazzi}@unipv.it

Abstract. Autism Spectrum Disorders (ASD) describe a heterogeneous set of conditions classified as neurodevelopmental disorders. Although the mechanisms underlying ASD are not yet fully understood, more recent literature focused on multiple genetics and/or environmental risk factors. Heterogeneity of symptoms, especially in milder forms of this condition, could be a challenge for the clinician. In this work, an automatic speech classification algorithm is proposed to characterize the prosodic elements that best distinguish autism, to support the traditional diagnosis. The performance of the proposed algorithm is evaluted by testing the classification algorithms on a dataset composed of recorded speeches, collected among both autustic and non autistic subjects.

Keywords: Speech Recognition · Machine Learning · Signal Classification · Autism

1 Introduction

Autism spectrum disorders (ASD) consist of a heterogeneous set of neurodevelopmental conditions characterized, at varying levels of complexity and severity, by persistent difficulties in verbal and non-verbal communication and in social interaction, and by patterns of repetitive behaviors and restricted interests [1]. ASD subjects represent a clinical condition with different levels of severity and whose features can be extremely heterogeneous [2].

The diagnosis of ASD is substantially clinical and it is formulated both in children and adults by physicians with significant expertise in ASD according to

This publication is part of the project NODES which has received funding from the MUR - M4C2 1.5 of PNRR funded by the European Union - NextGenerationEU (Grant agreement no. ECS00000036). The work was partially supported by Fondazione TIM under the Italian national project VOCE, call for proposals "Liberi di Comunicare".

international standardized criteria and supported by gold standard instruments (ADOS, ADI-R). Unfortunately, to date, there are no clear diagnostic biomarkers to support the clinician during the diagnostic process [3].

From their earliest characterizations [4], ASDs have been associated with particular speech tones and prosody disorders. Although 70–80% of individuals with ASD develop functional spoken language, at least half of the population with ASD develops atypical vocal patterns [5]. Specifically, verbal children with ASD often show some specific acoustic patterns [6]: prosodic features such as monotone tone, reduced stress, flat intonation, and even differences in the harmonic structure of their speech are among the first signs of the disorder [7].

To discuss the matter, it is useful to understand the mechanism behind speech production [8]. The organs of the vocal production system are the lungs (subglottal system), the larynx, and the vocal tract (supraglottal system). Lungs supply energy to the larynx in the form of an airflow that is modulated by the vocal cords. Vibration of the vocal cords turns the airflow into an almost periodic pressure variation or into a noisy sound depending on the action of the cords. This is used to excite the vocal tract system. This latter consists of oral, nasal and pharyngeal resonant cavities that further shape the signal spectrum of modulated airflow. The resulting signal is radiated through the lips. The vibration patterns of the vocal cords and the shape of the vocal tract system can produce different types of sounds. Therefore, the vocal signal generation system can be seen as consisting of an input excitation source to the vocal tract filters. This model is used in the source-filter theory of vocal production, which is based on the assumption that vocal outputs can be analyzed as the response of a series of vocal tract filters [8].

Specifically, the excitation signal for the vocal tract filter can be classified into one of the following list of options:

- Periodic glottal vibrations: quasi-periodic signal consisting of variable airflow cycles due to vocal cord vibration;
- Noise: source of aperiodic excitation generated when air flows rapidly through an open, non vibrating glottis (suction) or when air flows rapidly through a tight supra-laryngeal constriction (friction).
- Burst or pulse: short pulse of excitation caused by a rapid change in oral atmospheric pressure.

The input-output relationship of the vocal tract filter, where the input is the glottal airflow velocity and the output the airflow velocity through the vocal tract itself, can be approximated by a linear resonant filter. The resonant frequencies of the vocal tract are called formant frequencies or simply formants. The main objective of this work is to define appropriate algorithms for automatic extraction and classification of these speech features in order to correctly identify ASD subjects from the analysis of their recorded speech, partly building on previous results [11].

The rest of this work is organized as in the following: Sect. 2 shows the implemented algorithms from extraction of the speech features to subject classification. Section 3 is devoted to experimental results analysis, while in Sect. 4, we comment the obtained results and future research directions.

2   Feature Extraction and Classification Algorithms

In this section, we describe the signal processing chain designed to extract the vocal features of interest in order to correctly classify autistic subjects. Unless otherwise stated, all signal processing algorithms described here were implemented in Matlab [9]. The proposed algorithms were applied to the dataset [12], as detailed in the subsequent Sect. 3. Information on this dataset can be found in [13,14]. Figure 1 provides an overview of the implemented algorithm.

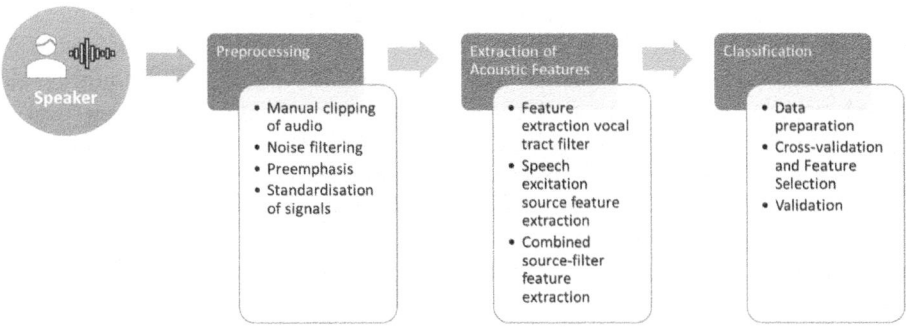

Fig. 1. Pipeline of the implemented algorithm

2.1   Preprocessing and Feature Extraction

Preprocessing were performed on each audio sequence, and include manual clipping of the signal, noise filtering, pre-emphasis, and signal normalization.

Manual clipping and noise filtering were done using the open source software Audacity [10], to remove the silent beginning and ending parts of each audio sequence and filter ambient noise. Regarding this latter, a part of the sequence containing only noise was selected, with a duration sufficient to guarantee good performance; for example, 0.05 s for an audio sequence sampled at 44.1 KHz. The noisy sample was selected to include different types of environmental noise, such as book page turning, and close-range buzzing of the microphone used for recording.

Once the noise profile had been analysed by the software, noise is reduced on the entire sequence of the audio waveform by setting suitable noise reduction parameters. Selection of parameter values was performed manually to avoid distortion of the speech sequences. The parameters include:

– Noise reduction set equal to 6 dB.
– Sensitivity: Audacity offers a range between 0 and 24 for this parameter. Higher values remove more noise, but with increasing likelihood of suppressing also a fraction of the useful speech signal. Lower values may however produce artefacts in the processed audio signal. We experimentally found the best tradeoff to be 6.

– Frequency damping: on a range between 1 and 6. The frequency damping operation consists of reducing the amplitude of selected frequency bands, in order to selectively filter noise in specific frequency ranges where it is thought to prevail. The width of each band is automatically selected according to the damping frequency of the audio sequence. It can be useful for reducing the effects of artifacts that may appear to the sensitivity parameter setting. The best compromise for this parameter was found to be 6, implying that selective suppression was very effective in noise reduction.

The subsequent preprocessing steps were implemented in Matlab [9]. Pre-emphasis was obtained through a high-pass finite impulse response (FIR) filter to increase the power of the high frequencies of the vocal signal while the low frequencies remain unaffected [15]:

$$H(z) = 1 - \alpha z^{-1} \tag{1}$$

where $0.9 \leq \alpha \leq 1$ is the pre-emphasis coefficient that fixes the cut off frequencies of the filter; it was set to 0.98.

Since the FIR filter (1) changes the distribution of energy among frequencies along with the overall energy level, which may impact on the energy-related acoustic characteristics [16], a normalization is applied to allow the comparison among speech signals independently from their amplitude variations. The i-th normalized sampled is defined as $S_{Ni} = (S_i - \mu)/\sigma$, where S_i is the i-th sample of the vocal signal, μ is the mean and σ is the standard deviation of the whole set of samples.

In order to extract the signal features used by the classification algorithms, the speech signal is here divided in vocal tract and vocal source to better discriminate the differences between the audio sequences of the autistic subjects and the ones recorded from neurotypical individuals. In the following, the employed techniques are described to extract the features of the vocal tract filter, of the excitation source, and of the combined source-filter [6].

Figure 2 shows a diagrammatic representation of the sequence of feature extraction methods used.

Among the features of the vocal tract filter, the first five formant frequencies (F1 to F5), and the first two dominant ones, FD1 and FD2, were extracted. The speech signal was divided into audio frames of 25 ms duration, with a frame shifting of 10 ms. In this way the original non-stationary speech signal is approximated with several shorter almost-stationary frames and Fourier analysis may be applied [17].

A Hamming window is then applied on each frame in order to minimize the signal discontinuity at the beginning and end of each segment and thus minimize the spectral distortion:

$$w(n) = 0.54 - 0.46 \ cos\left(\frac{2\pi n}{N-1}\right), \qquad 0 \leq n \leq N - 1 \tag{2}$$

where N is the number of samples per frame, so that the signal after the Hamming window is expressed as $y_k(n) = x_k(n)w(n)$ where n refers to the n-th sample in the considered k-th frame.

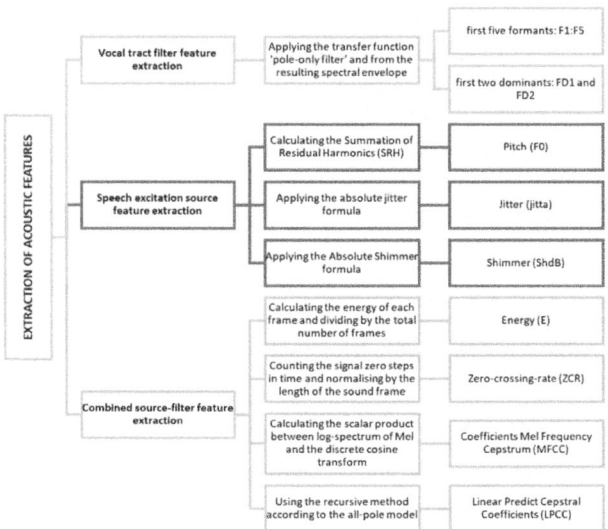

Fig. 2. Diagrammatic representation of the sequence of feature extraction methods used

After setting the framing of the signal, both the dominants and formants vocal tract features are computed following [6]. The envelope shape of the spectrum after passing a linear predictive (LP) filter is derived from each vocal frame and describes the features of the resonance frequencies of the vocal tract.

In further detail, the signal is resampled at 10 kHz, and divided into the frames as described above. An LP filter of order p equal to 10 is set to derive the formant frequencies. With these conditions, the frequency response of the filter has a maximum of five peaks corresponding to the frequencies of the first five formant ones, F1 to F5.

Figure 3 shows an example of an LP spectrum where the first 5 formant frequencies are highlighted.

If the filter order p is set equal to 5, the output of the filter shows only 2 peaks, which represent the dominant frequencies FD1 and FD2. Figure 4 represents an envelope of the LP spectrum where the dominant frequencies are highlighted. The filter is represented by

$$H(z) = \frac{1}{1 - \sum_{k=1}^{p} \alpha z^{-k}} \tag{3}$$

where p is the filter order and α_k are the LP coefficients for $k = 1, 2, ..., p$.

The excitation source features include pitch, closely related to fundamental frequency, shimmer and jitter. The method chosen to extract pitch is based on the summation of residual harmonics (SRH) [18]. It estimates an auto-regressive (AR) model of the spectral envelope of the speech signal $y(t)$ and derives the residual signal $e_r(t)$ by inverse filtering. For each frame, the amplitude of the

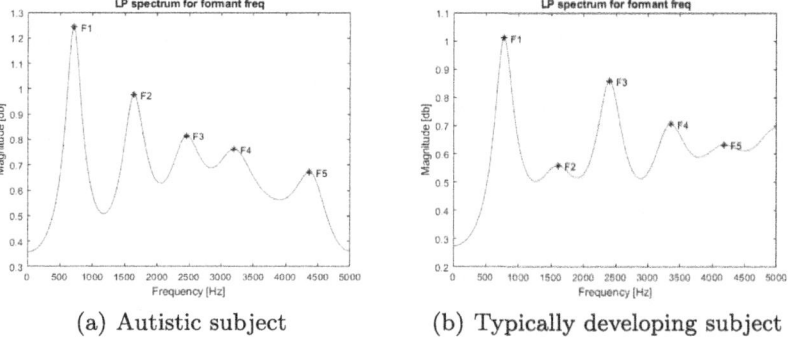

Fig. 3. LP spectrum showing the formant frequencies obtained from the audio signal of (a) an autistic subject, and (b) a neurotypical one.

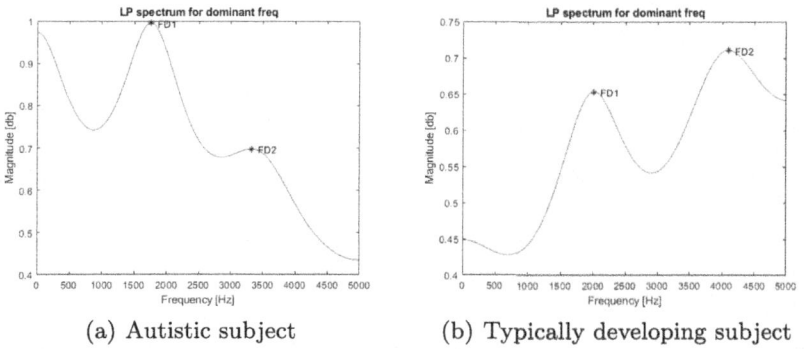

Fig. 4. LP spectrum showing the dominant frequencies obtained from the audio signal of (a) an autistic subject, and (b) a neurotypical one.

spectrum $E_r(f)$ is calculated, which has a relatively flat envelope for speech segments and has peaks at the harmonics of the fundamental frequency F_0. From this spectrum, and for each frequency in the range $[F_{0,min}; F_{0,max}]$, the SRH is calculated as:

$$SHR(f) = E_r(f) + \sum_{k=2}^{N_{harm}} \left[E_r(kf)E_r \left(\left(k - \frac{1}{2} \right) f \right) \right] \tag{4}$$

where N_{harm} is the number of the first harmonics taken into account, for instance $N_{harm} = 5$. The range of frequencies was set to $[70; 400]$ Hz to account for normal pitch ranges for both men and women. The estimated pitch value F_0 for a given frame is the frequency that maximizes $SRH(f)$.

The selected pitch extraction technique guarantees higher performance compared to other methods because of its robustness to interference and environmental noise.

Once the pitch for each subject's sound segment is estimated, the average F_0 is calculated and used to construct the input dataset for the classification methods.

Besides pitch, jitter and shimmer are calculated according to [18,19]. The absolute jitter $Jitt_a$, i.e., the absolute mean difference between consecutive glottal periods, measured in seconds, is defined as:

$$Jitt_a = \frac{1}{N_F - 1} \sum_{i=1}^{N_F-1} |T_i - T_{i-1}|$$ (5)

in which T_i is the extracted glottal period, corresponding to the instant of time when the maximum of $SRH(f)$ was detected, and N_F is the total number of sound frames.

The absolute shimmer $(ShdB)$ is calculated as:

$$ShdB = \frac{1}{N_F - 1} \sum_{i=1}^{N_F-1} \left| 20 \, log_{10} \left(\frac{A_{i+1}}{A_i} \right) \right|$$ (6)

where A_i is the amplitude associated with the pitch value F_0 of the i-th sound frame and N_F is the total number of sound frames.

Both jitter and shimmer are calculated only between consecutive sound frames.

The combined source-filter features analyzed in this work are energy, zero-crossing rate, Mel frequency cepstrum coefficient (MFCC) and linear prediction cepstrum coefficient (LPCC).

The energy for each frame is calculated as $E(i) = \frac{\sum_{n=1}^{N} |y_i(n)|^2}{N}$, with $i = 1, 2, ..., L$, where L is the total number of frames and N is the frame length. The energy of each frame is normalized to the maximum of its values.

The zero-crossing rate (ZCR) is computed for each frame, evaluating for each sample of the frame if its previous or following sample shows an opposite sign (Fig. 5).

To calculate MFCC coefficients, the audio signals were re-sampled at 10 kHz. Their power is calculated as $P(i) = \sum_{k=0}^{N-1} |X_i(k)|^2$, where k refers to the kth frequency sample of the spectrum of the ith frame and $X_i(k) = \sum_{n=0}^{N-1} x_i(n)e^{-\frac{2\pi jnk}{N}}$, $k = 0, 1, ..., N - 1$. Each mth triangular filter of the Mel filter bank is designed according to [20]:

$$H_m(k) = \begin{cases} 0, k < f(m-1) \\ \frac{k-f(m-1)}{f(m)-f(m-1)}, f(m-1) \le k < f(m) \\ 1, k = f(m) \\ \frac{f(m+1)-k}{f(m+1)-f(m)}, f(m) < k \le f(m+1) \\ 0, k > f(m+1) \end{cases}$$ (7)

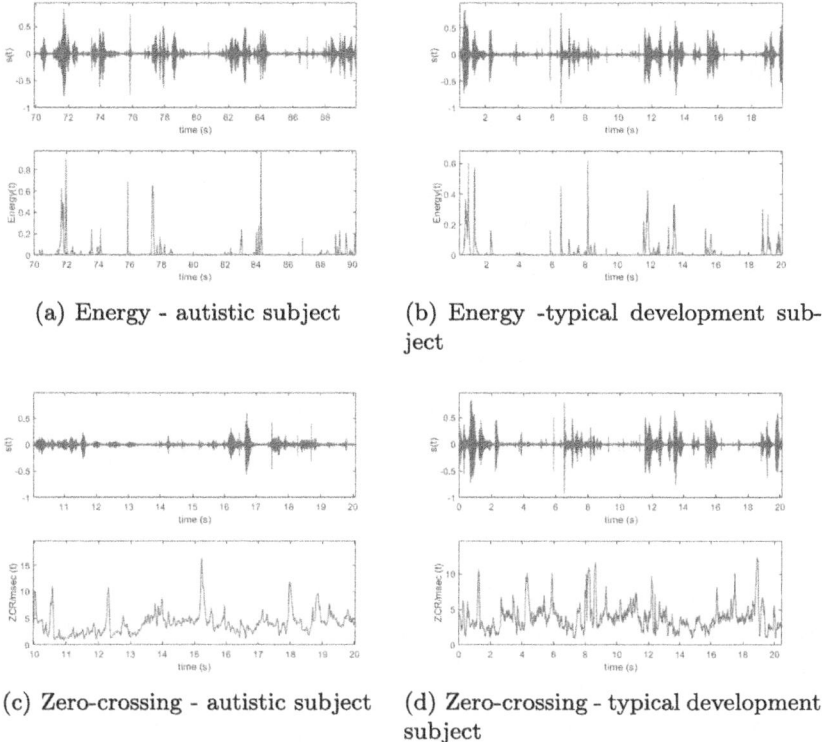

(a) Energy - autistic subject

(b) Energy -typical development subject

(c) Zero-crossing - autistic subject

(d) Zero-crossing - typical development subject

Fig. 5. Energy and zero-crossing rate of the audio signal for two different individuals.

where $m = 0, 1, ..., M - 1$, f is the normalized discrete frequency, $f(m)$ is the centre frequency of the triangular filter, and M number of triangular filters. M may be chosen between 4 and 160, and we set $M = 40$ as usual for speech recognition applications. The resulting filter bank is shown in Fig. 6. The figure shows the triangular filters that are linearly spaced from 0 to 1 kHz, and equally spaced in logarithmic scale after 1 KHz, following the typical filtering ability of the human ear.

The Mel spectrum is calculated as

$$S_{Mel}(m) = \sum_{k=0}^{N-1} |X_i(k)|^2 H_m(k), 0 \leq m \leq M - 1 \tag{8}$$

The Mel coefficients are calculated as

$$c(n) = \sum_{m=0}^{M-1} log_{10}(s_{Mel}(m)) cos \left(\frac{\pi n(m - 0.5)}{M} \right) \tag{9}$$

where $n = 0, 1, ..., C - 1$ with C the total number of MFCC filters. This operation converts the frequency spectrum into the time domain, keeping only the first C most significant coefficients: the first 12 Mel coefficients are considered here.

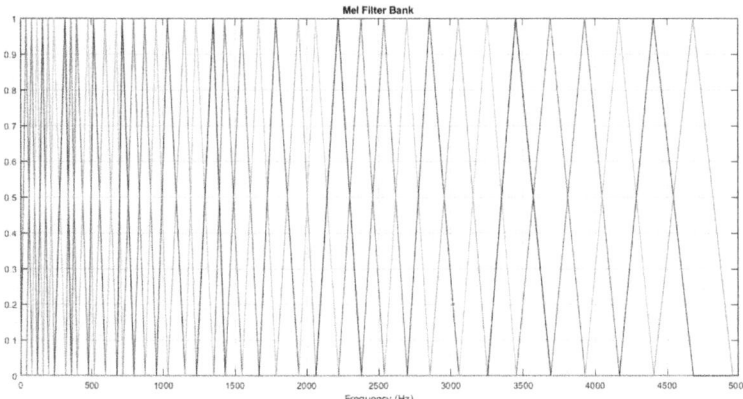

Fig. 6. Frequency response of the Mel filter bank in the range 0–5 KHz with triangular filter shape and M=40.

LPCC coefficients were calculated through a recursive method that allows to transform LPC filter parameters into the LPC cepstrum according to the all-pole model. The recursive method is described as

$$
c_n = \begin{cases} a_n, n = 1 \\[2mm] a_n + \sum_{k=1}^{n-1} \frac{k}{n} c_k a_{n-k}, 1 < n \leq p \\[2mm] \sum_{k=1}^{n-1} \frac{k}{n} c_k a_{n-k}, n > p \end{cases} \tag{10}
$$

where $a_1, a_2, ..., a_p$ are the coefficients of the LP filter with order $p = 12$.

2.2   Classification Algorithms

The dataset samples were classified according to the following 36 feature attributes: the fondamental frequency F_0, ZCR, the signal energy, the formant frequencies from $F1$ to $F5$, the dominant frequencies $FD1$ and $FD2$, the first 12 Mel-frequency Cepstrum coefficients, the first 12 LPC coefficients, shimmer, jitter.

Firstly, we considered a classification preprocessing phase in order to mage data normalization and select the best feature attributes for the main classification goal, i.e. to distinguish between autistic and non autistic recorded voices.

We focus on supervised classification, taking into accounts the random forest (RF), support vector machine (SVM), logistic regression (LR), and Naive Bayes (NB) algorithms [21].

In the next section, the implemented classification chain is described in detail, starting with a description of the experimental dataset used to provide the results obtained.

3   Experimental Results

In this section, we describe the dataset used for experimental validation of the proposed classification chain.

3.1   Dataset

In this work we analyze the speech sequences from ASDBank Dutch Asymmetries Corpus [12], and specifically the SK sub-corpus that comprises vocal samples of 46 children with ASD and 38 children with typical development (TD), both groups aged between 6 and 12 years (average 9 years). Most of them were boys and all were native Dutch speakers. These samples were produced between 2007 and 2012 in the framework of a research project at the University of Groningen, and are made available to the scientific community for research purposes [13,14].

The dataset consists of 84 examples in total, and there are no missing data. Two classes are defined: ASD with 46 subjects out of the total number of examples (54.76%) and TD with 38 (45.24%).

3.2   Data Preparation

As pointed out earlier, there are no missing data in the dataset. First, all 36 attributes were normalized in the range $[-1, 1]$, according to a min-max normalization procedure [21].

It is to be noted that a large number of attributes was defined, disproportionate to the number of available examples, hence classification algorithms may incur the so-called "curse of dimensionality" issue.

Following the rule of thumb that the number of features should be approximately equal to 1/10 of the number of examples that make up the dataset, a number of attributes equal to 8 should be selected. To reduce the number of features to the desired amount, the supervised feature selection strategy used was the T-test-based classification, which assigns a positive score to attributes whose difference in mean values between the two different classes is large.

The classification phase of this work was conducted on Orange, an open source toolkit for data visualization, machine learning and data mining [21]. Therefore, at each 5-fold cross-validation cycle, four folds are used as the training set and a ranking is performed on them. From the ranking, only the eight best variables are selected to form the reduced test set, the remaining fold, which represents the input of the classifiers. The features selected to compose the best set of features were the first eight:

- ZCR;
- the fundamental frequency F_0;
- the MFCC coefficients 3,4,6,8, and 12;
- the dominant frequency FD1

3.3   Automatic Classification

As stated above, we employed the following classification techniques: the RF, SVM, LR, and NB algorithms. Moreover, we validated the performance of classification algorithms by using the following metrics [22]:

$$Accuracy = \frac{TP + TN}{TP + TN + FP + FN} \tag{11}$$

$$Precision = \frac{TP}{TP + FP} \tag{12}$$

$$Recall = \frac{TP}{TP + FN} \tag{13}$$

where TP is the number of true positives, TN the number of true negatives, FP the number of false positives, and FN the false negatives.

A metric that combines the values of both of the above measures is the F measure, which is a harmonic mean between precision and recall:

$$F_{measure} = \frac{2 \cdot precision \cdot recall}{precision + recall} \tag{14}$$

3.4   Experimental Result Evaluation

Figure 7 shows the classification results. First we highlight the average results derived from the 5-fold cross-validation; at each cross-validation cycle we pinned the average results between ASD and TD classes and at the end of the procedure we extracted the average for Accuracy, $F_{measure}$, Precision and Recall. The best performing classifiers are SVM and RF.

Table 1 shows the confidence intervals of the punctual accuracy estimated so far. It turns out that SVM and RF show the same performance even in terms of confidence intervals.

However, Table 2 shows a difference between SVM and RF in terms of precision, which is higher for SVM, although all classifiers score high in precision.

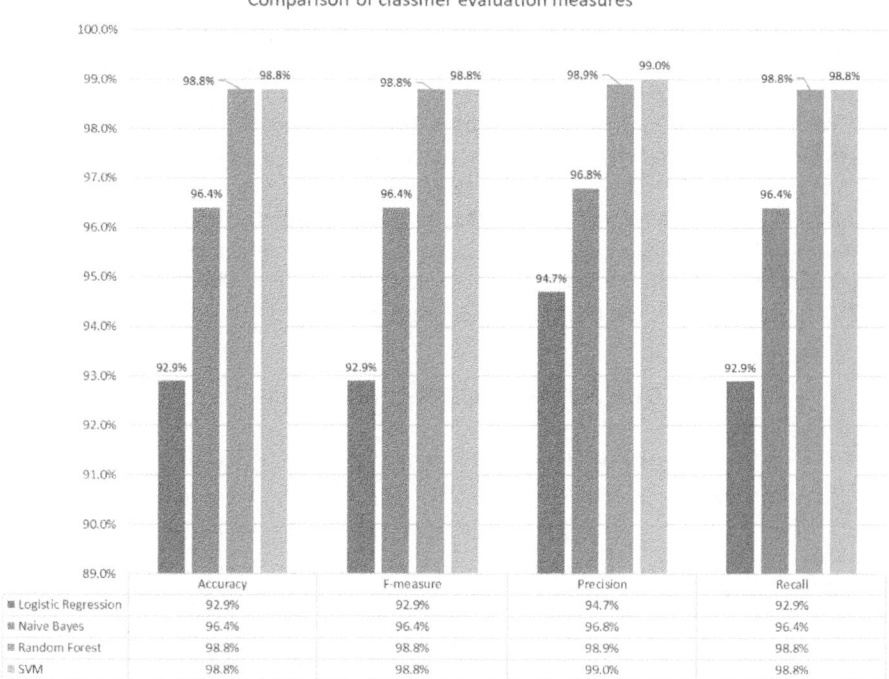

Fig. 7. Classification results.

Table 1. Confidence intervals of the classification algorithms.

Classifier	Lower limit	Estimated average accuracy	Upper limit
LR	0.8291	0.9294	1
NB	0.9326	0.9640	0.9954
RF	0.9632	0.9882	1
SVM	0.9632	0.9882	1

Table 2. ASD subjects: $F_{measure}$, *Precision* and *Recall*.

Classifier	F-measure	Precision	Recall
LR	0.932	0.976	0.891
NB	0.967	0.978	0.957
RF	0.989	0.979	1
SVM	0.989	1	0.978

3.5   Statistical Analysis

To validate the results obtained in terms of the quality of feature extraction, a parametric-type statistical test, the t-test, was performed, to assess the significance value by p-value. The starting hypothesis, called the null hypothesis H_0, is no difference in the averages of the distribution of attribute values between the "ASD" and "TD" classes; at the beginning of the test, the threshold value $\alpha = 0.05$ is then set, which indicates the level of significance with which to compare the p-value. If the p-value is less than α, then we reject the null hypothesis because there is a significant difference within the study. The closer the p-value is to 0, the more significant the test becomes.

Table 3. Statistical Analysis Results.

Features	ASD mean	TD mean	p-value	H_1 (5%)
ZCR	0.0987	0.167	<0.05	Accepted
F_0	289.124	272.247	<0.05	Accepted
MFCC12	−2.976	−3.784	<0.05	Accepted
MFCC16	−3.0188	−3.875	<0.05	Accepted
MFCC6	−3.0188	−3.875	<0.05	Accepted
MFCC3	−1.0186	−3.113	<0.05	Accepted
MFCC4	−5.0150	−6.360	<0.05	Accepted
MFCC8	−3.130	−3.792	<0.05	Accepted
FD_1	1853.942	1769.413	<0.05	Accepted
F_1	798.0834	820.146	0.00956	Accepted
F_2	1827.998	1817.923	0.206	Rejected

Table 3 shows that the alternative hypothesis H_1, according to which with 95% probability the null hypothesis H_0 can be rejected, is accepted and it can be confirmed with statistical significance that the differences between the two class means are different from 0. For completeness, we also reported statistics on the first two formant frequencies F_1 and F_2. It turns out that only the first formant frequency F_1 obtains a p-value less than 0.05.

4   Conclusions

Examining autistic prosody is essential because acoustic irregularities might contribute to the socio-communicative changes linked with the disorder. Our work aims to support the diagnosis of autism with more quantitative and objective assessments based on autistic speech. We attempted to create a clear and defined framework, both for the extraction part, exploiting more complex measures of speech recognition, such as MFCC and LPCC, and for the classification part, defining a systematic cross-validation and filtering of attributes, which is often missing inliterature. In the future our results will need to be validated by testing the classifiers on a larger number of examples and by generalising the models as much as possible by training and testing them on more languages, different ages or different tasks. Specifically, the focus will be on automatic voice classification of adult autistic individuals.

References

1. American Psychiatric Association. Diagnostic and statistical manual of mental disorders (5th edn. text rev.) (2022). https://doi.org/10.1176/appi.books.9780890425787
2. Di Volkmar, F.R.: Autism and Pervasive Developmental Disorders, 3rd edn. Cambridge University Press, Cambridge (2019)
3. Hodges, H., Fealko, C., Soares, N.: Autism spectrum disorder: definition, epidemiology, causes, and clinical evaluation. Transl. Pediatr. **9**(Suppl. 1), S55–S65 (2020). https://doi.org/10.21037/tp.2019.09.09. PMID: 32206584; PMCID: PMC7082249
4. Kanner, L.: Autistic disturbances of affective contact. Nervous Child **2**, 217–250 (1943)
5. Fusaroli, R., Lambrechts, A., Bang, D., Bowler, D.M., Gaigg, S.B.: Is voice a marker for Autism spectrum disorder? A systematic review and meta-analysis. Autism Res. **10**(3), 384–407 (2017). https://doi.org/10.1002/aur.1678. Epub 2016 Aug 8 PMID: 27501063
6. Mohanta, A., Mukherjee, P., Mirtal, V.K.: Acoustic features characterization of autism speech for automated detection and classification. In: 2020 National Conference on Communications (NCC), Kharagpur, India, pp. 1–6 (2020). https://doi.org/10.1109/NCC48643.2020.9056025
7. Asgari, M., Chen, L., Fombonne, E.: Quantifying voice characteristics for detecting autism. Front. Psychol. **7**(12), 665096 (2021). https://doi.org/10.3389/fpsyg.2021.665096. PMID: 34557127; PMCID: PMC8452864
8. Quatieri, T.F.: Discrete-Time Speech Signal Processing: Principles and Practice, 1st edn. Prentice Hall, Upper Saddle River (2001)
9. The MathWorks, Inc. MATLAB version: 9.13.0 (R2022b) (2022). https://www.mathworks.com. Accessed 01 Jan 2023
10. Audacity software is copyright 1999–2021 Audacity Team. https://audacityteam.org/ It is free software distributed under the terms of the GNU General Public License. The name Audacity is a registered trademark
11. Mohanta, A., Mittal, V.K.: Analysis and classification of speech sounds of children with autism spectrum disorder using acoustic features. Comput. Speech Lang. **72**, 101287 (2022). https://doi.org/10.1016/j.csl.2021.101287. ISSN 0885-2308
12. Hendriks, P., Koster, C., Kuijper, S.: ASDBank Dutch Asymmetries Corpus (2013). https://asd.talkbank.org/access/Dutch/Asymmetries.html
13. Hendriks, P., Koster, C., Hoeks, J.C.J.: Referential choice across the lifespan: why children and elderly adults produce ambiguous pronouns. Lang. Cogn. Neurosci. **29**(4), 391407 (2014). https://doi.org/10.1080/01690965.2013.766356
14. Kuijper, S.J., Hartman, C.A., Hendriks, P.: Who is he? Children with ASD and ADHD take the listener into account in their production of ambiguous pronouns. PLoS ONE **10**(7), e0132408 (2015). https://doi.org/10.1371/journal.pone.0132408. PMID: 26147200; PMCID: PMC4492581

15. Ai, O.C., Hariharan, M., Yaacob, S., Chee, L.S.: Classification of speech dysfluencies with MFCC and LPCC features. Expert Syst. Appl. **39**(2), 2157–2165 (2012). https://doi.org/10.1016/j.eswa.2011.07.065. ISSN 0957-4174
16. Vergin, R., O'Shaughnessy, D.: Pre-emphasis and speech recognition. In: Proceedings 1995 Canadian Conference on Electrical and Computer Engineering, Montreal, QC, Canada, vol. 2, pp. 1062–1065 (1995). https://doi.org/10.1109/CCECE.1995.526613
17. Muda, L., et al.: Voice Recognition Algorithms using Mel Frequency Cepstral Coefficient (MFCC) and Dynamic Time Warping (DTW) Techniques. arXiv abs/1003.4083 (2010)
18. Drugman, T., Alwan, A.: Joint Robust Voicing Detection and Pitch Estimation Based on Residual Harmonics. https://arxiv.org/abs/2001.00459
19. Teixeira, J.P., Oliveira, C., Lopes, C.: Vocal acoustic analysis - jitter, shimmer and HNR parameters. Procedia Technol. **9**, 1112–1122 (2013). https://doi.org/10.1016/j.protcy.2013.12.124. ISSN 2212-0173
20. Abdul, Z.K., Al-Talabani, A.K.: Mel frequency cepstral coefficient and its applications: a review. IEEE Access **10**, 122136–122158 (2022). https://doi.org/10.1109/ACCESS.2022.3223444
21. Demsar, J., et al.: Orange: data mining toolbox in Python. J. Mach. Learn. Res. **14**(Aug), 2349–2353 (2013). http://jmlr.org/papers/v14/demsar13a.html
22. Yalug, B.B., Arslan, D.B., Ozturk-Isik, E.: Chapter 19 - Prospect of data science and artificial intelligence for patient-specific neuroprostheses. In: Güçlü, B. (ed.) Somatosensory Feedback for Neuroprosthetics, pp. 589–629. Academic Press (2021). https://doi.org/10.1016/B978-0-12-822828-9.00005-8. ISBN 9780128228289

Channel Transfer Function Estimation of a Molecular-Electrical Communication Based on Redox

Karthik Reddy Gorla$^{(\boxtimes)}$ ⓘ and Massimiliano Pierobon ⓘ

University of Nebraska-Lincoln, Lincoln, USA
{kgorla2,maxp}@unl.edu

Abstract. The fusion of biological systems with electronic interfaces heralds a transformative era in the Internet of Bio-Nano Things (IoBNT), unlocking disruptive applications based on a network of biological and electrical nanoscale-based devices, especially within the human body. With recent advances in the field of Molecular Communication (MC), the propagation of information across interfaces that bridge biological and electrical domains can be modeled and characterized. Based on a pioneering proof-of-concept prototype that facilitates communication between biological entities and electrical circuits via redox chemical reactions, we describe the modeling of the interface as a molecular-electrical communication channel using the underlying diffusion and electrochemical principles. Using the linearity property within the analytical model, an empirical frequency analysis methodology is employed to extract the channel transfer function and the noise power spectral density through a simulation framework developed in MATLAB. In addition, we explore the behavior of the channel by varying a system design parameter, namely the length. Although preliminary, the combination of theoretical modeling, empirical analysis, and system design considerations informs a comprehensive framework for understanding and optimizing communication interfaces that are equipped to navigate the intricate landscape of the IoBNT paradigm.

Keywords: Internet of Bio-Nano Things · Molecular Communication · Frequency analysis · Channel transfer function · Redox reactions

1 Introduction

The Internet of Bio-Nano Things (IoBNT) is an emerging field of research on the seamless interconnected network of electrical components, such as implants

Supported by the National Science Foundation (NSF) through Grant No. ECCS-1807604 and Semiconductor Research Corporation (SRC) through Task No. 2843.001. Supported in part by the Italian Ministry of Foreign Affairs and International Cooperation, grant number US23GR04 (CUP: D43C23000350001).

M. Mizmizi et al. (Eds.): BodyNets 2024, LNICST 524, pp. 153–165, 2024.
https://doi.org/10.1007/978-3-031-72524-1_12

and biological components, both natural and synthetic within and outside the human body, which can then be connected to the Internet. To enable real-time integration between these components, an interface is needed that can facilitate the flow of information between them [1]. On the biological side of the interface, the flow of information can be characterized by using Molecular Communication, a field that uses the intrinsic properties of molecules to transmit information and further analyze natural systems that already exploit them at the nanoscale [2,6]. The other side of the interface is connected to the electrical domain, which is macroscopic in scale.

Recent years have seen an increase in modeling and characterizing of such interfaces using MC techniques [4,17]. Specifically, there has been work on an experimental proof-of-concept interface that uses a biochemical modality called redox to translate between biological information and electrical information [13–15,20].

In the scope of this paper, we analyze the interface as a communication channel from the Molecular domain to the Electrical domain, *i.e.,* a M2E communication channel. In our previous work, we have defined and characterized this redox-based M2E communication channel and then estimated the signal-to-noise ratio, limit of detection, and limit of quantification [10], followed by mutual information [11], and finally the water filling capacity [12]. Now, we want to estimate the transfer function of the channel and observe its behavior as a function of the size of the interface, specifically its length.

The rest of the paper is organized as follows. In Sect. 2, we detail the main concepts and analytical mathematical formulas of the M2E communication channel based on redox. The implementation of the simulation code and the methodologies adopted for frequency analysis are described in Sect. 3. Section 4 includes numerical results of the simulation model in terms of the empirical channel transfer function and noise power spectral density over varying channel length. Finally, we conclude the paper in Sect. 5.

2   System Model

In this section, we describe the system model of our M2E communication channel based on redox reactions. As seen in Fig. 1, the communication begins with a **Source** that releases a concentration of redox-active molecules which is modulated as the input signal as it is transmitted through the surface that acts as the **Molecular Transmitter**. These molecules diffuse through space via **Molecule Diffusion**, which is characterized by Brownian motion that is stochastic in nature. On reaching the electrode, these redox-active molecules react to undergo **Redox Reactions** that are influenced by an applied voltage signal and in turn cause electron exchange to produce electrical current, as measured at the **Electrical Receiver**, which is further connected to the **Destination**. As the name M2E suggests, in this model, we start with the Molecular domain at the beginning and end with the Electrical domain.

As a result of the stochastic behavior of the molecule diffusion, the system inherently has diffusion noise. In the scope of this paper, we have implemented the system to have a linear diffusion along the axis connecting the **Surface** and the **Electrode**. This helps to reduce complexity while still maintaining accuracy. When accounting for processes in only one dimension, we further implemented the following assumptions. The **Surface** is at the origin *i.e.*, $x = 0$ and the **Electrode** is at a distance H *i.e.*, $x = H$, which is used as a variable parameter to understand the behavior of the M2E communication channel, further explored in the Sect. 4. A more detailed explanation of the system model and its components is available in [12].

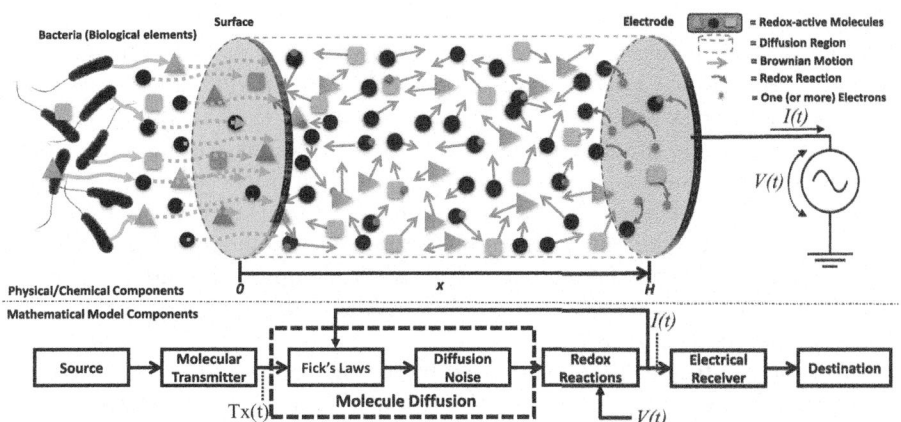

Fig. 1. System model of a M2E communication channel based on redox.

2.1 Molecular Transmitter

As observed from Fig. 1, the molecular transmitter can be defined as an emitter that modulates as the molecules from the source move through the surface, forming the transmitted signal. In our model, the transmitted signal can be mathematically described as the rate of input redox-active molecules into the communication channel and is expressed as

$$\text{Tx}(t) = \begin{bmatrix} C_{1,O}(0,t) \text{ .. } C_{m,O}(0,t) \text{ .. } C_{M,O}(0,t) \\ C_{1,R}(0,t) \text{ .. } C_{m,R}(0,t) \text{ .. } C_{M,R}(0,t) \end{bmatrix}, \tag{1}$$

where $\text{Tx}(t)$ is the transmitted signal as a function of time t, $C_{m,O}(0,t)$ and $C_{m,R}(0,t)$ are the concentrations of redox-active molecules in oxidized (O) and reduced (R) states respectively of species m at time t and on the **Surface**.

2.2 Molecular Diffusion

The transmitted redox-active molecules diffuse from the **Surface** to the **Electrode**, as observed from Fig. 1. The region where the diffusion occurs acts as the bridge between the molecular side and the electrical side of this channel. To reduce complexity without sacrificing accuracy, we assume diffusion to be one-dimensional, occurring along the axis perpendicular to the electrode surface. Using Fick's laws [7], the diffusion equation for our system is modeled as follows:

$$
\begin{cases}
\dfrac{\partial C_{m,S}(x,t)}{\partial t} = -\nabla \Big(-D_m \nabla C_{m,S}(x,t) \cdots \\
\qquad \cdots \pm \dfrac{I_m(t)}{n_m F Ar} \delta(x-H) \Big) \end{cases}_{m=1,2,\ldots,M;S=O,R} \tag{2}
$$

where $C_{m,S}(x,t)$ is the concentration of species m in a redox state S at time instant t and distance x from the **Surface**, $D_{m,S}$ is the diffusion coefficient of species m in a redox state S, $I_m(t)$ is the current at time instant t produced by species m, n_m is number of electrons transferred for species m, F is the Faraday constant, and Ar is the cross-sectional area of the reacting surface of the electrode. The inhomogeneous part that involves $I_m(t)$ is due to the change in the concentration of the redox-active molecules as they undergo redox reactions at the electrode. At the **Electrode**, we have a Neumann boundary condition where the sum of the fluxes of the oxidized and reduced species at any time during the reactions is zero [3].

The process of molecule diffusion is due to the rapid and continually irregular motion of molecules, known as Brownian motion. The stochasticity of the irregularity contributes as diffusion noise in our M2E communication channel. In our paper, we modeled diffusion noise as a volumetric Poisson counting process [18]. As such, we first estimate the actual number of molecules at the electrode $N'_{m,S}(t)$ to be

$$
N'_{m,S}(t) \sim Poiss\left(\nu N_A C_{m,S}(H,t) \right) \qquad , m=1,2,\ldots,M;S=O,R, \tag{3}
$$

where ν is an infinitesimal volume on the electrode, N_A is the Avogadro's number, and $C_{m,S}(H,t)$ is the concentration of molecules of species m in redox state S on the electrode surface at time instant t. Consequently, the effective redox-active molecule concentration at the electrode $C'_{m,S}(H,t)$ is estimated as

$$
C'_{m,S}(H,t) = \frac{N'_{m,S}(t)}{\nu N_A} \qquad , m=1,2,\ldots,M;S=O,R \tag{4}
$$

2.3   Redox Reactions

The redox-active molecules that diffuse until the electrode undergo redox reactions. During these reactions, they alternate between oxidized and reduced states through the exchange of electrons. A typical redox reaction is represented as seen below

$$
O + ne \underset{k_b}{\overset{k_f}{\rightleftharpoons}} R, \tag{5}
$$

where O is an oxidized species, R is a reduced species, e is an electron, n is the number of electrons transferred, k_f and k_b are the forward and reverse reaction rate constants, respectively. The conversion between the reduced and oxidized states of the redox-active molecules, being a reversible in nature, is regulated by these reaction rate constants. These rate constants can be expressed as a function of a applied voltage applied at the electrode as

$$k_{f_m}(t) = k_{0_m} e^{\frac{-\alpha_m n_m F}{RT}(V(t)-E_m^0)} , \tag{6}$$

$$k_{b_m}(t) = k_{0_m} e^{\frac{(1-\alpha_m)n_m F}{RT}(V(t)-E_m^0)} , \tag{7}$$

where k_{f_m} is the forward reaction rate constant of species m, k_{b_m} is the backward reaction rate constant of species m, k_{0_m} is the standard rate constant of species m, α_m is the charge transfer coefficient of species m, n_m is the number of electrons transferred per reaction of species m, F is the Faraday constant, R is the molar gas constant, T is the absolute temperature, $V(t)$ is the applied voltage applied at time t at the electrode, and E^0 is the standard potential of the species [3,5].

2.4 Electrical Receiver

The electrical receiver in our M2E communication channel model is composed of a voltage source and an ammeter connected to the **Electrode**. Specifically in the scope of this paper, the receiver is an electrochemical setup related to Cyclic Voltammetry (CV) [3]. In CV, by probing an electrochemical solution through a set of linear voltages in a periodic rhythm, we measure the generated current. This applied voltage in CV, is generally a triangular wave as seen in Fig. 2. We typically start at zero voltage, increasing linearly to reach a maximum voltage, decreasing linearly until a minimum voltage, and then increasing again to reach the initial zero voltage. The measured output is the electrical current that is generated by the redox reactions that occur at the electrode as the applied voltage changes. Figure 2 shows the measured electrical current and the corresponding applied voltage with respect to time, assuming a redox-active species named Ferrocene, with all molecules in an initial reduced state.

When the net voltage of $V(t) - E_m^0$ is positive, we can infer that the backward reaction rate constant is higher than the forward reaction rate constant, as seen from (6) and (7). This results in molecules in the reduced state being converted to the oxidized state *i.e.,* oxidation process, leading to a negative current. This is reflected in Fig. 2 where the current is mostly negative when the voltage is positive. As the net voltage goes negative, we have more reduction reactions, where the oxidized state molecules are converted into their reduced states, resulting in a positive current (loss of electron). The applied voltage in CV can be mathematically represented as

$$V(t) = \frac{2v_{Amp}}{\pi} \sin^{-1}(\sin(2\pi f t)) , \tag{8}$$

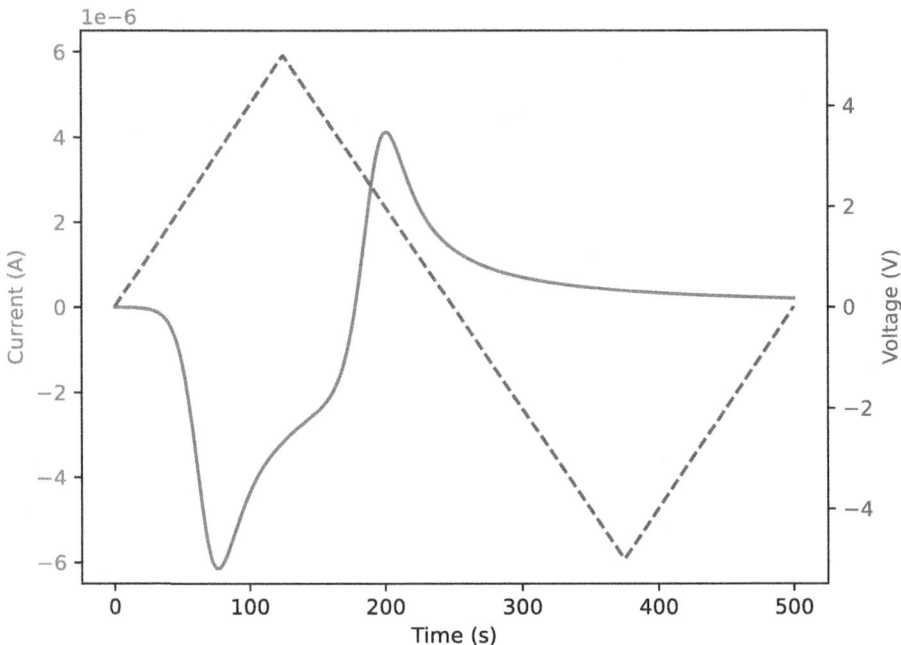

Fig. 2. Current and applied voltage (triangular wave) as functions of time in CV.

where $V(t)$ is a triangular signal with amplitude v_{Amp} and frequency f. The scan/sweep rate v is a parameter in electrochemistry, which translates into the rate of increase/decrease of the voltage at each time sample. With a higher scan rate, the voltage is varied more rapidly and this effectively forces redox reactions to occur faster, as observed from the relation between voltage and reaction rates in (6) and (7). The scan/sweep rate v, in terms of frequency f is expressed as

$$v = 2v_{Amp}f \tag{9}$$

The electrical current measured on probing with the applied voltage is calculated as follows:

$$I(t) = \sum_{m=1}^{M} n_m F Ar[k_{f_m}(t)C'_{m,O}(H,t)\cdots$$
$$\cdots - k_{b_m}(t)C'_{m,R}(H,t)], \tag{10}$$

where $I(t)$ is the total measured output current at time instant t, $C'_{m,S}(H,t)$ is the noise-affected concentration of species m in redox state S, at time instant t at the **Electrode**, n_m is number of electrons transferred for species m, F is the Faraday constant, Ar is the cross section area where reactions occur, $k_{f_m}(t)$ is the forward reaction rate constant of species m at time instant t, and $k_{b_m}(t)$ is the backward reaction rate constant of species m at time instant t.

3   Implementation

In this section, we briefly discuss the implementation of the M2E system model for simulation, followed by the frequency analysis methodology used in this paper to obtain the empirical channel transfer function. Due to the lack of an analytical closed-form solution, we opted to simulate the channel to observe and characterize it. In order to perform the simulation, we initiated the process by transforming the analytical equations provided in Sect. 2 into numerical equations based on finite difference methods. This allowed us to create a computational model of the channel. Building upon this model, we proceeded to develop the simulation framework using MATLAB code. The code implementation used for this paper can be found in the following GitHub repository - https://github.com/xneguvx7/RE-BIONICS-Code. For the implementation of the finite difference method, it is important to define the model sampling space Δx and the model sampling time Δt, as they influence the granularity of the simulation. The model sampling time is chosen on the basis of the sampling time window achievable by the CV setup, while maintaining the balance between simulation accuracy and complexity. The model sampling space is then calculated as follows [3]

$$\Delta x = \sqrt{\frac{\text{Max}(D_O, D_R).\Delta t}{DM}}, \tag{11}$$

where $\text{Max}(.)$ is a function that provides the maximum value among the input arguments, D_O is the diffusion coefficient of redox-active species in the oxidized state, D_R is the diffusion coefficient of redox-active species in the reduced state, Δt is the sampling time of the CV, and DM is the model diffusion coefficient (typically ≤ 0.45 [3]).

3.1   Frequency Analysis Methodology

Before performing a frequency analysis on a channel, it is important to verify its linearity. For a channel to be linear, it should satisfy the superposition principle, which is a combination of the homogeneity property and the additivity property. The M2E communication channel has a molecular input, an electrical current output, and an input probing voltage. While the relation between the input probing voltage and the electrical current output is nonlinear as observed through equations (6), (7), and (10), the relationship between the concentration of redox-active species and the electrical current output is linear, as can be observed in (10). Given a specific redox-active species and an auxiliary applied voltage signal, the output electrical current is proportional to the molecular species concentration at electrode, which in turn is proportional to the input molecular concentration according to Fick's laws of diffusion. As a consequence, the electrical current output signal (and its peaks) is proportional to the molecular concentration input signal.

Another theoretical proof of linearity for this system comes from the Randles-Sevchik equation, which calculates the peak current measured/achieved as a

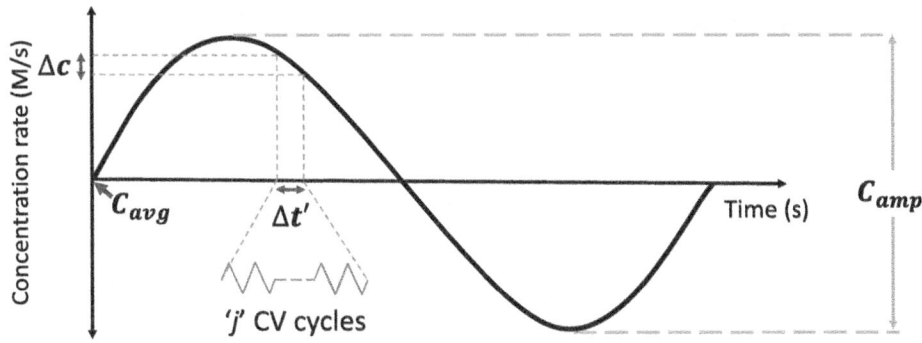

Fig. 3. Input sinusoidal signal.

function of the molecular concentration, diffusion coefficient, scan/sweep rate and other electrochemical-based constants [21]. Although the system has a Poisson-based noise, it can be approximated to Gaussian under specific constraints [8, 16, 19], allowing for channel linearity.

Given the linearity, we used a continuous input signal with varying frequencies to observe the corresponding electrical current measured and estimate the empirical transfer function of the M2E communication channel. Since the system is linear with respect to a molecular concentration input and the electrical current output, it would also be linear with respect to the rate of incoming molecular concentration and the rate of change in the corresponding peak electrical current measured. As such, we use a sinusoidal-based concentration rate signal as the input to be sent through the **Surface** seen in Fig. 1. The input signal as shown in Fig. 3 can be mathematically described as seen below.

$$\Delta C_S(0, t) = C_{avg} + C_{amp} \sin\left(2\pi \frac{1}{\tau j K} t\right), \qquad (12)$$

where $\Delta C_S(0, t)$ is the concentration rate at time t on the **Surface**, C_{avg} is the initial average concentration rate, C_{amp} is the amplitude of the sinusoidal concentration rate signal, τ is the time period of one CV cycle (triangular wave periods), j is the number of CV cycles that are performed within each sample interval $\Delta t'$, and K is the total number of samples across the input signal.

4   Results and Discussion

In this section, we provide the details specific to the simulations implemented, followed by the empirical frequency analysis on the simulated data to observe the channel transfer function and the noise power spectral density as a function of the length of the channel. In the scope of this paper, we use Ferrocene, a standard electrochemical compound [9] as the redox-active chemical species (resulting in $M = 1$ for all the equations in Sect. 2) along with the parameters tabulated

Table 1. Simulation Parameters

Parameter	Value
Oxidized Diffusion co-efficient (D_O)	$3.79 \times 10^{-6} \mathrm{cm}^2/\mathrm{s}$
Reduced Diffusion co-efficient (D_R)	$4.98 \times 10^{-6} \mathrm{cm}^2/\mathrm{s}$
Electrochemical rate constant (k_0)	$1.75 \times 10^{-2} \mathrm{cm}/\mathrm{s}$
Charge transfer co-efficient (α)	0.55
Standard potential (E_0)	0.247V
Electrons transferred per reaction (n)	1
Amplitude of voltage signal (v_{amp})	1V
Voltage scan rate (v $= \frac{2v_{amp}}{\tau}$)	0.01 V/s
Electrode surface area (Ar)	0.0314 cm^2
Model Sampling time (Δt)	0.1 s
Model Sampling space (Δx)	0.0011 cm
Number of Concentration Samples (K)	100
Average Concentration (C_{avg})	500 fM/s
Amplitude (C_{amp})	200 fM/s
Time Period of one CV cycle (τ)	20 s
Frequency $\frac{1}{\tau j K}$ Range	$\left[5e^{-6} - 5e^{-4} \right]$ Hz
Distinct Frequencies (N)	100

*Initial state of Ferrocene is reduced

in Table 1 that contain the species-specific parameters for Ferrocene and the simulation-specific parameters, including those related to the input signal.

To perform frequency analysis, we varied the frequency of the input signal $\frac{1}{\tau j K}$ by varying the number of CV cycles j performed between two consecutive input samples. We then simulated the code implemented 1000 times for each of the 100 distinct frequencies for the range mentioned in Table 1. The amplitude of the channel transfer function is obtained by extracting the average change in amplitude of the main frequency component from the output signal (at a frequency equal to the frequency of the corresponding input signal) for each probed frequency, and by dividing it by the corresponding input concentration rate. This can also be termed as the gain of the M2E communication channel. The noise power is instead obtained by dividing each change of the output signal by the corresponding sample of the input signal, *i.e.*, change in electrical current for a given input concentration rate, and then by computing the variance of the resulting values across all samples. To convert the noise power to the noise power spectral density (PSD), each noise sample is further divided by the corresponding frequency bandwidth. We then went a step further and evaluated the channel transfer function and the noise PSD when varying H, the distance between the **Surface** and the **Electrode** seen in Fig. 1 (length of the channel).

Figure 4 shows the magnitude of the channel transfer function of the M2E communication channel across the frequency range mentioned in Table 1 for dif-

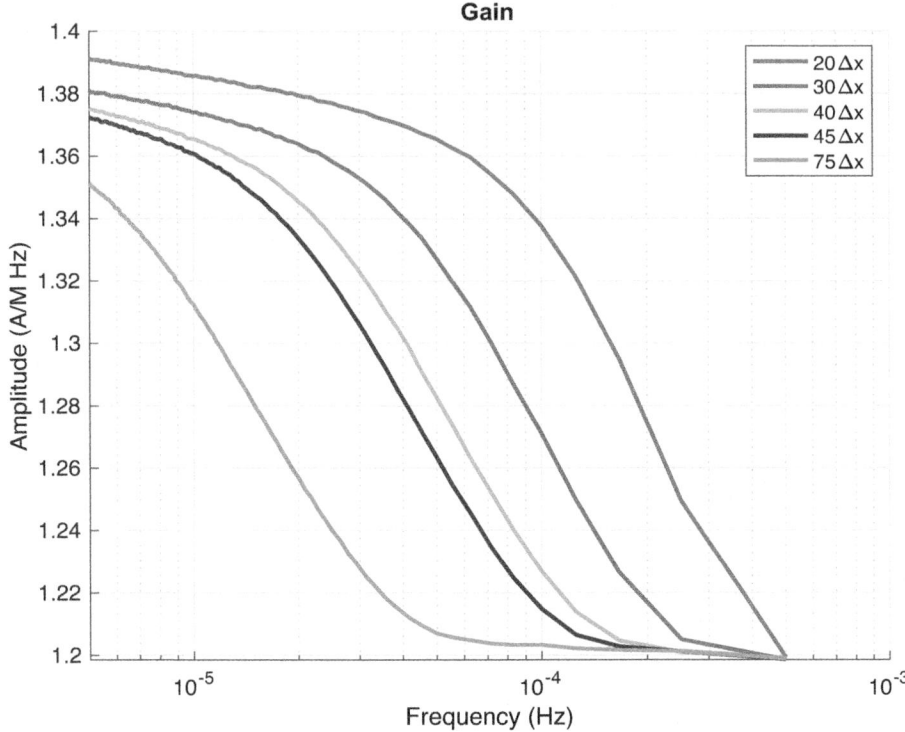

Fig. 4. Magnitude of the channel transfer function across a frequency range for varying channel lengths.

ferent channel lengths, which are described as multiples of the model sampling space Δx. It can be observed that, at a given frequency, as the length increases, the gain decreases. This is due to the fact that as the length increases, it takes longer for the molecules to disperse from the **Surface** to the **Electrode**, thus reducing the gain observed. It can also be noted from the gain plot that the channel behaves similarly to a low-pass filter. Interestingly, the phase obtained from the channel transfer function has been constant at a value of π radians in all scenarios, which needs to be further investigated.

Figure 5 shows the noise power spectral density (PSD) of the M2E communication channel across the frequency range mentioned in Table 1 for varying channel lengths, which are described as multiples of the model sampling space Δx. It can be observed that at a given frequency, as the length increases, the noise power decreases. This is more pronounced at lower frequencies. This is due to the fact that as the length increases, it takes longer for the molecules to disperse from the **Surface** to the **Electrode**, which in turn reduces the number of molecules at the **Electrode**. As the diffusion noise in this paper is a Poisson based on the count of molecules, the noise power correspondingly decreases.

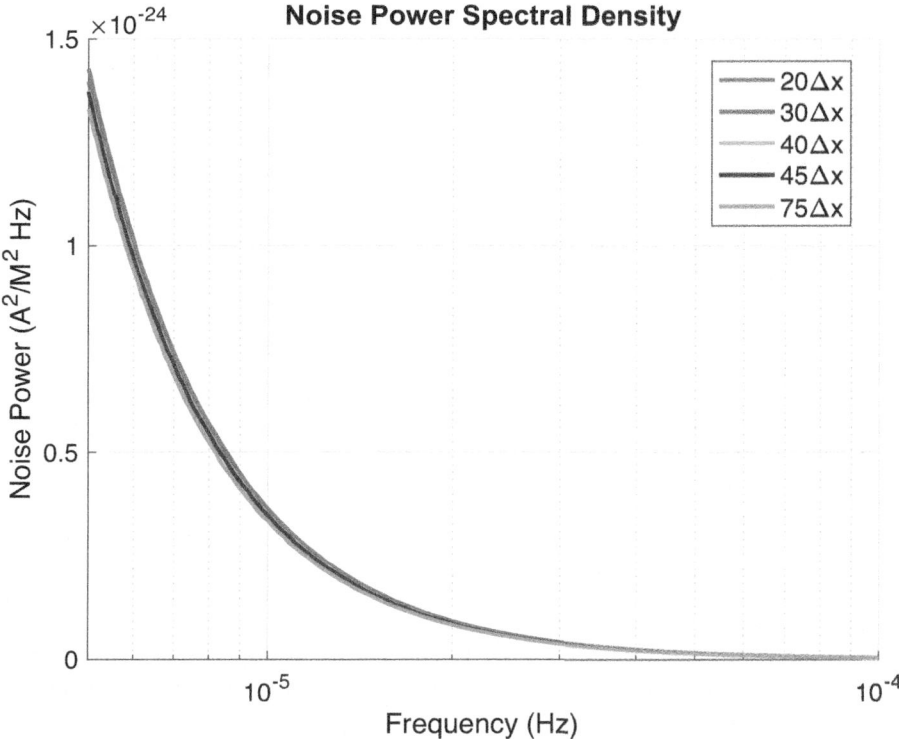

Fig. 5. Noise PSD across a frequency range for varying channel lengths.

5   Conclusion

In this paper, we analyzed a Molecular-Electrical (M2E) communication channel based on redox reactions. With the analytical equations derived from the underlying principles that define the M2E communication channel system model, we provided a simulation framework built in MATLAB and available on a GitHub repository. With the underlying linearity property of the channel, we used a sinusoidal input concentration signal with varying frequencies and performed an empirical frequency analysis. Using the frequency response data obtained from the simulations, we calculated the gain and phase of the channel transfer function and the noise power spectral density of the channel. We then varied the length of the channel in multiples of the model sampling space and observed the behavior of the channel in terms of the transfer function and the noise power spectral density. Though preliminary, this provides an insight into the trade-off between the design parameters and the performance of the system.

Acknowledgements. The authors acknowledge support and experimental setup knowledge from Dr. Gregory F. Payne and Dr. Eunkyoung Kim of Institute for Bioscience and Biotechnology Research (IBBR), University of Maryland.

References

1. Akyildiz, I., Pierobon, M., Balasubramaniam, S., Koucheryavy, Y.: The internet of Bio-Nano things. IEEE Commun. Mag. **53**(3), 32–40 (2015). https://doi.org/10.1109/MCOM.2015.7060516, http://ieeexplore.ieee.org/document/7060516/

2. Akyildiz, I.F., Pierobon, M., Balasubramaniam, S.: Moving forward with molecular communication: from theory to human health applications (2019). https://doi.org/10.1109/JPROC.2019.2913890

3. Bard, A.J., Faulkner, L.R.: Electrochemical Methods: Fundamentals and Applications. Wiley, Hoboken (2001)

4. Brand, L., et al.: Media modulation based molecular communication. IEEE Trans. Commun. **70**(11), 7207–7223 (2022). https://doi.org/10.1109/TCOMM.2022.3205949

5. Elgrishi, N., Rountree, K.J., McCarthy, B.D., Rountree, E.S., Eisenhart, T.T., Dempsey, J.L.: A practical beginner's guide to cyclic voltammetry. J. Chem. Educ. **95**(2), 197–206 (2018). https://doi.org/10.1021/acs.jchemed.7b00361

6. Farsad, N., Yilmaz, H.B., Eckford, A., Chae, C.B., Guo, W.: A comprehensive survey of recent advancements in molecular communication. IEEE Commun. Surv. Tutorials **18**(3), 1887–1919 (2016). https://doi.org/10.1109/COMST.2016.2527741

7. Fick, A.: On liquid diffusion. J. Membr. Sci. **100**(1), 33–38 (1995). https://doi.org/10.1016/0376-7388(94)00230-V, https://www.sciencedirect.com/science/article/pii/037673889400230V

8. Florence, K.A., et al.: Analytical challenges when sampling and characterising exhaled aerosol. Aerosol Sci. Technol. **56**(2), 160–175 (2022). https://doi.org/10.1080/02786826.2021.1990207

9. Gagne, R.R., Koval, C.A., Lisensky, G.C.: Ferrocene as an internal standard for electrochemical measurements. Inorg. Chem. **19**(9), 2854–2855 (1980). https://doi.org/10.1021/IC50211A080/ASSET/IC50211A080.FP.PNG_V03, https://pubs.acs.org/doi/abs/10.1021/ic50211a080

10. Gorla, K.R., Barker, T., Pierobon, M.: Modeling diffusion and chemical reactions to analyze redox-based molecular-electrical communication. In: ICC 2020 - 2020 IEEE International Conference on Communications (ICC), pp. 1–7 (2020). https://doi.org/10.1109/ICC40277.2020.9148750

11. Gorla, K.R., Pierobon, M.: A mutual information estimate for a redox-based molecular-electrical communication channel. In: Proceedings of the Eight Annual ACM International Conference on Nanoscale Computing and Communication. NANOCOM 2021, Association for Computing Machinery, New York (2021). https://doi.org/10.1145/3477206.3477474

12. Gorla, K.R., Pierobon, M.: Frequency analysis of a redox-based molecular-electrical communication channel. In: Proceedings of the 10th ACM International Conference on Nanoscale Computing and Communication, pp. 21–26. NANOCOM 2023, Association for Computing Machinery, New York (2023). https://doi.org/10.1145/3576781.3608724

13. Kim, E., et al.: Redox is a global biodevice information processing modality. Proc. IEEE **107**(7), 1402–1424 (2019). https://doi.org/10.1109/JPROC.2019.2908582

14. Liu, Y., et al.: Redox-enabled bio-electronics for information acquisition and transmission. IEEE Trans. Mol. Biol. Multi-Scale Commun. **9**(2), 146–166 (2023). https://doi.org/10.1109/TMBMC.2023.3274112

15. Liu, Y., et al.: Using a redox modality to connect synthetic biology to electronics: hydrogel-based chemo-electro signal transduction for molecular communica-

tion. Adv. Healthc. Mater. **6**(1), 1600908 (2017). https://doi.org/10.1002/adhm.201600908

16. Marcone, A., Pierobon, M., Magarini, M.: The Gaussian approximation in soft detection for molecular communication via biological circuits. In: 2017 IEEE 18th International Workshop on Signal Processing Advances in Wireless Communications (SPAWC), pp. 1–6 (2017). https://doi.org/10.1109/SPAWC.2017.8227764

17. Nariman, F., Guo, W., Eckford, A.W.: Tabletop molecular communication: text messages through chemical signals. PLOS ONE **8**(12), 1–13 (2013). https://doi.org/10.1371/journal.pone.0082935

18. Pierobon, M., Akyildiz, I.F.: Diffusion-based noise analysis for molecular communication in nanonetworks. IEEE Trans. Signal Process. **59**(6), 2532–2547 (2011). https://doi.org/10.1109/TSP.2011.2114656

19. Thomas, P., Spencer, D., Hampton, S., Park, P., Zurkus, J.: The diffusion-limited biochemical signal-relay channel. In: Thrun, S., Saul, L., Schölkopf, B. (eds.) Advances in Neural Information Processing Systems, vol. 16. MIT Press (2003)

20. VanArsdale, E., Pitzer, J., Payne, G.F., Bentley, W.E.: Redox electrochemistry to interrogate and control biomolecular communication. iScience **23**(9), 101545 (2020). https://doi.org/10.1016/j.isci.2020.101545, https://www.sciencedirect.com/science/article/pii/S2589004220307379

21. Zoski, C.G.: Handbook of Electrochemistry. Elsevier, Amsterdam (2007)

Real-Time and on-the-Edge Multiple Channel Capacitive and Inertial Fusion-Based Glove

Hymalai Bello[1,2]([✉]), Sungho Suh[1,2], Daniel Geißler[1], Lala Ray[1], Bo Zhou[1,2], and Paul Lukowicz[1,2]

[1] German Research Center for Artificial Intelligence (DFKI),
Kaiserslautern, Germany
[2] RPTU Kaiserslautern-Landau, Kaiserslautern, Germany
hymalai.bello@dfki.de

Abstract. Human-robot interaction (HRI) has become increasingly ubiquitous and pervasive, with hand gestures serving as a common means of communication between humans and robots. We present a glove-based wearable solution for classifying hand gestures. It is specifically designed for drone control applications. Our solution is a textile-based, low-power consumption (≤ 1.15 W), privacy-conscious, real-time, and on-the-Edge alternative, ensuring user comfort and data security. With a tiny memory footprint (≤ 2 MB), the proposed approach provides an efficient and sustainable approach to hand gesture recognition. To achieve high accuracy while maintaining low power consumption, we adopt a hierarchical lightweight neural network scheme. This fusion technique not only reduces energy consumption but also improves the overall performance of the system. During the offline evaluation of nine classes, including eight hand gestures and the null class, our system achieves an F1 score of 80%. In real-time and on-the-edge evaluation with one user, our wearable solution yields an F1 score of 67%, further highlighting its practicality and effectiveness in real-world scenarios.

Keywords: Real-time on-the-edge · TinyML · Capacitive Sensing · Gesture Recognition · Wearable Textile

1 Introduction

Designing interfaces to optimize user and robot interaction is the goal of human-robot interaction (HRI). The adoption of HRI in smart factories has led to improved efficiency and improved safety measures [6]. This integration also empowers workers through the implementation of human-centered artificial intelligence [16]. A specific application of HRI that has revolutionized smart factories is drone control. Drones are now extensively employed in various manufacturing processes, serving as infrastructure managers, ensuring rapid communication

M. Mizmizi et al. (Eds.): BodyNets 2024, LNICST 524, pp. 166–176, 2024.
https://doi.org/10.1007/978-3-031-72524-1_13

on construction sites, enhancing safety in hazardous workplaces, and providing real-time monitoring of production using sensors and cameras [21]. The use of drones in manufacturing has the potential to transform the industry, making it safer and more efficient [12].

Although camera-based solutions provide the most accurate option for drone operation [14,15,17,22,23], concerns over workers' privacy and technology protection in industrial environments have become paramount. In this context, alternative solutions that can provide good performance without the risk of technology leakage are highly encouraged. Non-camera-based wearables offer a convenient option for a privacy-aware and low-power robot control mechanism. An ideal wearable should be flexible and comfortable to ensure minimal disruption to the worker's schedule while maximizing efficiency.

To address these challenges, in this paper, we propose a real-time on-the-edge solution for drone control, leveraging textile-based sensing. The proposed approach offers flexibility, low power consumption, and cost-effectiveness, and holds potential applications in sign language, gaming, and robot control. We adopt lightweight neural network models to ensure a low memory footprint, resulting in an embedded and sustainable solution.

In this context, we introduce a glove-based textile solution for HRI, which holds particular significance within the wearable community [5]. Gloves, commonly used as protective equipment in various industries, offer unparalleled flexibility and dexterity, enabling the generation of various control patterns using fingers and wrist movements. Integration of textile sensors into gloves provides additional advantages, including softness, comfort, lightness, and air permeability. As a result, the glove-based textile solution presents a convenient wearable option for HRI applications.

The main contributions of our approach can be summarized as follows:

- We present a real-time on-the-edge solution for drone control that utilizes textile-based sensing, providing flexibility, low power consumption, and cost-effectiveness, with potential applications in sign language, gaming, and robot control.
- We employ lightweight neural network models to ensure a low memory footprint, providing an embedded and sustainable solution.
- We propose a hierarchical multimodal fusion to reduce power consumption and increase robustness against the null class, where the first stage detects movements and recognizes a non-null hand gesture using an inertial-based model. Then, using a capacitive-based model, the second stage classifies the dictionary shown in Fig. 1.
- Experimental results demonstrate that our approach is a step towards a wearable, textile, and privacy-friendly alternative for hand gesture recognition.

The paper is organized as follows; Sect. 2 presents a review of textile glove solutions for drone control. Section 3 provides detailed information on the hardware prototype. Section 4 introduces the details of the proposed multimodal fusion for hand gesture recognition, and Sect. 5 presents the experimental results

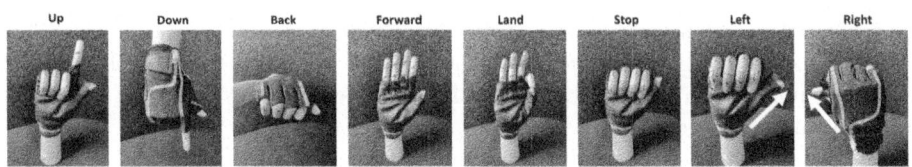

Fig. 1. Hand Gestures Dictionary for Drone Control [9]

and discussion. Finally, Sect. 6 concludes the article, highlighting potential future directions for this research.

2   Related Work

In this section, we focus on textile-based solutions for drone control. We can find several textile-based sensing modalities on gloves for drone control in the literature. Researchers have employed various sensing technologies, including textile pressure sensors, triboelectric nanogenerators (TENG), flexible capacitive pressure sensors, piezoresistive, and conductive fiber-based textile pressure sensors, among others [1,10,18,20]. A common practice among state-of-the-art textile wearable glove alternatives is to use different and limited gesture dictionaries compared to camera-based solutions, which mainly include going forward/backward and going to the left/right classes. For the capacitive or textile pressure sensor options, the textile is used as a soft push button, where each textile patch is an on/off instruction. Textile as binary actuators (push buttons) is a simple and effective way of HRI. However, it lacks robustness against the null class, and the number of control instructions is limited to the number of textile patches. This is an issue if the drone/robot requires performing more sophisticated tasks [8]. For example, in [10], the patches are placed on the fingertips, leading to the incorrect recognition of null activities, such as checking a smartphone, typing on a keyboard, or touching/grabbing tools, as control instructions for the drone/robot. In [1], the authors employed a capacitive textile sensor on the back of the palm of the right/left hand, and with the other left/right hand, the user touched the patches to generate the control signal for the drone. However, this solution does not account for the potential extension of gestures by including both hands in the pipeline. In [18], the authors used TENG to fabricate a sensing glove for gesture recognition, including sign language and drone control applications. However, their focus was mainly on introducing the technology and its futuristic applications, thus neglecting null activities and lacking information about user experimental evaluations.

To overcome these limitations, we introduce a capacitive and inertial fusion-based glove design for real-time on-the-edge hand gesture recognition. Our design incorporates textile capacitive electrodes as sensing channels on the fingers and an IMU sensor on the wrist. Textile capacitive sensing has demonstrated its effectiveness as a low-power consumption, cost-effective, and scalable technology for movement tracking in gesture and activity recognition [3,4,24]. Furthermore,

IMU sensors have been widely used to monitor wrist movements by researchers [7,11,19]. Our approach is an alternative solution for hand gesture recognition that addresses critical requirements, including minimal invasiveness, low power consumption, privacy preservation, flexibility, and scalability. While our focus is mainly on a gesture dictionary related to drone control, the same concept can be extended to hand-based HRI in various domains. The gesture dictionary is depicted in Fig. 1, which aligns with the gestures used in a camera-based solution [9], using MediaPipe for real-time recognition. The gesture majority are dominant by finger patterns.

3   Apparatus

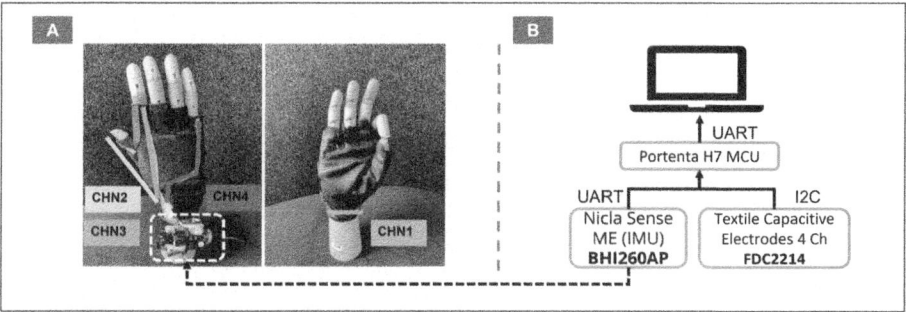

Fig. 2. (A) The Hardware Prototype Shows the Capacitive Channels and IMU Positions on the Sports Glove. **(B)** Depicts The Hardware Block Diagram with the Sensors Connections to the Main Board (Portenta H7) and PC.

Figure 2**A** presents the prototype showing the IMU and the capacitive channels (textile electrodes) on a sports glove. The hardware block diagram is in Fig. 2**B**. To monitor finger movements, we proposed to use textile conductive thin patches as capacitive channels. Moreover, the IMU-selected placement is on the wrist. This approach reduces the number of connections, and flexibility and comfort are considered. Noticeably, our glove does not cover the entire area of the fingers, minimally affecting the user's mobility.

The hardware has three blocks; a main board, an inertial and environmental sensing board, and a capacitive sensing board see Fig. 2**B**. The main board is a Portenta H7; the main processor is the dual-core STM32H747, including a Cortex M7 running at 480 MHz and a Cortex M4 running at 240 MHz. Portenta H7 offers 2 MB flash and 8 MB SDRAM and wireless data transmission options such as WiFi, Bluetooth classic, and BLE. The inertial board is a Nicla Sense with a 64 MHz ArmCortex M4 (nRF52832) and sensors such as; IMU, air pressure, humidity, temperature, and gas. The capacitive board is based on the state-of-the-art capacitance to digital converter FDC2214 with four channels. Four capacitive channels are distributed on the glove; channel one on the wrist, channel two on the thumb, channel three on the index finger, and channel four on

Table 1. Apparatus Component Highlights

Component	Benefits
Portenta H7	• Dual Core STM32H747 • Graphics Accelerator • 2 MB Flash, 8 MB SDRAM • WiFi/BT Module • NXP SE050C2 Crypto
Nicla Sense ME	• BHI260AP IMU • BMP390 and BME680, Pressure, Humidity, Temperature, and Gas • AI self-learning sensor
FDC2214	• 4 Channels 28-Bit Capacitance to Digital Converter • Single or Differential Mode • Proximity Detection • Liquids Sensing (Detergent, Soap, Ink) • Collision Avoidance • Rain, Fog, Ice, Snow Sensor
Textile Electrodes	• Shieldex Technik-tex P130+B • Knit type: Stretch-Tricot • Resistivity $\leq 2\Omega$ • Nitrile Rubber Protective Coating • Double Stretch Direction • Temperature Range of -30 to $90°C$

the little finger. The capacitive channels are textile electrodes based on Shieldex Technik-tex P130+B. The dimensions of the electrodes are 0.55 mm in thickness and between 11–15 cm long. The FDC2214 offers single-end and differential sensing modes. We use single-end mode to reduce the number of capacitive patches on the glove. Furthermore, the FDC2214 is configured using an external inductor of 18 uH and a capacitor of 33 pf to operate with an average frequency of 13.7 Mhz [24]. The sampling rate for the sensors is around 50 Hz. The highlights of our prototype are in Table 1.

4   Multimodal Sensor Fusion

As shown in Fig. 3, two collaborative models were deployed for the real-time and on-the-Edge (RTE) recognition of the gestures in Fig. 1. A pre-normalization $((x - x_{min})/(x_{max} - x_{min}))$ per window is applied to the inertial and capacitive signals. The window size is 2 s, and the window's step is 0.5 s. The first neural network model (NN) is the inertial model with three channels as input (linear acceleration). This model is used to distinguish the null class from gesture detection. The null class includes activities such as; walking and standing/sitting down, among others. The output of the acceleration model served as a trigger for the second model, the capacitive model. If an activity is classified as non-null, the capacitive model is activated. The second model fused the four capacitive channels as four independent input channels. The outputs of the capacitive model are the eight classes defined in the dictionary in Fig. 1 plus the null class (total of nine categories). The hierarchical approach reduces the complexity of the models, leveraging the information fusion with lightweight NNs (0.10–1.23 MB) to be deployed in tiny MCUs. The intermediate tensor space (Arena) is 16.66 KB for the inertial model and 130.56 KB for the capacitive model.

The Inertial Model: The NN structure comprises three convolutional layers (filters = 10, kernel = 10, ReLu). For each convolutional layer, batch normalization, max-pooling ((5,1)), and dropout (0.5) are applied. Then it is followed by a flattening layer, a fully connected (FC) layer of 10, and an FC with softmax and two outputs. The training ran for 100 epochs with early stopping (patience 30 and restoring weights). The number of parameters of the inertial model is 2882; thus, it is a lightweight design and less susceptible to overfitting.

The Capacitive Model: The NN structure comprises two convolutional layers (filters = 40, kernel = 10, ReLu). A normalization layer follows the first convolutional layers. For each convolutional layer, batch normalization, max-pooling ((5,1)), and dropout (0.3) are applied. Then it is followed by a flattening layer, a fully connected (FC) layer of 100, and an FC with softmax and nine outputs (gesture dictionary Fig. 1 + null class). The training ran for 200 epochs with early stopping (patience 30 and restoring weights). The number of parameters of the capacitive model is 49890; thus, it is a lightweight design and less susceptible to overfitting compared to a small network such as MobileNetV2 with 3.5 Million parameters.

For both models (inertial and capacitive), the NN optimizer is AdaDelta, with a learning rate of 0.9 and categorical cross-entropy as a loss function. The metric to monitor during training is accuracy. The NN models were trained using the TensorFlow/Keras 2.12.0 framework.

Real-Time and on-the-Edge (RTE): TensorFlow Lite for MCU was used to generate the embedded version of the NN models. For RTE recognition, a sliding window scheme is employed. A sliding window of 2 s (100 samples) with

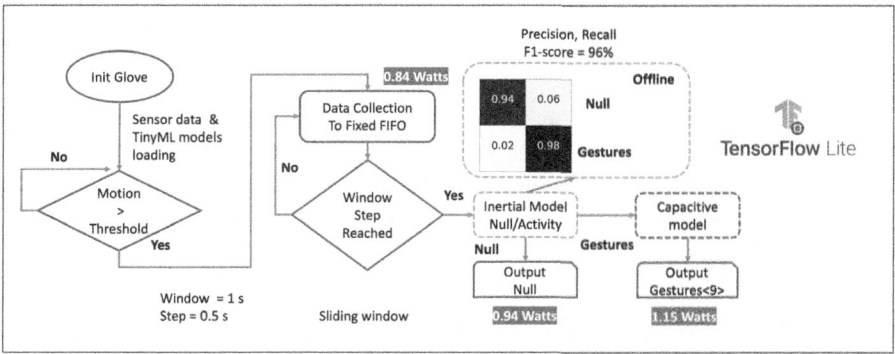

Fig. 3. Real-Time and on-the-Edge Implementation for Hand Gesture Recognition

a step size of 0.5 s is used as an input data frame to the NNs. The Fig. 3 depicts the real-time on-the-edge procedure. The first step consists of movement detection (using acceleration), reducing power consumption by 10%. The movement detection is based on a threshold condition ruled by $\Sigma_{n=0}^{5} = |a_x|_n + |a_y|_n + |a_z|_n$. Then, the inertial model will run and detect null or gesture cases. In the case of $activity \neq Null$, the capacitive model will output the recognized drone control gesture in Fig. 1. The power consumption (PC) when only the movement detection is activated (only sensor data acquisition) is 0.84 W. Then, if a movement is detected, the inertial model is triggered, and the PC increases by 0.10 W (0.94 W). If the inertial model detects a gesture, the capacitive model runs, and the PC increases to 1.15 W. Hence, the NN model PC adds 0.31 W to the system pipeline.[1]. For the real-time and on-the-Edge assessment, one volunteer performed five sessions with five repetitions of each gesture from our dictionary.

5   Results and Discussion

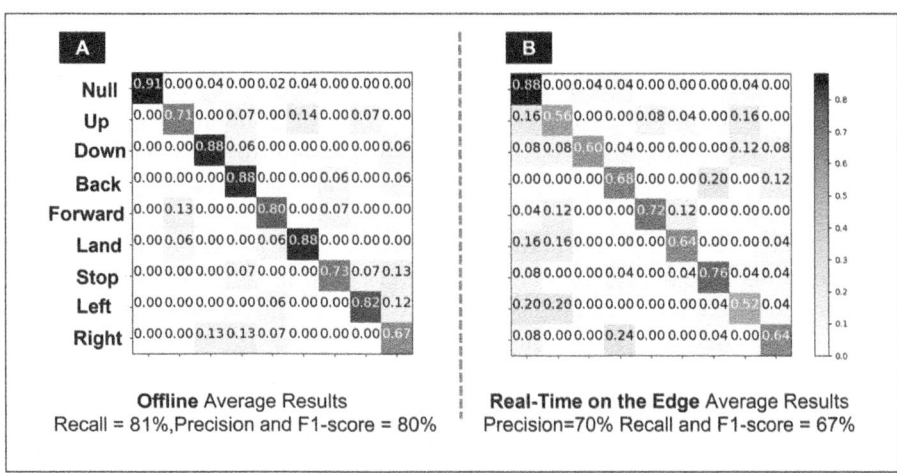

Fig. 4. Results of the offline Capacitive Model; Null(0), Up(1), Down(2), Back(3), Forward(4), Land(5), Stop(6), Left(7), Right(8) and F1-score = 80%(**A**). Real-Time on the Edge Results of Capacitive Model; F1-score = 67%(**B**)

Results: Figure 4 shows the offline results (10-fold cross-validation) for the collaborative approach; inertial model (Null vs. Activity) in Fig. 3 with F1-score = 96% and capacitive model (gesture dictionary) with an F1-score = 80% in Fig. 4**A**. For the training data (offline results), one volunteer (female) participated in mimicking (randomly ten sessions) the gesture dictionary in Fig. 1 while

---

[1] USB Digital Power Meter: https://www.az-delivery.de/en/products/charger-doktor DLA: December 13, 2024.

wearing the system. The sessions were recorded on different days to ensure our device was worn repeatedly. The offline evaluation scheme was 10-fold cross-validation with a leaving-one-session-out. Each session has four random tries per gesture.[2]

In Fig. 4**A** and in Fig. 4**B**, the confusion matrices for offline and online recognition are presented. In the offline results, we can observe confusion between the gestures, Up and Land (14%) and Forward and Up (13%); both pairs mainly differentiate by how the finger's upper parts move. The sports glove we employed does not cover the finger's upper parts to allow flexibility/comfort for the user. There is also confusion for the case of the pairs; Stop and Right (13%), Right and Down (13%), Right and Back(13%), and Left and Right (12%). All these pairs have in common that the fist is closed, and their main difference is how the thumb and the index finger move. For specific applications such as sign language gesture recognition, the glove can be extended to cover the fingers completely to reduce confusion. For applications where the finger flexibility/freedom does not want to be reduced, we proposed as a future work that the inertial data (including orientation) could be fused with the capacitive information to add the wrist position in space (earth navigation frame). As an example of such applications, in an industrial environment, when the worker is focusing on order and picking or assembling tasks, the worker can benefit from the help of a drone/robot to ease the workflow but still needs to handle tools comfortably. These future solutions will positively impact the online results presented in Fig. 4**B**. The real-time on-the-edge results (5 sessions, re-wearing, one volunteer) in Fig. 4**B** gave an F1-score = 67%. There was a reduction of 13% in the F1-score between the offline and the embedded solution. Noticeably, the RTE confusion matrix in Fig. 4**B** is based on cross-validation, shuffled, and without temporal smoothing between adjacent windows, which could improve the results in the future, as shown in Fig. 5.

Ground Truth → 0 0 1 1 1 1 1 1 1 0 0   **Prediction →** 0 0 1 1 0 1 3 1 1 0 0   **After Smoothing →** 0 0 1 1 1 1 1 1 1 0 0

Fig. 5. Example of Smoothing Temporal Windows for Continuous Recognition [13]

Discussion: Our system combines inertial and capacitive sensing modalities to recognize hand gestures used for drone control using a sports glove. The inertial information is employed as a movement detector (using a threshold). Later, using an inertial model, the inertial information is used again to recognize between null and gestures from the dictionary in Fig. 1. Then the inertial model triggers the gesture recognition with the capacitive information (nine classes). This is similar to the approaches applied in [4] and in [2], where the Radio Frequency Identification (RFID) signal is used as a trigger to begin gesture

---

[2] The participant signed an agreement following the policies of the university's committee for protecting human subjects and following the Declaration of Helsinki.

detection, reducing power consumption and model complexity while improving accuracy. The set of gestures is not very intuitive. The selected dictionary comes from [9]. And it could be improved to suit the target. We aimed to have a fair comparison between a real-time camera-based solution and our proposed method.

It is important to note that our system was tested for one participant. Thus, more participants are still required to make it generalizable. The solid hardware components (MCUs and IMU) position was limited to the wrist to reduce the negative impact on the user's movements. The capacitive electrodes used are stretchable and soft. We selected a sports glove that does not cover the entire fingers to maintain the user's mobility. The hierarchical fusion of the inertial and capacitive information impacts the power consumption reduction by about 27%. The fusion method also helps reduce model complexity and parameters to obtain lightweight neural networks to be deployed in embedded devices. Our approach is a step toward a textile, flexible, embedded solution for drone control. The main idea can be extended to other hand gesture-controlled applications where comfort, power consumption, and privacy are desirable.

On the other hand, our design has several limitations and possibilities for improvement. The hardware prototype can be reduced in size by doing a professional encapsulated electronic design. The latency of the recognition in real-time is not optimized. The main board offers two MCUs that can work in parallel, but in our design, we allocate the entire flash (2 MB) to the Cortex M7 core of the STM32H747, and the code is running only on the M7 at 480 MHz. The latency could be improved by using the M7 to run the neural network models and the Cortex M4 (at 240 MHz) for the sensor acquisition data. Special attention must be given to memory access to avoid collisions and bottlenecks. Additionally, our work transmits the recognition results to the PC using a universal asynchronous receiver/transmitter (UART) to focus on proving the idea. The main board can be configured to send the recognition results by wireless communication (Bluetooth or Wifi) to improve comfort and make the system ubiquitous. The Bluetooth/Wifi will require an external antenna and memory allocation for the wireless communication managing functions. For the case of the RTE results, the confusion matrix is calculated based on shuffled cross-validation over fine-granular windows, which does not consider continuous sequences of windows of a single gesture where the majority of windows are true positive with sparse false detection. Our result could be improved by merging temporal windows from simple gap filling and event-based smoothing to selective merging based on CNN [13]. Although temporal window smoothing techniques have been demonstrated in offline evaluations where the computation is performed on the PC, edge adaptation with resource-constrained embedded hardware is a task we will investigate in future work.

The power consumption reported in this work includes the complete pipeline. The pipeline comprehends sensor powering and data acquisition up to the RTE. For the worst-case power consumption, only 27% (0.31 W) is required for the real-time inference. Hence, the power consumption could be further reduced with techniques, such as lowering the data sampling rate and setting the sensors in sleep mode. In addition, the NNs can be pruned and trained with aware quantization to reduce size with minimal impact on the performance.

6 Conclusion

In this work, we have presented a glove-based design that provides a minimally obtrusive, low-power, privacy-friendly, flexible, and scalable solution for hand gesture recognition. By combining textile capacitive electrodes and inertial sensors, our system achieves real-time on-the-edge recognition of hand gestures for drone control.

A key contribution of our approach lies in the hierarchical fusion of inertial and capacitive information, which significantly reduces power requirements and enables the deployment of tiny memory models suitable for on-the-edge devices. This fusion technique improves the system's efficiency and performance, making it well-suited for practical applications.

Beyond drone control, our glove-based design holds great potential for various control-related applications, such as game control and assisting robot control in industrial settings. Moreover, its privacy-friendly nature and wearable form factor open up possibilities for broader adoption in human-robot interaction scenarios, sign language recognition, and gaming interfaces.

Acknowledgements. The research reported in this paper was partially supported by the German Federal Ministry of Education and Research (BMBF) in the projects SocialWear under grant agreement number 01IW20002 and by the European Union's Horizon 2020 program projects STAR under grant agreement number H2020-956573.

References

1. Agcayazi, T., Tabor, J., McKnight, M., Martin, I., Ghosh, T.K., Bozkurt, A.: Fully-textile seam-line sensors for facile textile integration and tunable multi-modal sensing of pressure, humidity, and wetness. Adv. Mater. Technol. **5**(8), 2000155 (2020)
2. Bello, H., Rodriguez, J., Lukowicz, P.: Vertical hand position estimation with wearable differential barometery supported by RFID synchronization. In: Mucchi, L., Hämäläinen, M., Jayousi, S., Morosi, S. (eds.) BODYNETS 2019. LNICST, vol. 297, pp. 24–33. Springer, Cham (2019). https://doi.org/10.1007/978-3-030-34833-5_3
3. Bello, H., Zhou, B., Suh, S., Lukowicz, P.: Mocapaci: posture and gesture detection in loose garments using textile cables as capacitive antennas. In: 2021 International Symposium on Wearable Computers, pp. 78–83 (2021)
4. Bello, H., Zhou, B., Suh, S., Sanchez Marin, L.A., Lukowicz, P.: Move with the theremin: body posture and gesture recognition using the theremin in loose-garment with embedded textile cables as antennas. Front. Comput. Sci. **4** (2022)
5. DelPreto, J., Hughes, J., D'Aria, M., de Fazio, M., Rus, D.: A wearable smart glove and its application of pose and gesture detection to sign language classification. IEEE Robot. Autom. Lett. **7**(4), 10589–10596 (2022)

6. Hentout, A., Aouache, M., Maoudj, A., Akli, I.: Human-robot interaction in industrial collaborative robotics: a literature review of the decade 2008–2017. Adv. Robot. **33**(15–16), 764–799 (2019)
7. Jiang, S., et al.: Feasibility of wrist-worn, real-time hand, and surface gesture recognition via sEMG and IMU sensing. IEEE Trans. Industr. Inf. **14**(8), 3376–3385 (2017)
8. Kangunde, V., Jamisola, R.S., Theophilus, E.K.: A review on drones controlled in real-time. Int. J. Dyn. Control, 1–15 (2021)
9. Kiselov, N.: Drone control via gestures using mediapipe hands (2021). https://developers.googleblog.com/2021/09/drone-control-via-gestures-using-mediapipe-hands.html
10. Lee, J.: Conductive fiber-based ultrasensitive textile pressure sensor for wearable electronics. Adv. Mater. **27**(15), 2433–2439 (2015)
11. Ma, Y., et al.: Hand gesture recognition with convolutional neural networks for the multimodal UAV control. In: 2017 Workshop on Research, Education and Development of Unmanned Aerial Systems (RED-UAS), pp. 198–203. IEEE (2017)
12. Maghazei, O., Netland, T.: Drones in manufacturing: exploring opportunities for research and practice. J. Manuf. Technol. Manag. **31**(6), 1237–1259 (2020)
13. Narayana, P., Beveridge, J.R., Draper, B.A.: Continuous gesture recognition through selective temporal fusion. In: 2019 International Joint Conference on Neural Networks (IJCNN), pp. 1–8. IEEE (2019)
14. Naseer, F., Ullah, G., Siddiqui, M.A., Khan, M.J., Hong, K.S., Naseer, N.: Deep learning-based unmanned aerial vehicle control with hand gesture and computer vision. In: 2022 13th Asian Control Conference (ASCC), pp. 1–6. IEEE (2022)
15. Natarajan, K., Nguyen, T.H.D., Mete, M.: Hand gesture controlled drones: an open source library. In: 2018 1st International Conference on Data Intelligence and Security (ICDIS), pp. 168–175. IEEE (2018)
16. Panagou, S., Neumann, W.P., Fruggiero, F.: A scoping review of human robot interaction research towards industry 5.0 human-centric workplaces. Int. J. Prod. Res. 1–17 (2023)
17. Patrona, F., Mademlis, I., Pitas, I.: An overview of hand gesture languages for autonomous UAV handling. In: 2021 Aerial Robotic Systems Physically Interacting with the Environment (AIRPHARO), pp. 1–7 (2021)
18. Shen, S., Xiao, X., Yin, J., Xiao, X., Chen, J.: Self-powered smart gloves based on triboelectric nanogenerators. Small Methods **6**(10), 2200830 (2022)
19. Siddiqui, N., Chan, R.H.: Multimodal hand gesture recognition using single IMU and acoustic measurements at wrist. PLoS ONE **15**(1), e0227039 (2020)
20. Su, M., Li, P., Liu, X., Wei, D., Yang, J.: Textile-based flexible capacitive pressure sensors: a review. Nanomaterials **12**(9), 1495 (2022)
21. Tosato, P., Facinelli, D., Prada, M., Gemma, L., Rossi, M., Brunelli, D.: An autonomous swarm of drones for industrial gas sensing applications. In: 2019 IEEE 20th International Symposium on "A World of Wireless, Mobile and Multimedia Networks" (WoWMoM), pp. 1–6. IEEE (2019)
22. Yoo, M., et al.: Motion estimation and hand gesture recognition-based human-UAV interaction approach in real time. Sensors **22**(7), 2513 (2022)
23. Yu, Y., Wang, X., Zhong, Z., Zhang, Y.: Ros-based UAV control using hand gesture recognition. In: 2017 29th Chinese Control And Decision Conference (CCDC), pp. 6795–6799. IEEE (2017)
24. Zhou, B., et al.: Mocapose: motion capturing with textile-integrated capacitive sensors in loose-fitting smart garments. In: Proceedings of the ACM on Interactive, Mobile, Wearable and Ubiquitous Technologies, vol. 7, no. 1, pp. 1–40 (2023)

Climbing Routes Clustering Using Energy-Efficient Accelerometers Attached to the Quickdraws

Sadaf Moaveninejad[1]([✉])[iD], Andrea Janes[2][iD], Camillo Porcaro[1][iD],
Luca Barletta[3][iD], Lorenzo Mucchi[4][iD], and Massimiliano Pierobon[5][iD]

[1] Department of Neuroscience and Padova Neuroscience Center,
University of Padova, Padova, Italy
{sadaf.moaveninejad,camillo.porcaro}@unipd.it
[2] FHV Vorarlberg University of Applied Sciences, Dornbirn, Austria
andrea.janes@fhv.at
[3] Department of Electronics, Information and Bioengineering,
Politecnico di Milano, Milan, Italy
luca.barletta@polimi.it
[4] Department of Information Engineering, University of Florence, Firenze, Italy
lorenzo.mucchi@unifi.it
[5] School of Computing, University of Nebraska-Lincoln, Lincoln, NE, USA
maxp@unl.edu

Abstract. One of the challenges for climbing gyms is to find out popular routes for the climbers to improve their services and optimally use their infrastructure. This problem must be addressed preserving both the privacy and convenience of the climbers and the costs of the gyms. To this aim, a hardware prototype is developed to collect data using accelerometer sensors attached to a piece of climbing equipment mounted on the wall, called quickdraw, that connects the climbing rope to the bolt anchors. The corresponding sensors are configured to be energy-efficient, hence becoming practical in terms of expenses and time consumption for replacement when used in large quantities in a climbing gym. This paper describes hardware specifications, studies data measured by the sensors in ultra-low power mode, detect patterns in data during climbing different routes, and develops an unsupervised approach for route clustering.

Keywords: Machine Learning · Artificial Intelligence · Internet of Things

1 Introduction

In the past two decades, sport climbing has become a highly popular sport [5]. Sport climbing refers to a form of climbing in which climbers use routes with prepared anchor points that prevent a climber from a ground fall. In this way, the

M. Mizmizi et al. (Eds.): BodyNets 2024, LNICST 524, pp. 177–193, 2024.
https://doi.org/10.1007/978-3-031-72524-1_14

challenge lies more in the mastery of the climbing route and less in maintaining safety.

In this paper, when talking about sport climbing, we refer to lead climbing, i.e., a form of sport climbing in which climbers are not secured by a rope hanging from the top, but in which climbers use the anchor points to attach the rope as they proceed to subsequent anchor points; one end of the rope is held by the belayer, the other end is attached at the climber.

In case of a fall, the rope is deflected on the last anchor point and the fall height of the climber minimized. On completion, climbers use the last (top) anchor point to secure the rope so that their partners on the ground can lower them. It can be carried out either outdoor on natural cliffs or indoor in climbing gyms. In the case of indoor, climbing gyms set up artificial walls with several routes with various difficulties. Along these routes, climbing gyms provide climbers with equipment and services which gives them the opportunity to challenge themselves and improve their skills without scarifying their safety. To this aim and similar to other sports (i.e. cycling, running), engineering and science have begun to help sport climbing [2].

The contribution of science in sports activities could take place in the form of collecting data from athletes using sensors embedded in electronic equipment such as smartwatches, smart bands, fitness trackers, and smartphones. These devices are attached to the body of the athletes (as in [3,4,9,10,12]). The corresponding measurements are time-series data used to visualize statistics of athletes and analyze their performance. Such analysis could be done either by a coach or through certain applications. Another way of acquiring data to analyze sports activities is based on the camera. In this approach, computer vision algorithms are developed to extract human 2-dimensional (2D) pose sequences from video frames and based on skeleton estimation of each person [6,16]. Instrumented climbing walls is the other approach for monitoring climbers which is inspected in [1,7].

The data acquisition methods based on wearable-sensors and camera are not always desirable for climbers. The former limits the convenience of the user when wearing an extra device during climbing, and the latter is against privacy. Keeping these issues in mind, for this paper data is collected from accelerometer sensors attached to a piece of climbing equipment mounted on the wall, called quickdraw. The sensor enhanced quickdraw hereinafter is referred to as smart-quickdraw (s-qd). To the best knowledge of the authors, the sensor enhanced quickdraws were studied the first time in our previous work [8]. We developed a hybrid system based on sensor and camera to detect rope-pulling activity. Apart from climbers, another concern for data collection relates to the climbing gyms. There is a large number of quickdraws in a climbing gym and regular changing batteries of the s-qds is expensive for the gym in terms of both time and costs. Hence, sensors attached to the quickdraws must be energy efficient such that their batteries do not need to be replaced in the short term.

The data collected from climbers helps both climbers and gyms in different ways. One goal is to improve the performance of the climbers, to achieve this, first must detect different activities during climbing i.e. ascending, resting, falling, lowering, and rope-pulling at the end of the climb. Then, the detected activities could be analyzed by experts and in off-line modes to provide recommendations for better performance, or in on-line mode to improve safety by early prediction of risk. Another goal is to improve the infrastructure of the gyms based on climbers' needs.

In this work, we investigated data from s-qds on the wall to differentiate between the different routes climbed in the same line. This reveals the most popular routes and helps the climbing gyms to better understand the needs of the climbers. Authors in [9] introduced a system to automatically detect the routes based on arm orientation from a single sensor. They collected data from wrist-worn Inertia Measurement Units (IMUs), extracted features from the sensor measurements, and finally evaluate the method by cross-validation. Our proposed method is an unsupervised algorithm based on clustering which does not need prior training of the model. This property makes our algorithm more general and less complex for the user since it could be easily adapted for new lines with different routes.

However, using sensors in energy-efficient mode and attaching them to the wall, instead of the body of the climber, introduces some challenges. Saving energy reduces the number of sensor samples. Moreover, different from algorithms based on wearable devices which mainly collect data through a single sensor on the body of the climber, we need to deal with multiple sensors when they are on the wall. Additionally, each sensor on the wall can provide us useful data only in a certain period during the climb.In the following, all these points are addressed in detail.

1.1 Contributions

Two male climbers participated in the experiment. The participants' skill levels were advanced i.e., self-estimated as a and 6b on-sight on the French Rating Scale of Difficulty (FRSD). The FRSD is a widely recognized system in the climbing community for grading the difficulty of routes. It ranges from easy levels (such as 1 or 2) to extremely challenging levels (like 9a). The scale progresses linearly: as the number increases, so does the difficulty. For example, a 6b route is more challenging than a 5c. A route graded 6b+ is a step above 6b, presenting even more complex and physically demanding challenges.

In our experiment, we selected routes graded 5c+, 6a+, and 6b+ to match the advanced skill levels of our participants. These grades ensured that the routes were challenging enough to test their abilities, yet within their competency range.

One participant was 27 years old with ten years of climbing experience and the other of 65 years old climbing for thirty years. For the purpose of data collection, the participants were asked to climb in the leading style on three different days. The three pre-selected routes were with difficulty levels of 5c+,6a+,and 6b+ (in French grading system). The routes were selected according to the skill levels of both climbers. The participants climbed at their usual speed, clipping the rope into every quickdraw, and were free to take resting time between climbs. The participant who climbed pulled the rope after each ascent. There was a person responsible for belaying.

On the first day, climber 1 was asked to climb a line with three routes nine times (each route three times). The order of climbing was: (5c+, 5c+, 5c+), (6b+, 6b+, 6b+), and (6a+, 6a+, 6a+). The following days, climber 1 practiced more and after one week he was asked to climb again the same line. In this experiment, which we refer to as 2nd-day of climber1, he climbed each route five times. This time we changed the order of climbing as (5c+, 6a+, 6b+) and repeated this process five times. Finally on the 3rd-day, we asked climber 2 to repeat a similar experiment as the 1st-day of climber1 but with different order as (5c+, 5c+, 5c+), (6a+, 6a+, 6a+), and (6b+, 6b+, 6b+). The aim of changing the climbers and the order of routes was to add different parameters *i.e.* age, tiredness, and provisioning to the data collected from the same routes.

Employing sensors in ultra-low-power mode enhances energy saving, but instead significantly reduces the number of samples. Considering this fact, we need to carefully understand the sensor functionality to analyze the received samples and find the more informative ones for our objective. To this aim, we described the details of our data acquisition system in Sect. 2. Afterward, in Sect. 3, the relevant features for route detection are extracted from sensor measurements. However, not all the features are necessary and a subset of features is selected through features optimization as in Sect. 4. In Sect. 5 the selected features are used for clustering the climbs to 3 different routes and the corresponding results are discussed in Sect. 4. Finally, the conclusion and future works are discussed in Sect. 7.

2   Data Acquisition System

Our data acquisition system is shown in Fig. 1 and consists of two main parts: 1- smart-quickdraws to measure 3-axis accelerations, 2- a base station to receive data from sensors and forwards them to the database in a remote server.

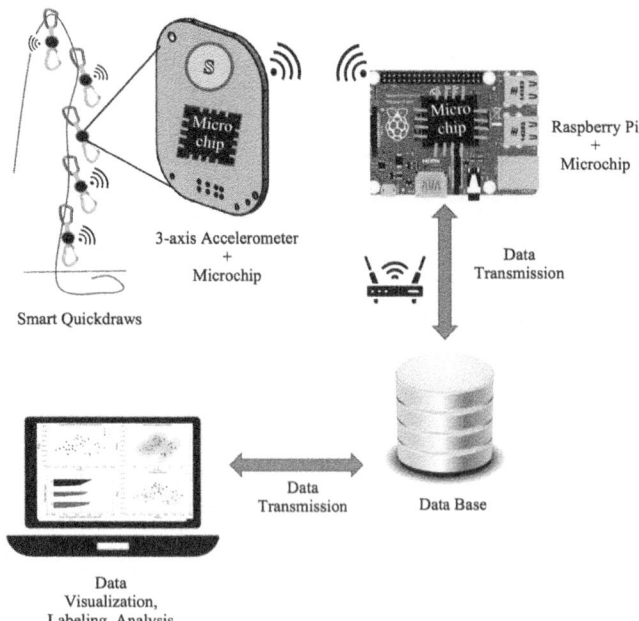

Fig. 1. Data acquisition system

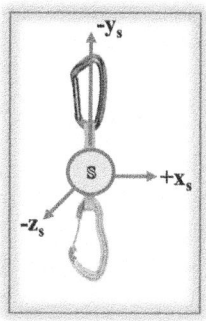

Fig. 2. x,y, z directions of 3-axis accelerometer sensor with respect to the climbing wall

2.1 Smart-Quickdraw

The so-called smart-quickdraw essentially refers to an in-house circuit board that is attached to the strip in the central part of the quickdraw. This board consists of an 3-axial accelerometer sensor to capture quickdraw movements along x, y, and z directions as shown in Fig. 2 and a microchip to control the accelerometer and communicate with the base station Fig. 1. For our application, energy efficiency is a primary issue as battery replacement of all smart-quickdraws in a climbing gym is both time and cost-consuming. In this regard, for the accelerometer, we selected LIS3DH by STMicroelectronics [17] which could be configured to operate in ultra-low-power modes through smart sleep-to-wake-up and return-to-sleep functions. Concerning the microchip, we used ATSAMR21G18A by Atmel [11] which combines a microcontroller unit (MCU) and an RF transceiver. The accelerometer sensor is controlled and configured via firmware which is developed inside the MCU, moreover, the smart-quickdraw communicates with the base station via the transceiver. In the following, some of our main settings for the accelerometer sensors are listed:

- **Full scale:** The LIS3DH has a dynamic user-selectable range of forces it can measure which are from ±2 g to ±16 g. Typically in accelerometers, the smaller the range, the more sensitive the readings will be. Hence, we selected 2 g as the full scale for our prototype.
- **Data rate:** The LIS3DH is capable of measuring accelerations with output data rates from 1 Hz to 5 kHz. For our energy-efficient system, we selected 10 Hz and 50 Hz for the inactive and active modes, respectively.
- **Output bits:** The analog to digital converter (ADC) of LIS3DH could have 8, 10, or 12 bits data output for operating in low-power, normal and high-resolution modes. Since our goal is to have an energy-efficient system, we selected 8-bit resolution for the sensor data output.
- **Range and resolution:** Accelerometers usually provide raw values which are not equivalent to meters per second squared. Consequently, we still need to scale the accelerometers' output based on our setting for full scale. In this

sensor's case, a signed 8-bit output data corresponds to a number ranging from -127 and 127. After scaling this range by ± 2 g full scale, sensor data output 127 is $+2$ g of force, and -127 is -2 g. The resolution of the data output after scaling is $\frac{2g}{127} \approx 16$ mg. Hence, knowing the range and scale is a key to deciphering the sensor's data output.

– **Noise reduction:** At a sampling rate of 50 Hz, there is still considerable noise in the sensor readings, which is the reason why a software averaging method has been implemented in our prototype. This simple method takes every subsequent set of 8 samples and calculates the average for the acceleration on each axis. Then, the corresponding averaged value is transmitted to the raspberry-pi.

– **Filter insignificant changes:** Regardless of whether there is movement or not, the accelerometer always provides sensor readings for the configured sampling rate. Since bandwidth is a premium for low-power devices, sensor values without any changes on any axis are not transmitted to the base station. However, even after averaging, hardly any sample is the same except if the sensor is completely still. Therefore a method has been implemented that prevents samples to be sent if there is no absolute change on any axis below a certain threshold. For this prototype, we set a threshold value equal to 15 units of the sensor's data output. The sensor does not consider any sample worth transmitting if the measured value of none of the axis has changed by at least 15 units. As mentioned above, the resolution of the data output for this sensor configuration is almost 16 mg, therefore the 15 units threshold is equivalent to the acceleration of 15×16 mg $= 240$ mg. This value is chosen because 240 mg represents a significant enough movement to be relevant for analysis, while also being large enough to filter out minor fluctuations that could be attributed to noise.

– **Grouping samples:** To save even more power (the radio of the smart-quickdraw is always off while no data is being sent) all sensor values are sent to the base station as a batch of values, i.e., grouped. We set this value to two samples, meaning that no sample is sent out individually, except before going to sleep after inactivity, in that case, any sample that was held back is being sent out. This may have the effect that sensor data is not received to the base station in real-time, but with a delay. However, since every sensor value has a timestamp this should not be an issue for analysis use-cases.

2.2 Base Station

The base station of our system comprises a board with the microchip, similar as in the smart-quickdraw, mounted on a raspberry-pi [14]. The raspberry-pi is used as a powerful CPU and hosts the application programming interface (API) that allows communication with the devices, as well as a web-server and possibly other services. In addition, the raspberry-pi CPU communicates with its board via the serial line. The firmware of the board within the base station performs the "network translation" to the radio network that is used amongst the boards (inside the base station and smart-quickdraws).

2.3   Ultra-Low-Power Data Acquisition:

In our system, the power-saving features are primarily managed by the CPU within each smart-quickdraw, which is a part of the Microcontroller Unit. This CPU is responsible for configuring the sensor's operation modes between sleep and active modes and is distinct from the CPU in the base station, which has a different role and does not interact directly with the sensor or its configuration settings. The s-qd CPU functions as follows:

- **Sleep mode:** When the sensor is stationary, the CPU sets the sensor to sleep mode, sampling data at a lower rate (10 Hz). This conserves power as less data is processed and transmitted.
- **Activation and inactivity detection:** If the sensor detects movement exceeding the threshold (15 units of sensor data), the CPU switches the sensor to active mode (50 Hz sampling rate) for more frequent data collection.
- **Inactivity Detection:**
  1. If the sensor data exceeds the threshold (15 units of sensor data), indicating significant movement, the CPU switches the sensor to active mode, increasing the sampling rate to 50 Hz for more frequent data collection.
  2. Conversely, if the measured values in all three axes are consistently lower than the threshold, the CPU filters out these readings as insignificant, preventing unnecessary data processing.
- **Transition Back to Sleep Mode:** While in active mode, the CPU averages every 8 samples and sends them to the base station. If the averaged data falls below the threshold for 0.8 s, the sensor is considered inactive. If this inactivity continues for 20 s, the CPU switches the sensor back to sleep mode.

In contrast, the base station CPU primarily manages data reception and network communication, without influencing the sensor's power-saving configurations.

3   Features Engineering

After visually keeping track of the climbers in the gym, we assume that the most relevant information for route identification are: 1- statistical features of quickdraws accelerations, 2- the moment when the climber reaches each quickdraw. Accordingly, we extract statistical and temporal features from sensor measurements as stated in the following.

3.1   Statistical Features

The sensor embedded in smart-quickdraw works in ultra-low-power mode, hence the s-qd does not continuously send data to the base station. Instead, transmits samples when it is in active mode and the change in the movement of the corresponding quickdraw exceeds a certain threshold. In our experience, all quickdraws of the line are sensor enhanced, and i, j refer to the position of two different s-qds in the line. During climb c, each sensor at position i transmits samples with timestamp t_{i_k}:

$$T_i^c = \{t_{i_k} | k \geq 1\} \tag{1}$$

where k refers to the index of the samples and T_i^c is the set of timestamps of all samples transmitted from s-qd at position i to the base station. These samples are measured when the s-qd is clipped till shortly afterward, while the climber's movement still causes tangible changes in the acceleration of the s-qd. On this assumptions, a vector of statistical features could be extracted from the N_i^c samples measured by each s-qd in a period between the moment when s-qd is activated through clipping at $t_{i_{k=1}}$, till clipping the next sensor at $t_{(i+1)_{k=1}}$. In addition to the 3-axis accelerations along the x,y, z axis, for each sample we can have a new value g corresponds to the sum of the energy of that sample along the three axes:

$$g_{i_k}^c = \sqrt{(x_{i_k}^c)^2 + (y_{i_k}^c)^2 + (z_{i_k}^c)^2}, \ \ 1 \leq k < N_i^c \tag{2}$$

Accordingly, we have four data sets for each s-qd:

$$X_i^c = \{x_{i_k}^c \mid 1 \leq k < N_i^c\} \tag{3}$$
$$Y_i^c = \{y_{i_k}^c \mid 1 \leq k < N_i^c\} \tag{4}$$
$$Z_i^c = \{z_{i_k}^c \mid 1 \leq k < N_i^c\} \tag{5}$$
$$G_i^c = \{g_{i_k}^c \mid 1 \leq k < N_i^c\} \tag{6}$$

For each s-qd at position i, the following statistical features are calculated over X_i^c, Y_i^c, Z_i^c, and G_i^c: 1-mean, 2- minimum, 3- maximum, 4- variance, 5- standard deviation, 6- root mean square, 7- the pth percentile where $p = \{5, 25, 75, 95\}$, 8- kurtosis, 9- skew, 10- Pearson correlation (between $x_{i_k}^c y_{i_k}^c$, $x_{i_k}^c z_{i_k}^c$, and $y_{i_k}^c z_{i_k}^c$), 11- number of peaks.

3.2   Temporal Features

Knowing the moment of clipping the rope to each s-qd, a vector of temporal features could be extracted from the timestamps of the received samples as follows:

1. Δts^c: a set of numbers which represents the time the climber spends in short-segments of the route between every two subsequent s-qds at positions i and $i + 1$:

$$\Delta ts^c = \{\Delta t_{i_k, i+1_k}^c | i = 2, \cdots, (ie - 2), k = 1\} \tag{7}$$

where ie is the position of the s-qd at the end of the line.

2. Δtl^c: a set of numbers which represents the time a climber spends between starting point of the climb $i = 2$ and each s-qd j. These time-deltas correspond to long-segments of the route and excludes $j = i + 1$ which is already considered in (7):

$$\Delta tl^c = \{\Delta t_{i_k, j_k}^c | i = 2, j = (i + 2), \cdots, (ie - 2), k = 1\} \tag{8}$$

3. Δtc^c: the duration of the climb c which is equivalent to the time difference between clipping the rope to the s-qds in the beginning and at the end of the climb. This is the extreme case of (8) where $j = ie - 1$.

$$\Delta tc^c = \left\{ \Delta t^c_{i_k, j_k} | i = 2, j = ie - 1, k = 1 \right\} \tag{9}$$

4. Statistical features of Δts^c: a set of features including minimum, maximum, mean, and standard deviation of Δts^c (the time a climber spends in short segments of a route in each climb).

4   Features Optimization

In the previous section, we introduced the features which are intended to be used for route clustering. Before clustering, features are optimized in two steps: 1- feature scaling, 2- feature selection.

4.1   Features Scaling

Many machine learning algorithms (*i.e.* Linear Regression, Logistic Regression, K-Means clustering) which calculate the similarities based on Euclidean distance do not give a reasonable recognition to the smaller feature [15]. Accordingly, features must be pre-processed through scaling to normalize them within a particular range. For instance, if not scaled, the time-delta of longer segments Δtl^c dominate the ones corresponding to shorter segments Δts^c.

There are different scaling techniques, the most common ones are Standards scaling, Min-Max scaling, Robust scaling, and Quantile transform. We selected Quantile Transform scaler since this scaler converts the variable distribution to a normal one and spread out the most frequent values and reduces the impact of outliers [13].

4.2   Feature Selection

The length of the features vector depends on the number of s-qds. As shown in the Fig. 3, features vector of each climb consists of sub-vectors extracted from s-qds. We ignored the sub-vectors related to the first and last s-qds. Because, the first sensor is mainly affected by the performance of the belayer. In addition, the last sensor measures the movements of the last s-qd when the climber finished climbing and is preparing for lowering. Consequently, our features vector consists of sub-vectors 2 to 7. However, some of these features (and corresponding s-qds) are redundant because different routes in the same line differ in certain parts and have similar difficulties in the rest of the line. In this regard, the features vector must be optimized not only to reduce the number of features and increase the efficiency and effectiveness of the algorithm but also to simplify the hardware by removing sensors that provide irrelevant features.

In this work, we utilized univariate feature selection to find features that can cover data related to different climbers, or the same climber on different days. This approach works by assigning a score to all features, based on univariate statistical tests, then selects a specific number of features with the highest scores [13]. Various score-functions are available *i.e.* ANOVA F-value, mutual information, chi-square, etc., each of which is suitable for a specific type of data. We selected ANOVA (analysis of variance) F-test to calculate the ratio between variances values and find a score for each feature saying how well this feature discriminates between three routes. Thereupon, remove the features with low scores that are independent of the routes.

5   Routes Clustering

Given a set of features for each climb, we can use a clustering model to make a certain number of clusters and group similar data from different climbs to the same cluster.

K-Means clustering is a common algorithm and is widely used in literature. We set the number of clusters equal to three (equal to the number of routes), then the model initialized with three random center points in features space. Each data point (climb) is classified by computing the distance between that point and each group center. In other words, this model assigns cluster membership to each data point based on distance from cluster center [13]. Since cluster centers

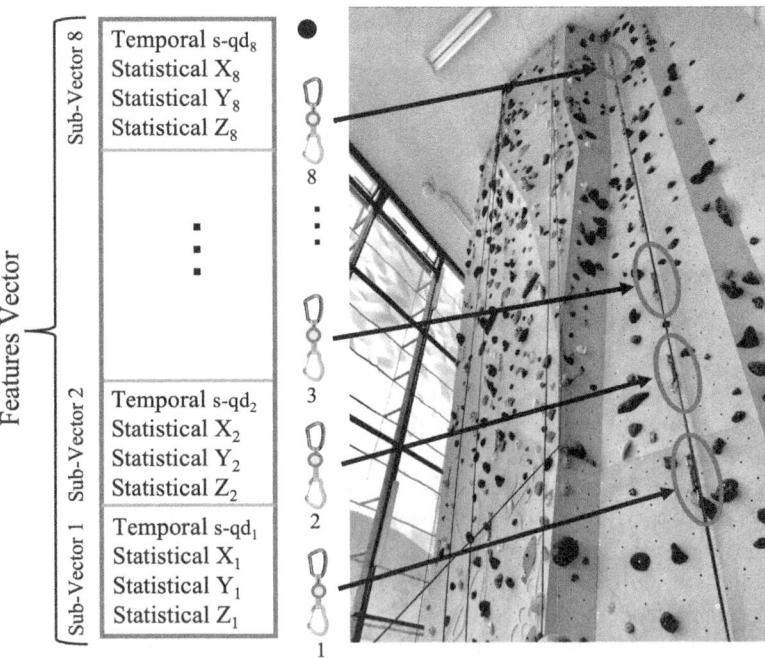

Fig. 3. Features vector of one climb composed of sub-vectors of temporal and statistical features of each s-qds

are randomly selected, this model does not give us a single answer. Hence, with only one model realization we can not have a definitive result and the algorithm must be verified through iterations. In the following for each set of features, K-Means clustering is evaluated over 100 iterations.

Given the knowledge of the ground truth class assignments route-labels and our clustering algorithm assignments of the same samples predicted-labels, the (adjusted or unadjusted) rand-index is a function that measures the similarity of the two assignments, ignoring permutations. The average, maximum, and minimum value of rand-index over 100 iterations of K-Means clustering is shown by gray bars, blue lines, and solid lines respectively. Our reference for selecting the optimum number of features is based on a minimum number of features which leads to the highest value for the minimum rand-index. This way we consider the worst case, while the average and maximum rand-index could be much higher.

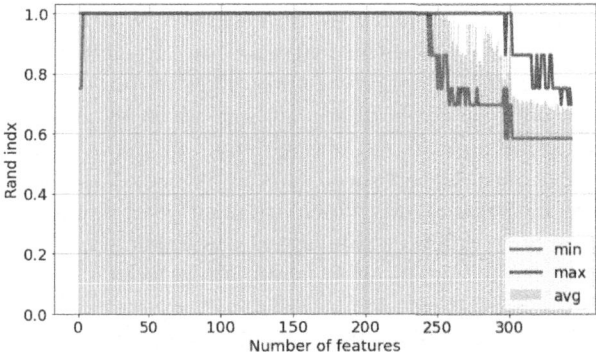

Fig. 4. Feature optimization for K-Means clustering over 100 iterations for data from climber 1 on 1st-day, features scaled by QuantileTransform and selected by ANOVA f-test

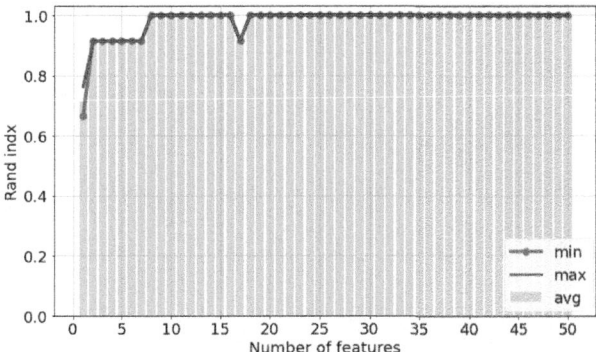

Fig. 5. Feature optimization for K-Means clustering over 100 iterations for data from climber 1 in 2nd-day, features scaled by QuantileTransform and selected by ANOVA f-test

- **Same climber in 1st day (without prevision):** climber 1 on 1st-day. Figure 4 shows that with only three features, K-Means model clusters all climbs of climber 1 in 1st-day with rand-index = 1 in all 100 iterations. One feature is temporal and the other two are acceleration statistics. The temporal one is the time difference between clipping the 2nd and the 5th quickdraws: $\Delta t^c_{i_k, j_k}$ where $i = 5$, $j = 2$, and $k = 1$. The two statistical features belongs to the acceleration along y-axis of s-qd at position 7: 1- $(Y^c_7)_{max}$ maximum value of acceleration, 2- $(Y^c_7)_{95^{th}}$ the 95th percentile of acceleration. Similar results were obtained for climber 2.

- **Same climber in 2nd day (with prevision):** climber 1 in 2nd-day. Figure 5 demonstrates that despite the reordering of routes on the second day of the experiment (as described in Subsect. 1.1), it is still possible to cluster the climbing data points for the same climber with a rand-index of 1. This clustering is achievable due to the climber's prior experience on these routes. However, factors like provisioning and fatigue alter the data in a way that, in contrast to Fig. 4, more features are necessary to achieve a rand-index of 1. These eight features are seven features from acceleration statistics of 5th and 7th s-qds and one temporal feature. The temporal feature is the average time spent between two subsequent s-qd given by $\overline{\Delta ts^c} = mean\{\Delta ts^c\}$. Hence, temporal features are not enough anymore and acceleration statistical features are of utmost importance. This implies that the selected statistical features belong to certain s-qds which are positioned in part of the line where different routes have different difficulties. As expected, the difficult part of the route is not at the beginning to avoid falling from a short distance to the ground and serious injuries.

- **Same climber in different days:** climber 1 on 1st and 2nd days. In this case, the best performance is rand-index equal to 0.94 obtained through 37 features. These features are extracted from s-qds at positions 2, 4, 5, and 7 and includes 35 acceleration statistical features and two temporal feature $\Delta t^c_{4_1, 2_1}$, $\Delta t^c_{5_1, 2_1}$. In Fig. 6, the first peak of minimum rand-index is 0.82 and

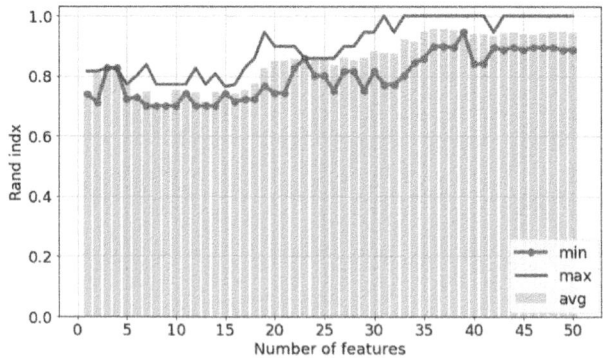

Fig. 6. Feature optimization for K-Means clustering over 100 iterations of mixing attempt 1 and 2 of climber 1, with features scaled by QuantileTransform and selected by ANOVA f-test

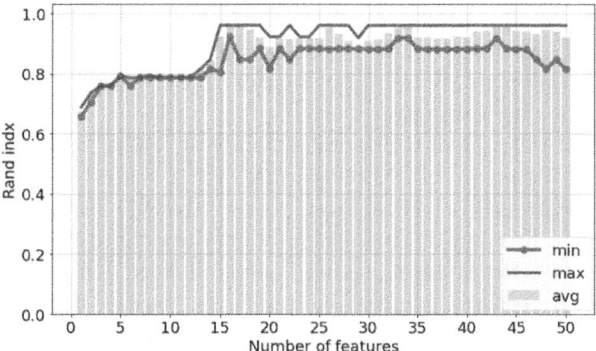

Fig. 7. Feature optimization for K-Means clustering over 100 iterations of mixing all attempts of two climbers, with features scaled by QuantileTransform and selected by ANOVA f-test

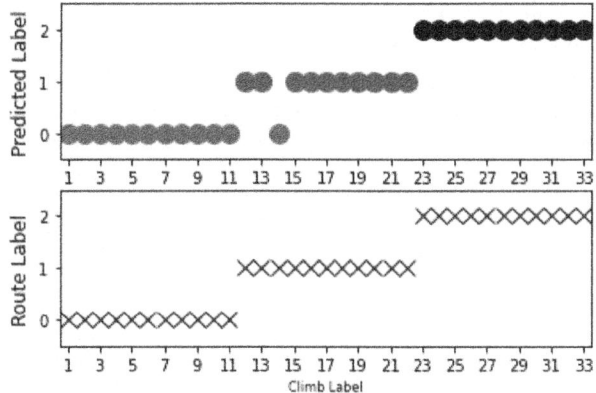

Fig. 8. K-Means clustering of climbing data points belongs to different climbers in different conditions

obtained through 3 statistical features belonging to accelerations of s-qds at positions 5, and 7.

- **Different climbers:** climber 1 on 1st and 2nd days and climber 2. The optimum performance in Fig. 7 is obtained with 16 features: 14 acceleration statistics of s-qds at positions 5, 4, and 7 and two temporal features $\Delta t^c_{4_1,2_1}$, $\Delta t^c_{5_1,2_1}$.

6   Visualization of Clusters:

Figure 8 represents the outcome of clustering data points that correspond to climbing three different routes by different climbers in different conditions. For better visualization, the data points are sorted based on their labels from 0 to

2. Based on the results of the previous section, for each data point, 16 features are given to the K-Means model. As could be seen, only 1 climb (from route 1) out of 33 climbs has a predicted label (as for route 0) different from the other points belonging to the same route.

Figure 9 depicts Principle Component Analysis (PCA) of data points in conjunction with K-Means and GMM clusterings. PCA is used to reduce the dimension of the selected features vector from 16 to 2. In 2-D PCA features space we can visualize how climbing data points are clustered by different models. However, for each climb, the K-Means model needs at least 5 features from PCA to have the optimum performance obtained with 16 selected features and without PCA. Here 2-D PCA slightly decreases the performance of the K-Means model and leads to one more mistake in data points clustering. Four subplots of Fig. 9 contains the following information:

– **top-left:** shows the ground truth in the 2-D features space (PCA1 and PCA2) as 33 data points refer to 33 climbs corresponding to 3 different routes identified by three colors (red, violet, black) and labels (0,1,2).
– **top-right:** we can see the three clusters' center points and the data points assigned to each of them. Despite the slight overlap between clusters 0 and 2, most of the data points are well-separated in the 2-D features space. Thus, the K-Means model finds suitable clustering results based on distance from

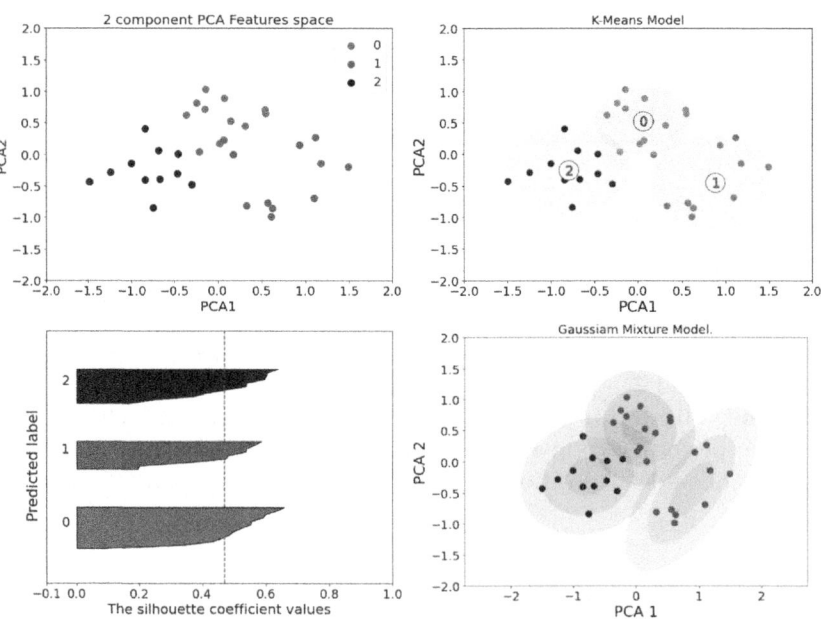

Fig. 9. Visualization of data points from different climbers in 2-D PCA feature space (top left), K-Means clustering (top right), silhouette scores for K-Means clusters (bottom left), and GMM clusterings (bottom right)

centers. Here, with 2 features obtained from PCA, we have two data points from cluster 1 (violet) which are wrongly assigned to cluster 0 (red).

- **bottom-left:** The quality of the clusters is evaluated by silhouette score (on the left side) and shows how well climbing data points are grouped with other similar points within a cluster and separated from data points of other clusters. To do so, first, we compute the silhouette score for each data point. Then, sort the silhouette scores for data points belonging to each cluster. Consequently, for each cluster, we have a thick line with upper and lower limits along a vertical axis which refers to the maximum and minimum silhouette scores of its data points, respectively. The other samples fill the space between these two lines. It is evident that for each cluster, the thickness of different parts of the line depends on the number of points that have that specific silhouette score. The low value of the silhouette score means that the data point lies between two clusters. This is evident for cluster 0 and cluster 1 with silhouette scores less than 0.2 and 0.4, respectively which indicates their overlap in some of their samples.

- **bottom-right:** In addition to the K-Means algorithm, the same data points are clustered through the Gaussian mixture model (GMM) and the result is depicted on the bottom right of Fig. 9. Similar to K-Means, GMM clustering is also based on random initialization. But, clusters in GMM have flexible shapes based on a mixture of multi-dimensional Gaussian probability distributions that best fits all data points. While in K-Means each cluster is associated with a hard-edged sphere [13]. In this figure for each cluster, we have three ellipses of different sizes. The dimension of the smallest ellipses depends on the eigenvalues of the covariance matrix of the corresponding cluster and the other two ellipses are twice and three times bigger than the smallest one. The intensity of the color of each ellipse depends on the weight of the cluster evaluated by the GMM model. The higher the density of data points, the darker the ellipse.

7 Conclusion and Future Work

In this work, we utilized 3-axis accelerometer sensors working in ultra-low power mode and attached them to the quickdraws hanging from climbing walls. Features are extracted from sensors data which were measured while different climbers were climbing three different routes. Feature optimization reveals redundant features and corresponding s-qds, hence reducing the complexity of the algorithm and the hardware. The corresponding features are given to the K-Means algorithm to cluster data points to three different groups.

The results show that when there is the possibility to identify the climber, we have perfect clustering with few features. However, the algorithm requires more features for detecting the routes climbed by the climber with prior practice, compared to the situation when the climber is without provisioning. But if data obtained from more than one climber and the climbers are not identified, then we need more features and the clustering algorithm may not be 100%

correct although the performance of the algorithm is still very high with only 1 mistake out of 33 climbs. In this case, the features are mainly statistical features obtained from the acceleration of s-qds which are positioned in the second half of the line. In addition to accelerations statistics, we need two temporal features as the time the climber spent to reach these s-qds. The position of these selected s-qds corresponds to the part of the line where different routes have different difficulties. Another reason why the statistical features obtained from the acceleration of lower sensors do not have any impact on clustering could be related to the behavior of the belayer. During each climb, the belayer pulled the rope tightly to prevent the climber from falling. Therefore, the s-qds at the beginning of the line can not move freely.

As the next step, we aim first to collect more data from more climbers climbing other routes and improve the current algorithm. The second goal is to develop another algorithm based on a new type of feature which is the orientation of quickdraws. These features could be utilized to detect activities during climbing such as lowering.

Acknowledgments. This work has been partly supported by the project "Sensors and data for the analysis of sport activities (SALSA)", funded by the EFRE-FESR programme 2014–2020 (CUP: I56C19000110009). This work was supported in part by the Italian Ministry of Foreign Affairs and International Cooperation, grant number US23GR04 (CUP: D43C23000350001).

References

1. Aladdin, R., Kry, P.: Static pose reconstruction with an instrumented bouldering wall. In: Proceedings of the 18th ACM Symposium on Virtual Reality Software and Technology, pp. 177–184 (2012)
2. Association, I.S.E., Moritz, E.F., Haake, S., et al.: The Engineering of Sport 6, vol. 6. Springer, Cham (2006)
3. Boulanger, J., Seifert, L., Hérault, R., Coeurjolly, J.F.: Automatic sensor-based detection and classification of climbing activities. IEEE Sens. J. **16**(3), 742–749 (2015)
4. Boulanger, J., Seifert, L., Herault, R., Coeurjolly, J.F.: Automatic sensor-based detection and classification of climbing activities. IEEE Sens. J. **16**(3) (2016)
5. Committee, I.O.: History of sport climbing. https://olympics.com/en/sports/sport-climbing/
6. Einfalt, M., Dampeyrou, C., Zecha, D., Lienhart, R.: Frame-level event detection in athletics videos with pose-based convolutional sequence networks. In: Proc. of the 2nd International Workshop on Multimedia Content Analysis in Sports. Association for Computing Machinery (2019)
7. Fuss, F.K., Niegl, G.: Instrumented climbing holds and performance analysis in sport climbing. Sports Technol. **1**(6), 301–313 (2008)
8. Ivanova, I., Andrić, M., Moaveninejad, S., Janes, A., Ricci, F.: Video and sensor-based rope pulling detection in sport climbing. In: Proceedings of the 3rd International Workshop on Multimedia Content Analysis in Sports, pp. 53–60 (2020)

9. Kosmalla, F., Daiber, F., Krüger, A.: Climbsense: automatic climbing route recognition using wrist-worn inertia measurement units. In: Proceedings of the 33rd Annual ACM Conference on Human Factors in Computing Systems - CHI 2015. ACM Press, New York (2015)

10. Ladha, C., Hammerla, N.Y., Olivier, P., Plötz, T.: ClimbAX. In: Proceedings of the 2013 ACM International Joint Conference on Pervasive and Ubiquitous Computing - UbiComp 2013. ACM Press (2013)

11. Microchip: Atsamr21g18a - wireless modules (2023). https://www.microchip.com/wwwproducts/en/ATSAMR21G18A. Accessed 24 Apr 2023

12. Pansiot, J., King, R.C., McIlwraith, D.G., Lo, B.P.L., Yang, G.Z.: ClimBSN: climber performance monitoring with BSN. In: 2008 5th International Summer School and Symposium on Medical Devices and Biosensors. IEEE (2008)

13. Pedregosa, F., et al.: Scikit-learn: machine learning in python. J. Mach. Learn. Res. **12**, 2825–2830 (2011)

14. Raspberry Pi Foundation: Raspberry pi: Technical specifications (2023). https://www.raspberrypi.org/products/. Accessed 24 Apr 2023

15. Saha, A., Das, S.: Feature-weighted clustering with inner product induced norm based dissimilarity measures: an optimization perspective. Mach. Learn. **106**(7), 951–992 (2017)

16. Sasaki, K., Shiro, K., Rekimoto, J.: Exemposer: predicting poses of experts as examples for beginners in climbing using a neural network. In: Proceedings of the Augmented Humans International Conference, pp. 1–9 (2020)

17. STMicroelectronics: LIS3DH Datasheet (2023). https://www.st.com/resource/en/datasheet/lis3dh.pdf. Accessed 24 Apr 2023

Finding Beauty in Mobile EEG When Visiting Art Exhibitions

Maurizio Palmieri[(✉)] [iD], Marco Avvenuti[iD], Alejandro Luis Callara[iD],
Francesco Marcelloni[iD], and Alessio Vecchio[iD]

Department of Information Engineering, University of Pisa, 56122 Pisa, Italy
{maurizio.palmieri,marco.avvenuti,alejandro.callara,
francesco.marcelloni,alessio.vecchio}@unipi.it

Abstract. Neuroaesthetics studies the biological bases of aesthetic experiences. In this paper, we describe a method, based on EEG signals, aimed at recognizing the experience of beauty when users are exposed to art. The method is evaluated on a public dataset collected from the visitors of an art exhibit in a museum, where signals were collected by means of mobile EEG solutions, thus ensuring a naturalistic setting. Besides presenting the results, characterized by good accuracy, we also describe the main problems, and the related solutions, found during the different stages of the method.

Keywords: EEG · classification · neuroaesthetics

1 Introduction

The notion of beauty is inherently subjective, influenced by individual preferences, cultural upbringing, and personal experiences. Nevertheless, numerous studies suggest the possibility of common neural patterns underlying beauty perception. Technological advancements have empowered neuroaesthetic research, with EEG signal analysis offering unique insights into neural responses during aesthetic encounters. EEG enables non-invasive monitoring of brain activity, providing real-time access to the cognitive processes during art appreciation. In particular, mobile EEG solutions allow the collection of data in a natural setting, without imposing constraints on the involved subjects.

This paper describes a method for classifying EEG signals originating from exposure to art pieces. The method is based on a public dataset, which was collected using mobile EEG systems on a number of subjects when visiting an art exhibition [16]. Subjects were asked to identify the most beautiful art piece and the most emotionally stimulating one. The dataset is highly naturalistic, as signals were collected imposing very limited restrictions on the subjects, who were free to move within the exhibition and to look at art pieces according to their will. Such a naturalistic setting increases the significance of collected data, which is obviously closer to a real user experience, but at the same time makes the

M. Mizmizi et al. (Eds.): BodyNets 2024, LNICST 524, pp. 194–206, 2024.
https://doi.org/10.1007/978-3-031-72524-1_15

problem harder. EEG signals are known to be disturbed from non-physiological and physiological sources. Examples include power-line interference or electrode pops, which are more likely to occur when the user moves in a realistic setting, or ocular motions and muscle activations, which again are more abundant and difficult to record in a realistic setting.

The proposed method is described incrementally, in order to highlight the impact, in terms of accuracy, of the adopted techniques. In particular, this paper quantifies the improvements obtained when facing the dataset unbalance and removal of artifacts. Results show that it is possible to classify the pieces in special (beautiful or emotionally pleasing) or normal with good accuracy.

2 Related Work

The main topic of this work is related to EEG analysis of users' exposure to art. The most relevant papers are [3–5]. All these articles focus on EEG data acquisition of users visiting a museum exhibit. Similar work is performed by [12] to evaluate the performance of two EEG headsets for the task of capturing the emotions arising from musical stimuli. Moving toward the topic of machine learning, [31] has proposed an interesting review that combines different aspects of neuroscience, aesthetics, and computer science, including topics such as image quality assessment and machine learning. Other interesting reviews have been presented by [38] and [24] with more emphasis on emotion recognition. In [6], the authors provide a comparative analysis of different machine learning algorithms to recognize different emotional states. [14] and [15] have both studied the usage of machine learning approaches for emotion recognition from the EEG, using the same dataset. The first paper reports on the comparison of different types of classifiers, showing that Random Forest is better than KNN and Naive Bayesian, while SVM has computational limitations. The second paper reports on the usage of deep machine learning, comparing different classification algorithms showing that gcForest, tailored for EEG analysis, achieves the best results. [17] and [40] both report on their experiment on emotion recognition with deep learning mechanism, obtaining more than 90% of accuracy for valence and arousal classification. [37] uses a Random Forest algorithm to classify EEG data using only 3 channels (F3, Fz, F4 according to the extended 10–20 international system) into two different classes of mental effort. The work shown in [25] considers different approaches to include the baseline in the analysis process, highlighting the good results obtained with the subtraction approach extended with partial least squares analysis. Finally, [36] compares different preprocessing methods and evaluates their impact on the EEG analysis, claiming that small changes in the preprocessing phase have a significant impact on the analysis and that the best practice is to combine different approaches. Early work on the neural correlates of beauty also adopted functional MRI (fMRI) instead of EEG. In particular, in [28] 10 subjects were monitored through fMRI when exposed to paintings that they were asked to classify as beautiful, ugly, or neutral. Results show that a functional specialization lies at the base of the aesthetic classification and that the classification of a painting as beautiful or not is correlated with specific brain structures (the orbito-frontal cortex and the motor cortex). Subsequent experiments, again based on fMRI, showed that one area, located in the medial orbito-frontal cortex, was characterized by an activity level proportional to the intensity of beauty declared by subjects, both when exposed to visual stimuli and auditory stimuli [27].

3   Materials and Methods

3.1   Ethics Statement

The study does not involve direct human participants, thus informed consent was not required. Fully detailed description of the dataset can be found in [16].

3.2   Dataset Description

The dataset used in this study has been already published and is freely available at [1]. It consists of EEG traces collected from 431 participants (208 males/223 females; age range 6–81 years) using five mobile EEG caps (four dry ones and a gel-based one) during a visit at the Menil Collection (Houston, Texas, US) in 2014. EEG systems were purposely chosen to let the volunteers freely move through the exhibit 'The Boundary of Life is Quietly Crossed' by Dario Robleto. Among the total, 207 subjects completed a questionnaire with personal information (age, gender, nationality, etc.) and with their art preference, by pointing out the most aesthetically pleasing piece and the most emotionally stimulating one. However, due to technical issues resulting from the unconstrained and unsupervised nature of the study (e.g., poor wireless communication, file corruption, sensor disconnection, low system battery, etc.), the final dataset contains EEG data from only 134 individuals (77 males/53 females; age range 15–77 years). The dataset was originally acquired to evaluate the feasibility of using a dry EEG headset, in terms of usability, when subjects are free to move while watching art pieces by means of a Power Spectral Density (PSD) analysis [16]. Additional analysis on these data was performed in [29], where the subset related to the 32-channel Brain Products actiCAP is analyzed.

This work is focused on a subset of the full dataset, only exploiting the 8-channel (F3, Fz, F4, C3, C4, P3, Pz, P4) Neuroelectrics Starstim headset dataset, as it was the one with the higher number of participants (n=32). The dataset is organized as a collection of MATLAB files, where each file represents a pair Visitor-Piece (or Visitor-Baseline) and contains the related EEG. The dataset consists of 157 files (please note that some pair Visitor-Piece are not available for the analysis). The baseline consists of 60 s interval of EEG data captured while the visitor was staring at a white wall. The Visitor-Piece consists of roughly 20 s of EEG data collected when the subject was looking at one of the art pieces included in the collection. Based on the questionnaire's outcome, each couple Visitor-Piece was labeled as: **Beautiful** (the visitor marked the related piece as the most aesthetically pleasing), **Emotional** (the visitor marked the related piece as the most emotionally stimulating), **Piece** (none of the above). It is important to note that for some visitors, the EEG data corresponding to the most aesthetically pleasing or most emotionally stimulating piece was not available. Among the 157 files, 32 are related to the baselines of the 32 visitors, 24 have been labeled **Beautiful**, 18 **Emotional**, and 83 **Piece**.

3.3 General Purpose EEG Data Preprocessing and Feature Extraction

EEGs were analyzed offline using MATLAB R2022b. The raw EEG data were filtered in the 1–50 Hz frequency range with a 4th-order Butterworth passband filter to remove DC components and high-frequency noise not related to brain activity, as well as to suppress undesired signals caused by the electrical grid. Then, the 20 s data records were divided into 4-seconds segments without overlap and, for each segment and for each channel, the mean value (**Mean value**), standard deviation (**Std**), maximum value (**Max value**), kurtosis distance (**Kurt**), and the Shannon entropy (**Entr**) from the time domain, the first mel frequency cepstral coefficient [32] (**Cesp**) from the mel-frequency domain, and the mean Power Spectral Density (PSD) in the five relevant frequency bands: δ (1–4 Hz), θ (4–8 Hz), α (8–12 Hz), β (12–30 Hz), and γ (30–50 Hz) were computed. Accordingly, there is a total of 11×8 features for each segment.

3.4 Statistical Analysis

To evaluate whether subjects exposed to art pieces exhibited physiological changes in the EEG signal, a 1×4 ANOVA (ANalysis Of VAriance) on the spatial average (i.e., over channels) of each feature was performed. Post-hoc comparisons were performed with paired t-tests. Multiple hypothesis testing was adjusted with Bonferroni correction. Figure 1 reports the outcome of the statistical analysis. It is possible to observe that **Std**, **Max value**, **Kurt**, **Entr** and **Ceps** significantly differed between the resting baseline and each type (according to subject's specific rating) of aesthetic exposure. However, it is not possible to observe any significant difference between **Piece**, **Beatiful**, and **Emotional**. The remaining features did not show any significant change during the experiment.

3.5 Classification Procedure

The results of the statistical analysis suggest that the problem of predicting the aesthetic response of users facing an art piece is not a simple task and can benefit from the application of machine learning approaches. The Classification Learner MATLAB application is exploited to compare different classification strategies in terms of accuracy, namely, Tree, Discriminant, Naive Bayesian, KNN, SVM, Ensemble, and Kernel, including parameter variations. The aim was to correctly classify beauty assessment. The first step consists of splitting the dataset into a

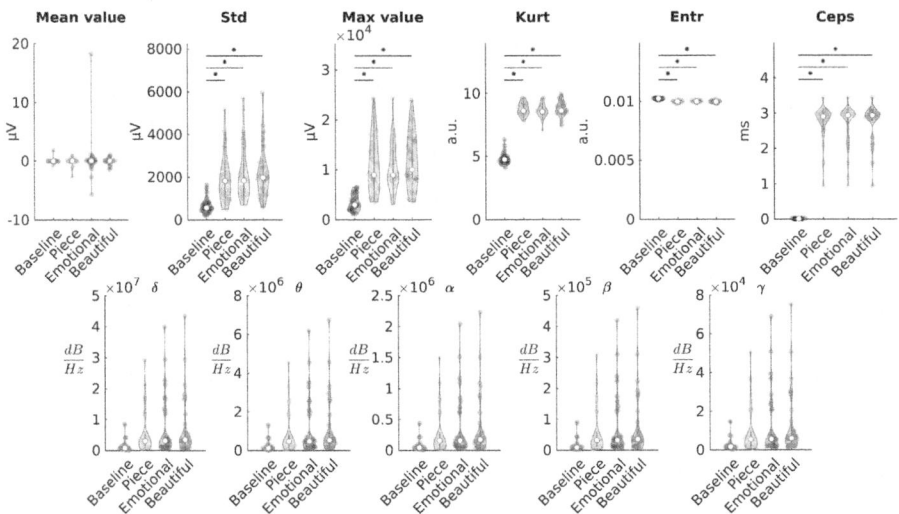

Fig. 1. Violin plot for each feature. Significant differences ($p < 0.05$, Bonferroni corrected) are marked with an asterisk * and the black horizontal segment identifies the couple of classes. For the units, a.u. is used as a short version of arbitrary units.

training set (90%) and a testing set (10%), the second step consists of applying a stratified 5-fold cross-validation to assess the best classification strategy, sorting the strategies based on the F-measure obtained during the validation phase, and the last step, consists of evaluating the performance of the best strategy against the test set.

4   Results

This section reports on the main problems encountered during the analysis of the dataset, the effects of the chosen mitigation techniques, and the reasoning about possible choices to improve the quality of the classifier.

4.1   Effect of the Unbalanced Data on Classification Accuracy

It is easy to notice that the selected dataset suffers from the problem of unbalanced classes: 66.4% of the data belongs to the majority class (**Piece**) against 14.4% (**Emotional**) and 19.2% (**Beautiful**). Figure 2 clearly shows the effect of the unbalanced dataset: the best classifier obtained with the chosen classification procedure, in this case, an Ensemble based on boosted trees, achieves a 64.5% of accuracy but it is clearly biased to assign the label **Piece** to most of the input test data and never assigns the label **Emotional**.

Given the small size of the available dataset (625 entries), the sub-sampling of the majority class has been ruled out, as it would lead to the usage of a very small

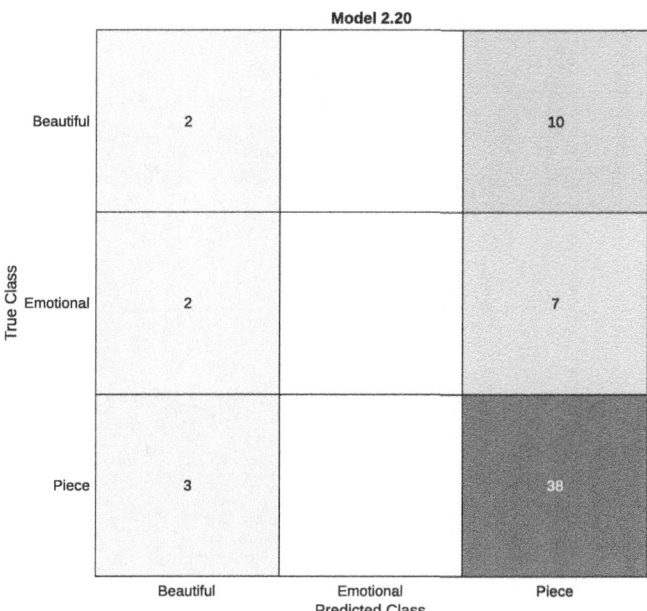

Fig. 2. Biased classifier confusion matrix

dataset. Re-sampling both the minority classes, to match the size of the majority class, led to a decrease in the accuracy to 51% because the resulting dataset is composed of more synthetic entries than real ones. In order to implement the re-sampling it is possible to use the SMOTE [13] algorithm to increase the size of the training set while perfectly balancing all the classes.

A couple of mitigation techniques to cope with the unbalanced dataset have been enacted; first, the combination of the two minority classes into one class named **Special**, and second, the doubling the cost of mislabelling of the minority class w.r.t. the cost of mislabelling the majority class; the results shown in Fig. 3 prove that the best classifier, that is an Ensemble based on KNN, is less biased towards the majority class and achieves the same accuracy (64.5%).

4.2 Effect of EEG Artifacts on the Classification Accuracy

The performance of the classifier is tightly related to the capability of the pre-processing phase to correctly clean the data, removing artifacts that can hinder the performance of the classifier. In the domain of brain measurements, data are usually affected by natural artifacts (e.g. eye movement and blinking) that require specific algorithms for detection and correction. The adopted pre-processing only involves a bandpass filter to clean the data, without taking into account brain artifacts, and therefore it should be combined with known algorithms for brain artifacts detection to improve the accuracy of the classifier. One such algorithm is the Artifact Subspace Reconstruction (ASR) [30], which is

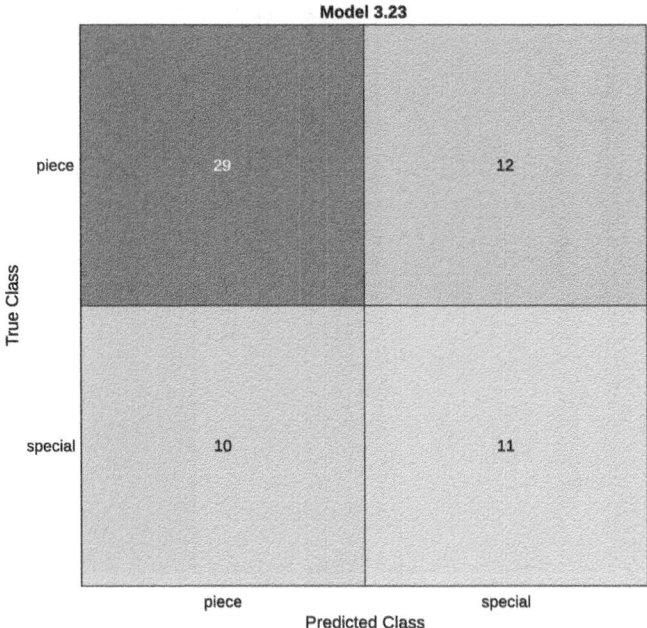

Fig. 3. Unbiased classifier confusion matrix

included in the EEGLAB [18] extension for MATLAB. ASR exploits clean portions of EEG (in our case the 60 s baselines) as references to detect and reject (or reconstruct) data afflicted by artifacts.

The ASR has been included in the proposed pre-processing, using a conservative cutoff parameter of 20, leading to the results shown in Table 1 where it is possible to see a comparison of the considered strategies applied to the ASR-corrected, pre-processed dataset. The values in the table have been computed as the average over 10 different applications of the classification procedure and they are sorted by F-measure. It is possible to notice that Naive Bayesian approaches are not suited for computational neuroaesthetics as they achieved lower-than-chance performances. The most promising strategy is the one based on the Ensemble approach that achieves a 70.4% Accuracy with an F-measure of 65.9.

Figure 4 shows the confusion matrix of the best classifier, a KNN-based Ensemble, that achieves a 74.1% of accuracy without bias, which is significantly higher than the 64.5% achieved without the ASR.

4.3 Effects of Data Re-sampling on Classification Accuracy

Another possible approach to improve the performance of the classifier is a more aggressive technique to cope with the unbalanced dataset: the re-sampling of the minority class. Given the mitigation enacted in Sect. 4.1, the minority class

Table 1. Comparison of different strategies

Strategy	Accuracy	F-measure	Precision	Recall
Ensemble	70.4	65.9	67.0	66.0
KNN	69.0	64.7	65.3	64.7
SVM	67.9	62.4	63.4	62.1
Kernel	64.00	60	60.6	60.7
Tree	63.2	59.6	59.6	59.8
Discriminant	58.3	56.6	57.3	58.08
Naive Bayes	34.0	27.8	44.4	48.5

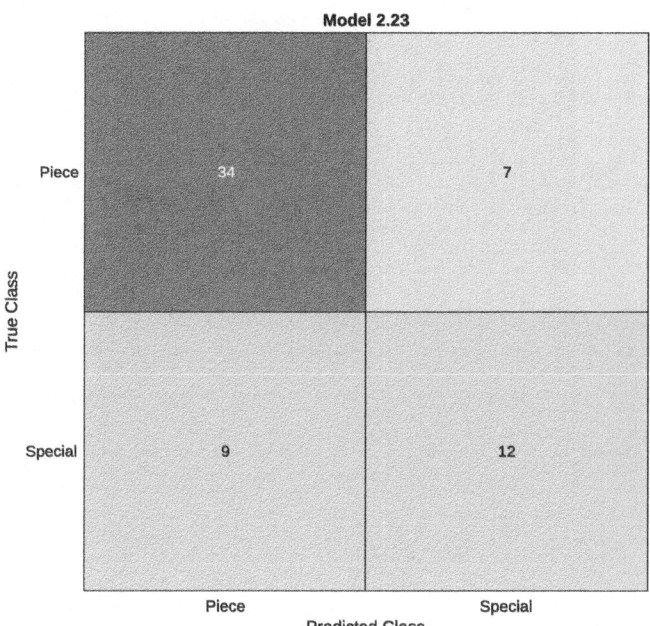

Fig. 4. Best confusion matrix with ASR

(**Special**) is roughly half the size of the majority class (**Piece**) and therefore the re-sampling of the minority class is now a viable option.

The classification procedure, empowered with the SMOTE re-sampling algorithm achieves the results shown in Table 2, where it is possible to see higher values for the metrics of the three top strategies (Ensemble, KNN and SVM) with respect to the results shown in Table 1 and lower values for the other strategies.

Figure 5 shows the confusion matrix of the best classifier, a KNN-based Ensemble, that achieves a 79% of accuracy without bias.

Table 2. Comparison of different strategies with re-sampling

Strategy	Accuracy	F-measure	Precision	Recall
Ensemble	72.7	70.0	70.0	70.5
KNN	70.9	68.6	68.5	69.4
SVM	67.9	65.6	66.1	67.0
Tree	62.5	59.4	59.5	60.0
Kernel	59.3	58.6	61.2	62.1
Discriminant	54.5	54.1	60.3	60.0
Naive Bayes	36.4	31.1	53.9	50.5

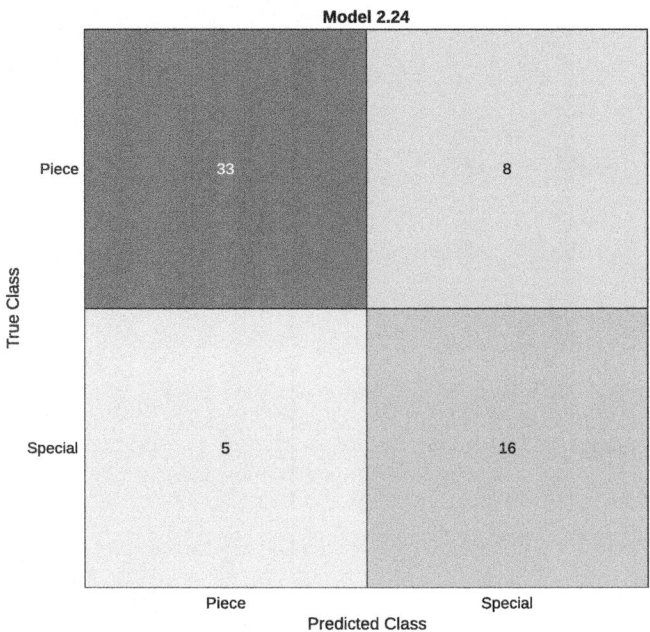

Fig. 5. Best confusion matrix with re-sampling

5 Discussion and Conclusion

This work has shown that the application of machine learning approaches to the field of neuroaesthetics requires a deep knowledge in the specific domain of EEG analysis as the general-purpose approach for data pre-processing yields poor performances and biased classifiers. General validity mitigation techniques can improve the quality of the classifiers but it is only thanks to the EEG-specific cleaning algorithm ASR that it is possible to achieve an accuracy above the 70%. The preliminary results shown in the previous section suggest that the Ensemble classification strategy, especially the one based on KNN sub-spacing, is the most promising one for EEG data analysis.

Data re-sampling is only able to produce a small improvement in the performance of the classifier, while the enhancement of the pre-processing with the application of the ASR algorithm has introduced a more interesting improvement, therefore future directions of this work should focus on improving the pre-processing phase.

It is worthwhile mentioning that this paper focused on relatively simple features of the EEG based on signal statistics and power measures. However, more sophisticated analyses could include other features, as for instance those derived from connectivity analysis [21,23]. Indeed, emotions involve complex interactions in the brain [33,34], which may be properly captured by this kind of analysis [10,20]. In turn, such interactions may change based on the psychophysiological state of the subject, as well as between healthy and pathology [9,26,35]. As a result, including other physiological signals such as the heart-rate-variability [19] and the electrodermal activity [8] may provide additional relevant information about the state of the subject [2,11,20,22]. Finally, collecting movement data by means of wearable sensors could be helpful in identifying and discarding less significant segments from the EEG trace [7,39].

Future work will also concern the analysis of the data belonging to the same dataset but collected using other EEG collection systems. The goal is to understand if the use of a different EEG collection system, possibly with an increased number of electrodes or a different interface (gel-based), provides some benefits in terms of accuracy. In this light, future works will also focus on complementary features, for instance, those obtained from connectivity analysis.

Acknowledgments. Research partly funded by the European Union - Next Generation EU, in the context of The National Recovery and Resilience Plan, Investment 1.5 Ecosystems of Innovation, Project Tuscany Health Ecosystem (THE), Spoke 3 "Advanced technologies, methods, materials and health analytics" CUP: I53C22000780001 and partially supported by the Italian Ministry of Education and Research (MIUR) in the framework of the FoReLab project (Departments of Excellence).

References

1. Mobile EEG recordings in an art museum setting (2017). https://doi.org/10.21227/H2TM00
2. Appelhans, B.M., Luecken, L.J.: Heart rate variability as an index of regulated emotional responding. Rev. Gen. Psychol. **10**(3), 229–240 (2006)
3. Babiloni, F., et al.: The great beauty: a neuroaesthetic study by neuroelectric imaging during the observation of the real michelangelo's moses sculpture. In: 2014 36th Annual International Conference of the IEEE Engineering in Medicine and Biology Society, pp. 6965–6968 (2014). https://doi.org/10.1109/EMBC.2014.6945230
4. Babiloni, F., et al.: Neuroelectric brain imaging during a real visit of a fine arts gallery: a neuroaesthetic study of xvii century Dutch painters. In: 2013 35th Annual International Conference of the IEEE Engineering in Medicine and Biology Society (EMBC), pp. 6179–6182 (2013). https://doi.org/10.1109/EMBC.2013.6610964

5. Babiloni, F., et al.: The first impression is what matters: a neuroaesthetic study of the cerebral perception and appreciation of paintings by titian. In: 2015 37th Annual International Conference of the IEEE Engineering in Medicine and Biology Society (EMBC), pp. 7990–7993 (2015). https://doi.org/10.1109/EMBC.2015.7320246

6. Bălan, O., Moise, G., Petrescu, L., Moldoveanu, A., Leordeanu, M., Moldoveanu, F.: Emotion classification based on biophysical signals and machine learning techniques. Symmetry **12**(1) (2020). https://doi.org/10.3390/sym12010021, https://www.mdpi.com/2073-8994/12/1/21

7. Bonsignori, C., et al.: Estimation of user's orientation via wearable UWB. In: 2020 16th International Conference on Intelligent Environments (IE), pp. 80–83 (2020). https://doi.org/10.1109/IE49459.2020.9154983

8. Boucsein, W.: Electrodermal Activity. Springer Science & Business Media (2012)

9. Callara, A.L., Morelli, M.S., Hartwig, V., Landini, L., Giannoni, A., Passino, C., Emdin, M., Vanello, N.: LD-EEG effective brain connectivity in patients with cheyne-stokes respiration. IEEE Trans. Neural Syst. Rehabil. Eng. **28**(5), 1216–1225 (2020)

10. Callara, A.L., Greco, A., Frasnelli, J., Rho, G., Vanello, N., Scilingo, E.P.: Cortical network and connectivity underlying hedonic olfactory perception. J. Neural Eng. **18**(5), 056050 (2021)

11. Callara, A.L., Sebastiani, L., Vanello, N., Scilingo, E.P., Greco, A.: Parasympathetic-sympathetic causal interactions assessed by time-varying multivariate autoregressive modeling of electrodermal activity and heart-rate-variability. IEEE Trans. Biomed. Eng. **68**(10), 3019–3028 (2021)

12. Chabin, T., Gabriel, D., Haffen, E., Moulin, T., Pazart, L.: Are the new mobile wireless EEG headsets reliable for the evaluation of musical pleasure? PLOS ONE **15**(12), 1–19 (2021). https://doi.org/10.1371/journal.pone.0244820

13. Chawla, N.V., Bowyer, K.W., Hall, L.O., Kegelmeyer, W.P.: Smote: synthetic minority over-sampling technique. J. Artif. Intell. Res. **16**, 321–357 (2002). https://doi.org/10.1613/jair.953

14. Chen, P., Zhang, J.: Performance comparison of machine learning algorithms for EEG-signal-based emotion recognition. In: Lintas, A., Rovetta, S., Verschure, P.F.M.J., Villa, A.E.P. (eds.) ICANN 2017. LNCS, vol. 10613, pp. 208–216. Springer, Cham (2017). https://doi.org/10.1007/978-3-319-68600-4_25

15. Cheng, J., et al.: Emotion recognition from multi-channel EEG via deep forest. IEEE J. Biomed. Health Inform. **25**(2), 453–464 (2020). https://doi.org/10.1109/JBHI.2020.2995767

16. Cruz-Garza, J.G., et al.: Deployment of mobile EEG technology in an art museum setting: evaluation of signal quality and usability. Front. Hum. Neurosci. **11** (2017). https://doi.org/10.3389/fnhum.2017.00527, https://www.frontiersin.org/articles/10.3389/fnhum.2017.00527

17. Cui, H., Liu, A., Zhang, X., Chen, X., Wang, K., Chen, X.: EEG-based emotion recognition using an end-to-end regional-asymmetric convolutional neural network. Knowl.-Based Syst. **205**, 106243 (2020). https://doi.org/10.1016/j.knosys.2020.106243

18. Delorme, A., Makeig, S.: EEGLAB: an open source toolbox for analysis of single-trial EEG dynamics including independent component analysis. J. Neurosci. Methods **134**(1), 9–21 (2004). https://doi.org/10.1016/j.jneumeth.2003.10.009

19. Electrophysiology, T.F.O.T.E.S.O.C.T.N.A.S.O.P.: Heart rate variability: standards of measurement, physiological interpretation, and clinical use. Circulation **93**(5), 1043–1065 (1996)

20. Engelen, T., Buot, A., Grèzes, J., Tallon-Baudry, C.: Whose emotion is it? perspective matters to understand brain-body interactions in emotions. Neuroimage **268**, 119867 (2023)
21. Friston, K.J.: Functional and effective connectivity: a review. Brain Connectivity **1**(1), 13–36 (2011)
22. Greco, A., et al.: Acute stress state classification based on electrodermal activity modeling. IEEE Trans. Affect. Comput. (2021)
23. He, B., et al.: Electrophysiological brain connectivity: theory and implementation. IEEE Trans. Biomed. Eng. **66**(7), 2115–2137 (2019)
24. Houssein, E.H., Hammad, A., Ali, A.A.: Human emotion recognition from EEG-based brain-computer interface using machine learning: a comprehensive review. Neural Comput. Appl. **34**(15), 12527–12557 (2022). https://doi.org/10.1007/s00521-022-07292-4
25. Hu, L., Xiao, P., Zhang, Z., Mouraux, A., Iannetti, G.D.: Single-trial time-frequency analysis of electrocortical signals: Baseline correction and beyond. Neuroimage **84**, 876–887 (2014). https://doi.org/10.1016/j.neuroimage.2013.09.055
26. Ishii, R., et al.: Healthy and pathological brain aging: from the perspective of oscillations, functional connectivity, and signal complexity. Neuropsychobiology **75**(4), 151–161 (2018)
27. Ishizu, T., Zeki, S.: Toward a brain-based theory of beauty. PLoS ONE **6**(7), e21852 (2011)
28. Kawabata, H., Zeki, S.: Neural correlates of beauty. J. Neurophysiol. **91**(4), 1699–1705 (2004). https://doi.org/10.1152/jn.00696.2003
29. Kontson, K., et al.: 'Your Brain on Art': emergent cortical dynamics during aesthetic experiences. Front. Hum. Neurosci. **9** (2015) https://doi.org/10.3389/fnhum.2015.00626, https://www.frontiersin.org/articles/10.3389/fnhum.2015.00626
30. Kothe, C.A.E., Jung, T.P.: Artifact removal techniques with signal reconstruction (2016). uS Patent App. 14/895,440
31. Li, R., Zhang, J.: Review of computational neuroaesthetics: bridging the gap between neuroaesthetics and computer science. Brain Inform. **7**, 1–17 (2020). https://doi.org/10.1186/s40708-020-00118-w
32. Molau, S., Pitz, M., Schluter, R., Ney, H.: Computing mel-frequency cepstral coefficients on the power spectrum. In: 2001 IEEE International Conference on Acoustics, Speech, and Signal Processing. Proceedings, vol. 1, pp. 73–76 (2001). https://doi.org/10.1109/ICASSP.2001.940770
33. Pessoa, L.: On the relationship between emotion and cognition. Nat. Rev. Neurosci. **9**(2), 148–158 (2008)
34. Pessoa, L., Adolphs, R.: Emotion processing and the amygdala: from a'low road'to'many roads' of evaluating biological significance. Nat. Rev. Neurosci. **11**(11), 773–782 (2010)
35. Pievani, M., Filippini, N., Van Den Heuvel, M.P., Cappa, S.F., Frisoni, G.B.: Brain connectivity in neurodegenerative diseases-from phenotype to proteinopathy. Nat. Rev. Neurol. **10**(11), 620–633 (2014)
36. Robbins, K.A., Touryan, J., Mullen, T., Kothe, C., Bigdely-Shamlo, N.: How sensitive are EEG results to preprocessing methods: a benchmarking study. IEEE Trans. Neural Syst. Rehabil. Eng. **28**(5), 1081–1090 (2020). https://doi.org/10.1109/TNSRE.2020.2980223
37. Sciaraffa, N., et al.: Mental effort estimation by passive BCI: a cross-subject analysis. In: 2021 43rd Annual International Conference of the IEEE Engineering in Medicine & Biology Society (EMBC), pp. 906–909. IEEE (2021). https://doi.org/10.1109/EMBC46164.2021.9630613

38. Suhaimi, N.S., Mountstephens, J., Teo, J., et al.: EEG-based emotion recognition: a state-of-the-art review of current trends and opportunities. Comput. Intell. Neurosci. **2020** (2020). https://doi.org/10.1155/2020/8875426
39. Vecchio, A., Mulas, F., Cola, G.: Posture recognition using the interdistances between wearable devices. IEEE Sens. Lett. **1**(4), 1–4 (2017). https://doi.org/10.1109/LSENS.2017.2726759
40. Yang, Y., Wu, Q., Qiu, M., Wang, Y., Chen, X.: Emotion recognition from multichannel EEG through parallel convolutional recurrent neural network. In: 2018 international joint conference on neural networks (IJCNN), pp. 1–7. IEEE (2018). https://doi.org/10.1109/IJCNN.2018.8489331

An Unsupervised Approach to Speed Up the Training of Multiple Models on Biomedical KGs

Leonardo De Grandis, Guido W. Di Donato$^{(\boxtimes)}$, and Marco D. Santambrogio

DEIB, Politecnico di Milano, Milan, Italy
leonardo1.degrandis@mail.polimi.it,
{guidowalter.didonato,marco.santambrogio}@polimi.it

Abstract. Knowledge Graphs (KGs) are powerful tools to represent complex networks with their interactions. This is especially true in the biomedical domain, where improvements in data collection techniques have enabled the construction of large networks combining information from heterogeneous data sources. Such biomedical KGs can be used to train different supervised Graph Machine Learning (GML) models for different predictive tasks. However, training multiple supervised GML models on massive KGs can result in prohibitive cumulative training time and costs, which hinders the adoption of such techniques.

For this reason, this work presents a methodology to reduce the cumulative time of multiple predictive models trained on the same KG, by leveraging an unsupervised GML approach. Our methodology consists of learning, in an unsupervised way, general representations of the graph's entities and relationships in the form of numerical vectors (i.e., embeddings), and then feeding such vectors to multiple classical machine learning models, each trained for a specific predictive task. We evaluated the proposed methodology on two relevant tasks, namely link prediction and multi-class link classification, on the open `ogbl-biokg` graph dataset. Experimental results show how our approach can reduce the cumulative training time for the two tasks by 27%, while also improving the prediction accuracy of 4% and 13% when compared to a classical supervised GML approach.

Keywords: Unsupervised Learning · Graph Representation Learning · Knowledge Graph Embedding

1 Introduction and Motivation

Recent trends in Big Data are leading to a massive amount of data collection and storage, with major research and development for tools and models that are able to provide insightful analyses. In particular, access to more and more healthcare data surely provides an unprecedented opportunity for data science technologies to derive data-driven insights and improve the quality of care delivery. For

M. Mizmizi et al. (Eds.): BodyNets 2024, LNICST 524, pp. 207–221, 2024.
https://doi.org/10.1007/978-3-031-72524-1_16

instance, Machine Learning (ML) techniques are being used in the biomedical context to achieve new research findings, but also to support diagnosis [9] and therapeutic planning [28]. Nonetheless, handling a massive amount of biomedical data of various kinds still constitutes an open challenge.

In this context, *Knowledge Graphs (KGs)* emerge as a powerful tool, given their ability to represent large volumes of heterogeneous data in a structured way (i.e., complex networks of entities and their relations), constituting a promising base for clinical decision support systems. Biomedical KGs are capable of modeling proteins' interactions, the reactions between drugs and diseases, and chemical effects, to name a few examples. One relevant application of KGs to this domain is the understanding of interactions between chemicals in many areas, from Drug Repurposing (DR) [26] to Drug-Target Interaction (DTI) to predict the binding of proteins to the ligands [7]. Indeed, in the context of drug development, experimental tests and validation require different time-consuming and costly stages. Therefore, automatically identifying promising interactions through the analysis of biomedical KGs can provide significant advantages, resulting in shorter time-to-market and reduced costs.

KGs enable different levels of automatic analysis. On the one hand, it is possible to implement *rule-based* decision systems that extract insights from the KG through structured queries and combine the results of such queries according to imperative rules. The main advantage of such an approach is the interpretability of the results. However, rule-based systems require running many specific queries on massive KGs; thus they do not scale well with the amount of data to be processed, and they strongly depend on the target application and the underlying graph ontology. Moreover, the different rules can generate conflicts that are hard to manage; this leads to significant difficulties in generating new complex rules that can provide better results and advance the state of the art.

On the other hand, *Graph Machine Learning (GML)* techniques allow us to automatically recognize inner patterns and perform predictions given the features of the input network. GML models can learn low-dimensionality representations (called *embeddings*) of nodes, links, or the whole graph, and use such representations for different predictive tasks. The main advantage of GML is that it provides a general approach that can be employed for many different applications. Moreover, GML-based methods are easily extensible to new data, thus providing great research opportunities. In particular, aggregating heterogeneous data in a KG can also benefit the GML models by adding depth to their internal representations. This means that a single KG, adequately constructed, can be utilized as input for different predictive tasks.

This is particularly important because one of the main drawbacks of KGs is that their construction is a burdensome job, which requires intensive human supervision and domain experts' knowledge. Fortunately, recent developments in Natual Language Processing (NLP) and Data Mining techniques enable to simplify and speed up this process, showing great potential for future developments. Examples are numerous in the biomedical and healthcare domain, where the help of language models is capable of recognizing chemical relations from literature with an average precision of 70% [6], or in network medicine to expand available datasets with new research developments [1]. However, the performance of automatic approaches is not good enough yet to completely handle the KG construction, which remains a time-consuming job requiring manual intervention. Thus, leveraging the same KG for different predictive tasks is an important opportunity to reduce the development time of GML-based applications.

Another critical factor to consider is that traditional GML models are *supervised*, which means that the models, and thus their internal representations, are specific to the task assigned. This allows developers to achieve good prediction performance but implies limited flexibility. Indeed, to perform different predictive tasks, different supervised GML models must be trained on the same data, one for each task. However, training a GML model is a time-consuming and compute-intensive task. Subsequently, training multiple supervised models on massive KGs can lead to prohibitive cumulative training time and costs. Such a problem is also well-known in other Deep Learning (DL) areas involving complex models that require lengthy and expensive training. To tackle such a challenge, *unsupervised learning* techniques have been proposed in the literature as a potential solution to reduce the training time of some DL models but, to the best of our knowledge, they have not largely investigated in the context of Graph Machine Learning [18].

For these reasons, this work proposes a methodology that uses unsupervised GML to reduce the *cumulative training time* of different predictors that leverage the same underlying KG. According to our methodology, unsupervised GML models are used as a pre-training routine, able to learn general *Knowledge Graph Embeddings (KGEs)*, without the need for explicit labeling. The obtained embeddings, which represent the original knowledge of the network in a low-dimensional latent space, can then be fed to classical supervised ML models for multiple downstream prediction tasks. Indeed, these classical models, such as Random Forests (RF) [3], XGboost [8], or Feed-Forward Neural Networks (FFNN) [21], can be trained in much less time than supervised GML models, resulting in lower cumulative training time. In this paper, we provide an experimental validation of the proposed approach on the open `ogbl-biokg` graph dataset. In particular, we validate our methodology on two relevant tasks: Drug-Disease Interaction (DDI) identification, crucial in Drug Repurposing applications [26], and Protein-Protein Interaction (PPI) classification, important in biological and medical research [7].

2 Background and Related Works

A KG is a representation of *heterogeneous entities and the relations among them*. The entities are the *nodes* of the network and they can have features, while their interactions are the *edges* of the network. This structure is capable of reconstructing a complex and multi-domain semantic that can be fed to GML models to formulate predictions [16].

Current GML models perform an embedding of the input data, learning a meaningful representation of the KG in a low-dimensionality feature space that encapsulates the information contained in the dataset [2,25]. In this process, the scoring function, the embedding dimension, the model's choice, and the considered features, play a relevant role in the obtained KGEs. At each iteration, the embeddings are fed to the last layers of the models to obtain the desired predictions. These predictions are involved in the feedback mechanism and will influence the next iteration of the training procedure. This is the underlying mechanism of supervised GML models, where the generation of the embeddings is trained together with the prediction layers, so the process is specialized for a single task. If multiple tasks, such as link prediction and classification are required, the embeddings must be learned multiple times, requiring intensive resources and time.

Alternatively, as we propose in this work, the embeddings can be learned in an unsupervised way and then used as input to multiple classical supervised ML models to generate the predictions. Such an approach has the advantage that the *representation learning* phase, which learns how to compress the knowledge included in the network into mathematical vectors, is done only once in an unsupervised manner. In this case, the loss function - to be minimized during the training - is simply a graph reconstruction error, which does not require any external labels. The obtained representations in the latent space are then general and not task-specific, so they can be used as input to multiple ML predictive models, that need a much shorter training time [18,19].

It is also important to notice that, despite all recent developments, the understanding of the learning process of a DL architecture remains an open problem. In this area, extensive research has been carried out by Ehran et al. [10,11] to understand how *unsupervised routines can help the optimization process*. Their findings show that the unsupervised pre-training successfully guides the supervised training towards minima that support better generalization. When starting from random initialization (without unsupervised pre-training), as the complexity of deep models grows, they show a higher probability of finding poor apparent local minima. Instead, with the pre-training, deep models proved to be more robust in their behavior. Moreover, the pre-training phase brings us to a more favorable region of the parameters space, close to deeper basins of attraction, and it also has a regularization effect, providing not necessarily better training error but systematically better test error. Thus, the procedure seems to be able to guarantee better generalization capabilities for deep models. This technique became well-known in various fields, such as Computer Vision [5,23] and NLP [27]. More and more methods are adopting this procedure to cope with poorly labeled data or to augment available information [7,18,19,24].

In this work, we propose a similar methodology in the context of Graph Machine Learning. We show that by leveraging the proposed methodology, with the proper choice of downstream ML models for end-tasks, it is possible to obtain similar or even higher performance compared to a classical supervised GML pipeline, while also achieving a significant reduction in the overall training time. Moreover, for the final predictive tasks, simple models such as RF or XGBoost produce remarkable performance while being available in common development frameworks and code libraries, providing an off-the-shelf, easy-to-use, and time-saving solution.

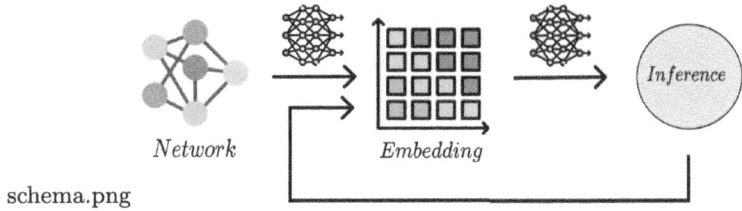

schema.png

Fig. 1. GML training schema. Supervised training has a feedback mechanism based on label predictions to update model parameters.

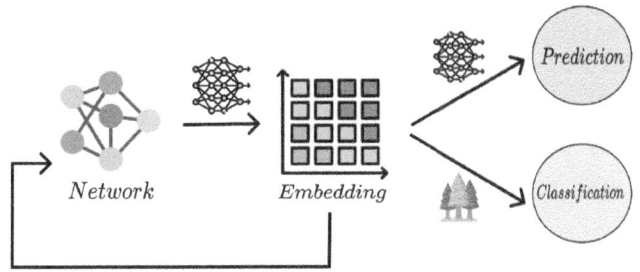

Fig. 2. Unsupervised training schema. Unsupervised training has a feedback mechanism based just on input data to generate the embedding vectors.

3 Data and Methods

As illustrated in the previous section, traditional supervised GML models are generally based on a Neural Network with some Message Passing Layers [15] that reduce network topology and features into embedding vectors of desired dimension. The final layers instead are used to perform inference tasks, such as binary prediction or multi-class classification. Thus, such models require proper training for every task, as shown in Fig. 1.

The alternative approach, proposed in this work and shown in Fig. 2, consists of learning only one set of embedding vectors (one for each entity in the graph), which has to be general and represent the knowledge of the entire network. Common techniques for unsupervised learning on graphs are *DeepGraphInfomax* [30] or the *Variational Grah Auto Encoders* (VGAEs) [20], which are specifically adopted in this work. With VGAEs, the embeddings are obtained by training the model to compress the graph and reconstruct its adjacency matrix, so no labels are needed for the procedure. Once this step is completed, the final different prediction tasks can be performed with ML models such as XGBoost, RF, or NNs. The overall computational advantage consists of having only one representation learning phase, which is computationally demanding since it has a lot of parameters to optimize, and relying on classical ML models (easier to implement and faster to train) for the different downstream predictive tasks.

In the remainder of the section, we present the graph dataset employed in this work and an overview of the processing steps we implemented to leverage such a

Table 1. Distribution of nodes across the classes in the `ogbl-biokg`.

Node type	Number of nodes
Disease	10687
Drug	10533
Protein function	45085
Protein	17499
Side effect	9969

Table 2. Distribution of Protein-Protein Interaction links across the classes in the `ogbl-biokg`, after merging.

Class	Number of links
0	115846
1	292253
2	303433
3	352507

dataset as the input to GML models. Then, we provide a detailed description of how we implemented both the proposed methodology, leveraging unsupervised GML for pre-training and supervised ML for the predictive tasks, and different baselines leveraging the classical supervised ML and GML approaches.

3.1 Dataset Description and Predictive Tasks Formulation

In this work, we used the open `ogbl-biokg` [17], a graph containing information obtained from many different biomedical repositories. Such a database allows users to get insights into human biology and guide biomedical developments, proving to be a relevant instrument for the research field. The `ogbl-biokg` is an heterogeneous KG composed of 93773 nodes and 4762678 links. Nodes and edges represent the entities in the graph and their relationships, and they are subdivided into 5 and 51 classes respectively. Table 1 shows the distribution of the nodes among the 5 classes in the graph.

For what concerns the investigated predictive tasks, we chose two applications that are relevant in the biomedical context. The first task is the Drug-Disease Interaction (DDI) prediction, which is critical in Drug Repurposing applications. DDI prediction can be easily formulated as a binary link prediction on the `ogbl-biokg`, targeting Drug-Disease links. In detail, the DDI edges present in the network are 5147. The same number of negative samples is generated from non-existing links to provide negative examples for balanced training. They have been then split in $80\% - 10\% - 10\%$ for training, validation, and test sets respectively.

The second task, instead, is the classification of Protein-Protein Interactions (PPIs), which is critical in computational biology research. This task can be formulated as a multi-class classification of the link between two proteins. In this case, the number of total PPI links is 1064039, and they are split into 8 different classes in the original dataset. Since these 8 categories are not uniformly distributed, the 5 less numerous classes have been merged to balance the data and obtain an easier classification task. This choice is motivated by our intent not to provide the best solution for PPI prediction or any other specific task. Instead, we want to demonstrate that, when there is the need for numerous predictive tasks on the same KG, learning embeddings in an unsupervised way and feeding them to multiple downstream ML models is more convenient than using multiple supervised GML models. The result of our choice is an easier 4-labels classification task, whose distribution is shown in Table 2. A stratified sampling strategy is then applied to obtain a split of $80\% - 10\% - 10\%$ for training, validation, and test sets respectively, to be used in the training and evaluation of the models.

It is important to note that, in the `ogbl-biokg`, neither nodes nor edges have numerical features associated with them. The only information related to nodes and edges is the label that provides the class of each entity and relation. To leverage such information during the representation learning phase, we transformed the heterogeneous `ogbl-biokg` graph to a homogeneous network by one-hot encoding the classes of the entities and relations as features. This allows us to exploit simpler homogeneous GML models without losing the information contained in the dataset. In the case of the PPI classification task, we omitted the edges' types from the feature vectors to avoid an information leak in the training that would have caused overoptimistic performance estimations.

3.2 The Proposed Methodology

Before presenting the details of our approach, we describe the different baselines employed in our study. A first immediate baseline is obtained by performing both the DDI and PPI tasks with traditional ML models. In particular, we used a simple NN and XGBoost. To implement such a baseline, we manually created the embedding vectors of the links by simply concatenating the head and tail nodes' feature vectors. This strategy, intuitively, cannot produce valuable results since the only information encoded in the embedding vectors are the types of the related nodes, while the structural topology of the network is not taken into account.

Therefore, we attempted another strategy to obtain a more significant classical ML baseline. In order to provide the models with relevant topology information, we performed data augmentation by appending structural metrics to each node's feature vector. In particular, the chosen metrics are different forms of centrality, i.e. *closeness, betweenness, harmonic,* and *degree centrality,* and two other topological metrics, i.e. the *clustering coefficient* and the *number of triangles* per node. Given the size of the `ogbl-biokg` network, the computation of such metrics would not be feasible in a reasonable time with classical graph processing libraries, such as NetworkX [13]. Thus, to speed up the metrics computation, we exploited the functionalities offered by GRAPE [4]. GRAPE is a

Table 3. GML link prediction GCN model parameters.

Parameter	Value
GCN layers	2
GCN sizes	64
Training epochs	200
Loss function	BinaryCrossEntropy
Learning rate	$1e-3$
Optimizer	Adam

Table 4. GML link classification GCN and GAT model parameters.

Parameter	Value
Layers	2
Sizes	64
Training epochs	750
Loss function	CrossEntropy
Dropout	0.2
Learning rate	$1e-3$
Optimizer	Adam

high-performance graph analysis library developed in Rust with Python bindings, which is a much faster alternative than more common libraries available in Python. This choice allowed us to expedite the computation of the shortest paths involved in the feature calculations, which would have been a bottleneck when processing a big graph such as `ogbl-biokg`.

Supervised Graph Machine Learning Approach. The direct GML baseline is implemented by adopting the PyTorch Geometric library [12]. This approach allows us to leverage both feature vectors and the network's topology for our predictive tasks, resulting in great predictive performance improvement at the cost of increased computation time. In particular, the model for DDI link prediction implements Graph Convolutional Network (GCN) layers. On the other hand, for the PPI classification task, we investigated both GCN and Graph Attention Network (GAT) layers to compare their performance in such a more challenging task. Table 3 and 4 respectively provide a summary of the parameters of the link prediction and link classification GML models.

Unsupervised Pre-training Approach. To perform the unsupervised embedding of nodes and links of the graph, we adopted an encoder-decoder architecture with a VGAE model [14]. This model does not require any label during the training since it learns a meaningful representation of the network by

Table 5. VGAE unsupervised model parameters.

Parameter	Value
Layers	2
Sizes	64
Training epochs	200
Loss function	Graph reconstruction error
Dropout	0.2
Learning rate	$1e - 2$
Optimizer	Adam

compressing the input data into a low-dimensionality feature space z with the encoder module, and then reconstructing the adjacency matrix A of the graph with the decoder module. The total reconstruction loss also includes a component based on the Kullback-Leibler divergence, shown in Eq. (1), to make the overall procedure more robust to noise.

$$loss = Sigmoid(Sum(z * z')) + KL_{loss} \qquad (1)$$

The power of this methodology is that, without any explicit labeling, the learned vectors are already capturing relevant knowledge about the structure and topology of the KG. The VGAE has been tested with different layers, such as GCN, GAT, and Sample and Aggregation (SAGE), while the training settings remained unchanged and are shown in Table 5.

After the embedding vectors are obtained with this method, we perform the two tasks of prediction and classification using them as input. The adopted models are again XGBoost and a NN, the same used for the ML baseline. The Random Forest algorithm was also tested, but we are not reporting the related results since XGBoost performed better in all the tasks.

4   Experimental Results

This section presents the results related to the previously presented methodologies. The considered evaluation metric is the *F1-score* for both the link prediction and classification tasks. All the reported results are obtained by running experiments on a virtual machine equipped with an Intel Xeon Platinum $8167M$, 12 core, $72GB$ RAM, and one NVIDIA Tesla $P100$ with $16GB$ RAM, as available on the Oracle Cloud Infrastructure (OCI). The training procedure has been accelerated by leveraging the GPU through the Pytorch+CUDA framework.

Classical Supervised Machine Learning. As shown in Table 6, the first ML baseline, as expected, cannot produce significant results (due to the lack of informative features in addition to the node types. Moreover, Table 7 shows

Table 6. Experimental results of the baseline ML approach.

Task	F1-score
Link prediction	0.5 ± 0.00
Link classification	0.33 ± 0.00

Table 7. Experimental results of the baseline augmented ML approach.

Task	Model	F1-score
Link prediction	NN	0.57 ± 0.02
	XGB	0.77 ± 0.03
Link classification	NN	0.33 ± 0.00
	XGB	0.33 ± 0.00

Table 8. GML models training time and their prediction scores.

Task	Layer	Time [s]	F1-score
Prediction	GCN	431.2 ± 12.4	0.88 ± 0.03
Classification	GCN	545.6 ± 13.9	0.45 ± 0.04
	GAT	590.5 ± 18.1	0.45 ± 0.05

how data augmentation with network topology metrics helps improve the performance of the ML models. We can notice how the more challenging task of PPI classification is still not benefiting from the augmentation process. On the other hand, for the simpler task of DDI prediction, combining the data augmentation strategy with a state-of-the-art classifier, like XGBoost, provides a significant improvement.

Supervised Graph Machine Learning. Adopting a GML approach allows us to complete both tasks with a significant performance improvement, as shown in Table 8. This method benefits from both node features and network topology information, capturing the inner knowledge contained in the KG. Again, we can notice the same pattern of the previously exposed results. The link prediction task is now performing properly, while classification is still struggling, even if the performance gain is noticeable. These results can be used as a proper baseline to evaluate the results of the proposed unsupervised approach.

Our Methodology. The training, according to the proposed methodology, can be divided into two phases. The first one is the representation learning phase, which consists of optimizing the VGAE model until it generates informative embeddings. This phase is the longest one, and it took $701.3\,s \pm 21.2$ to complete, on average. The second phase is the training of downstream predictors using

Table 9. Link prediction results from the unsupervised embeddings.

Embedding layer	Neural Network	XGBoost
GCN	0.89 ± 0.03	0.92 ± 0.02
SAGE	0.86 ± 0.04	0.88 ± 0.02
GAT	0.80 ± 0.05	0.85 ± 0.03
Average train time [s]	3.71 ± 0.16	0.72 ± 0.02

Table 10. Link classification results from the unsupervised embeddings.

Embedding layer	Neural Network	XGBoost
GCN	0.42 ± 0.03	0.51 ± 0.02
SAGE	0.37 ± 0.05	0.34 ± 0.04
GAT	0.39 ± 0.04	0.34 ± 0.04
Average train time [s]	278.47 ± 8.17	7.09 ± 0.28

classical supervised ML models, whose training times are shorter than their GML counterparts, as shown in Table 9 and 10.

Table 9 and 10 show that the performance of the unsupervised + NN strategy is, in general, comparable to the GML baseline, with a $+1\%$ in prediction and a -7% in classification. The choice of adopting a different classifier, XGBoost, provides instead a relevant improvement, with $+4.5\%$ and $+13\%$ respectively. This proves that XGBoost is the most suitable model for such a classification problem, leveraging as input the embedding vectors computed through the VGAE. Another significant result relates to the cumulative training time of the two predictive tasks. As the tables show, the unsupervised GML + NN approach requires comparable cumulative training times with the GML baseline, $983.4s$ and 976.8 respectively, for an overall $+1\%$ of total computational time. Instead, XGBoost proves to be very efficient in the training, even with a large training sets (as in the case of the PPI classification task), resulting in a cumulative training time of $709s$ and, thus, providing a -27% reduction of the total time when compared to the GML baseline.

4.1 Discussion

To interpret and understand the results obtained by the models, we performed a dimensionality reduction of the embeddings with t-SNE [22]. From an embedding vector of length of 64, as generated by the unsupervised VGAE, we extracted compressed representations made of only 2 and 3 features. Figure 3 shows the 2D representation associated with the labels of the DDI prediction task, and the 3D representation associated with the labels of the PPI classification tasks. In both cases, we can notice a visible separation of the samples with different labels. This means that the VGAE proved to be an effective algorithm in learning a meaningful representation of the KG that, in turn, can lead to good performance of the end tasks as well.

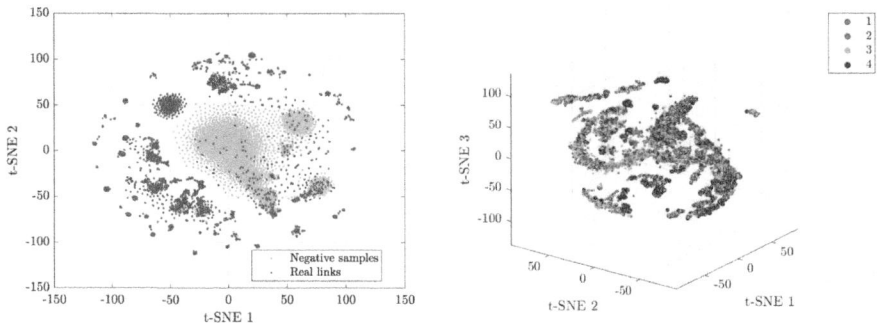

Fig. 3. t-SNE dimensionality reduction of the embedding generated from VGAE with GCN layers, for both the link prediction (left) and link classification (right) tasks.

As suggested by Erhan et al. [10,11], the unsupervised contribution can lead the overall training process to minima with better generalization capabilities. We applied the same procedure based on a functional approximation, comparing input-output functions rather than directly comparing model parameters, which produced similar results. To visualize the training trajectories, the outputs of the models in the test set were concatenated to form a vector representing the function space. This vector is generated for every iteration of the training process and the full trajectory can be mapped in a lower-dimensionality space with feature reduction techniques, such as ISOMAP [29]. In Fig. 4, the color from dark blue to cyan indicates the progression of the training trajectories of 50 GML models for link prediction and 50 unsupervised + NN models.

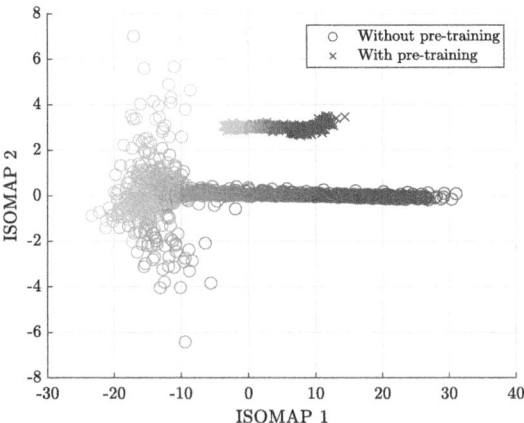

Fig. 4. Functional space approximation during training evolution reduced with ISOMAP.

As we can see, the trajectory of the model without pre-training shows greater variability in the final endpoints of the learning. With the pre-training, the learning moves in a different and much narrower function space, which also implies different model parameters. This evidence supports the hypothesis that the unsupervised routine acts like a regularizer during the training, constraining the parameters in a more favorable region.

5   Conclusions

In this work, we proposed a methodology that uses unsupervised Graph Machine Learning to reduce the cumulative training time of different predictors that leverage the same underlying Knowledge Graph. Experimental results showed how eliminating the redundancy in the representation learning phase, by using an unsupervised approach, can significantly reduce the total training time while also providing improvements in the predictive scores. Our results show also an important dependency on the choice of an adequate classifier for downstream tasks, such as XGBoost in the investigated cases. Another important consideration is that GCN layers performed generally better both in GML predictions and unsupervised embedding generation. This is probably due to the presence of few relevant features for the nodes. We believe that more complex layers, such as SAGE and GAT, could provide better performance than GCN layers in the case of KG containing many numerical features for each entity.

Possible future developments include the research and optimization of adequate cost functions related to the unsupervised embedding procedure. Another area of improvement could be an investigation of how data augmentation with relevant features can affect embedding results. Finally, it is worth noticing how the proposed methodology is domain-agnostic and can be applied to other contexts where using the same graph database for multiple predictions is a valuable opportunity. Thus, we plan to validate our methodology in different domains, beyond the biomedical one, to demonstrate how it can be beneficial for many GML-based applications.

References

1. Barabási, A.L., Menichetti, G., Loscalzo, J.: The unmapped chemical complexity of our diet. Nature Food **1**(1), 33–37 (2020)
2. Bonner, S., et al.: Understanding the performance of knowledge graph embeddings in drug discovery. Artif. Intell. Life Sci. **2**, 100036 (2022)
3. Breiman, L.: Random forests. Mach. Learn. **45**, 5–32 (2001)
4. Cappelletti, L., et al.: Grape for fast and scalable graph processing and random-walk-based embedding. Nature Comput. Sci. **3**(6), 552–568 (2023)
5. Caron, M., Bojanowski, P., Mairal, J., Joulin, A.: Unsupervised pre-training of image features on non-curated data. In: Proceedings of the IEEE/CVF International Conference on Computer Vision, pp. 2959–2968 (2019)

6. Cenikj, G., Strojnik, L., Angelski, R., Ogrinc, N., Koroušić Seljak, B., Eftimov, T.: From language models to large-scale food and biomedical knowledge graphs. Sci. Rep. **13**(1), 7815 (2023)
7. Chatterjee, A., et al.: Improving the generalizability of protein-ligand binding predictions with AI-bind. Nat. Commun. **14**(1), 1989 (2023)
8. Chen, T., Guestrin, C.: XGBoost: a scalable tree boosting system. In: Proceedings of the 22nd ACM SIGKDD International Conference on Knowledge Discovery and Data Mining, pp. 785–794 (2016)
9. D'Arnese, E., di Donato, G.W., del Sozzo, E., Santambrogio, M.D.: Towards an automatic imaging biopsy of non-small cell lung cancer. In: 2019 IEEE EMBS International Conference on Biomedical & Health Informatics (BHI), pp. 1–4 (2019). https://doi.org/10.1109/BHI.2019.8834485
10. Erhan, D., Courville, A., Bengio, Y., Vincent, P.: Why does unsupervised pre-training help deep learning? In: Proceedings of the Thirteenth International Conference on Artificial Intelligence and Statistics, pp. 201–208. JMLR Workshop and Conference Proceedings (2010)
11. Erhan, D., Manzagol, P.A., Bengio, Y., Bengio, S., Vincent, P.: The difficulty of training deep architectures and the effect of unsupervised pre-training. In: Artificial Intelligence and Statistics, pp. 153–160. PMLR (2009)
12. Fey, M., Lenssen, J.E.: Fast graph representation learning with PyTorch geometric. In: ICLR Workshop on Representation Learning on Graphs and Manifolds (2019)
13. Hagberg, A., Conway, D.: NetworkX: network analysis with python (2020). https://networkxgithub.io
14. Hamilton, W.L., Ying, R., Leskovec, J.: Representation learning on graphs: methods and applications. arXiv preprint arXiv:1709.05584 (2017)
15. Hamilton, W.L., Ying, R., Leskovec, J.: Representation learning on graphs: methods and applications (2018)
16. Hogan, A., et al.: Knowledge graphs. ACM Comput. Surv. (CSUR) **54**(4), 1–37 (2021)
17. Hu, W., et al.: Open graph benchmark: datasets for machine learning on graphs. Adv. Neural. Inf. Process. Syst. **33**, 22118–22133 (2020)
18. Hu, W., et al.: Strategies for pre-training graph neural networks. arXiv preprint arXiv:1905.12265 (2019)
19. Hu, Z., Fan, C., Chen, T., Chang, K.W., Sun, Y.: Unsupervised pre-training of graph convolutional networks. In: ICLR 2019 Workshop: Representation Learning on Graphs and Manifolds (2019)
20. Kipf, T.N., Welling, M.: Variational graph auto-encoders. arXiv preprint arXiv:1611.07308 (2016)
21. LeCun, Y., Bengio, Y., Hinton, G.: Deep learning. Nature **521**(7553), 436–444 (2015)
22. Van der Maaten, L., Hinton, G.: Visualizing data using t-SNE. J. Mach. Learn. Res. **9**(11) (2008)
23. Paine, T.L., Khorrami, P., Han, W., Huang, T.S.: An analysis of unsupervised pre-training in light of recent advances. arXiv preprint arXiv:1412.6597 (2014)
24. Pellegrini, C., Navab, N., Kazi, A.: Unsupervised pre-training of graph transformers on patient population graphs. Med. Image Anal. **89**, 102895 (2023)
25. Pradipta Gema, A., et al.: Knowledge graph embeddings in the biomedical domain: Are they useful? A look at link prediction, rule learning, and downstream polypharmacy tasks. arXiv e-prints, pp. arXiv–2305 (2023)

26. Ramalli, E., Parravicini, A., Di Donato, G.W., Salaris, M., Hudelot, C., Santambrogio, M.D.: Demystifying drug repurposing domain comprehension with knowledge graph embedding. In: 2021 IEEE Biomedical Circuits and Systems Conference (BioCAS), pp. 1–5. IEEE (2021)

27. Schneider, S., Baevski, A., Collobert, R., Auli, M.: wav2vec: unsupervised pretraining for speech recognition. arXiv preprint arXiv:1904.05862 (2019)

28. Stoppa, E., Di Donato, G.W., Parde, N., Santambrogio, M.D.: Computer-aided dementia detection: how informative are your features? In: 2022 IEEE 7th Forum on Research and Technologies for Society and Industry Innovation (RTSI), pp. 55–61. IEEE (2022)

29. Tenenbaum, J.B., Silva, V.D., Langford, J.C.: A global geometric framework for nonlinear dimensionality reduction. Science **290**(5500), 2319–2323 (2000)

30. Veličković, P., Fedus, W., Hamilton, W.L., Liò, P., Bengio, Y., Hjelm, R.D.: Deep graph infomax. arXiv preprint arXiv:1809.10341 (2018)

Privacy and Security in Wireless Body Area Networks

Performance Evaluation of Distance-Based Random Mean Shift Clustering and Humpback Whale Optimization Algorithm for Sink Node Placement in WBAN

Maria Hanif[1], Rizwan Ahmad[1]([envelope]), Waqas Ahmed[2], Micheal Drieberg[3], and Muhammad Mahtab Alam[4]

[1] School of Electrical Engineering and Computer Science (SEECS), National University of Sciences and Technology (NUST), Islamabad 44000, Pakistan
{mhanif.phdcs20seecs,rizwan.ahmad}@seecs.edu.pk

[2] Department of Electrical Engineering, Pakistan Institute of Engineering and Applied Sciences (PIEAS), Islamabad 44000, Pakistan
waqas@pieas.edu.pk

[3] Department of Electrical and Electronic Engineering, Universiti Teknologi PETRONAS, Seri Iskandar 32610, Malaysia
mdrieberg@utp.edu.my

[4] Thomas Johann Seebeck Department of Electronics, Tallinn University of Technology, 12616 Tallinn, Estonia
muhammad.alam@taltech.ee

Abstract. Wireless Body Area Networks (WBANs) have transformed human life, bringing about notable advancements in healthcare, fitness, entertainment, and sports applications. Sink node placement in WBANs has an impact on network connectivity, power efficiency, and overall network performance. Designing the placement of sinks in Wireless Body Area Networks (WBANs) poses two significant challenges: ensuring energy efficiency and establishing robust connectivity. To track a patient's vital signs, sensor nodes of a WBAN are implanted in various locations throughout the patient. Additionally, a sink node receives the physiological data sent by the WBAN sensor nodes. As a result, choosing the best position for the central hub node turns out to be essential for minimizing node energy consumption during data transmission. Considering the hardness of the problem, this paper presents Distance-based random mean shift clustering(D-RMS). In D-RMS we apply: a) Random coordinator placement and b) Mean shift clustering algorithm to compute optimal position and compare it with the state-of-the-art approaches i.e.; Humpback Whale Optimization Algorithm (HWOA) for sink node placement. The best position of coordinator placement using D-RMS and HWOA is $(97.9175, 115.76)$ and $(97,100)$. The results demonstrate that the suggested approach (D-RMS) is more stable and has lower localization errors than earlier ones. Overall, the residual energy of D-RMS is 92% and HWOA is 90%. Moreover, the

M. Mizmizi et al. (Eds.): BodyNets 2024, LNICST 524, pp. 225–245, 2024.
https://doi.org/10.1007/978-3-031-72524-1_17

Average localization error (ALE) of D-RMS and HWOA is *0.568* m and *0.619* m.

Keywords: Wireless body area network · Humpback Whale optimization algorithm (HWOA) · Node placement · D-RMS shift clustering

1   Introduction

Wireless Body Area Networks (WBANs) use wireless communication technologies to connect wearable or implantable devices or a central monitoring system. These devices are commonly positioned either on or inside the human body, capable of measuring diverse physiological parameters, including heart rate, blood pressure, temperature, and oxygen saturation. WBANs have many potential applications, particularly in the healthcare industry. They can be used to monitor patients with chronic diseases, such as diabetes, heart disease, and hypertension, in real-time, allowing for early diagnosis and timely intervention. WBANs can also be used to monitor the health of athletes, soldiers, and workers in hazardous environments, such as mines and factories [1]. The design and implementation of WBANs present many challenges, particularly in terms of power management, data transmission, and security. Due to their proximity to the human body, WBANs must be designed to be safe, comfortable, and unobtrusive. Moreover, the data transmitted by WBANs must be reliable and accurate, and the network must be secure to prevent unauthorized access or tampering [2,3]. Despite these challenges, WBANs have garnered significant interest and attention from researchers and developers, with many innovative solutions and technologies being developed in recent years. Several technologies employed in Wireless Body Area Networks (WBANs) encompass Bluetooth, Zigbee, and WiFi. Additionally, more specialized protocols like Medical Implant Communication Service (MICS) and Wireless Medical Telemetry Service (WMTS) play crucial roles in this domain [4,5]. WBANs are a promising technology with many potential applications in healthcare and beyond [6,7]. As research and development continue to progress, we can expect to see many exciting and innovative WBAN-based solutions being developed in the years to come. The strategic placement of coordinator nodes in a Wireless Body Area Network (WBAN) is pivotal for ensuring optimal, dependable, and secure communication among sensor nodes. This placement significantly influences key aspects such as network performance, energy efficiency, and the quality of collected data, underscoring its critical importance in the design and deployment of WBANs. In reference [8], the placement of body nodes on the human body considers three distinct positions: waist (Location 1), upper limb (Location 2), and head (Location 3). In [9], a node is positioned in one of three different locations due to the frequent changes in posture of human legs. Specifically, the central node is placed on the head instead of the lower leg. In our "Distance-based Random Mean Shift algorithm", we position six sensors at fixed locations and introduce (25, 50, 75, 100) coordinators on random body parts. Subsequently, we apply a mean shift clustering algorithm to identify cluster centers, which represent the average positions of the combined nodes, converging to a local mode. The BNC placement scheme in Wireless Body Area Networks (WBANs) employing Multi-Objective Particle Swarm Optimization (MO-PSO) demonstrates the capability to identify the optimal location for the Body Node Coordinator (BNC). This leads to a decrease in network energy consumption and an extension of the network lifetime, as mentioned in the work by [10]. In the "Humpback Whale Optimization Algorithm", certain whales exhibit an "encircling prey" behavior during their search. This behavior entails a group of whales making random movements around potential prey, aiming to discover an improved position for sink placement.

1.1 Background and Overview of WBAN

Wireless Body Area Networks (WBANs) comprise a collection of small, low-power, and wearable sensors positioned on or near the human body. These sensors are engineered to observe diverse physiological parameters, including heart rate, body temperature, blood pressure, and blood glucose levels. Subsequently, the gathered data is transmitted to a central monitoring station for in-depth analysis, as referenced in [12] and [13]. The architecture of a WBAN typically Comprises three main components: sensors, a wireless communication channel, and a central monitoring station as shown in Fig. 1.

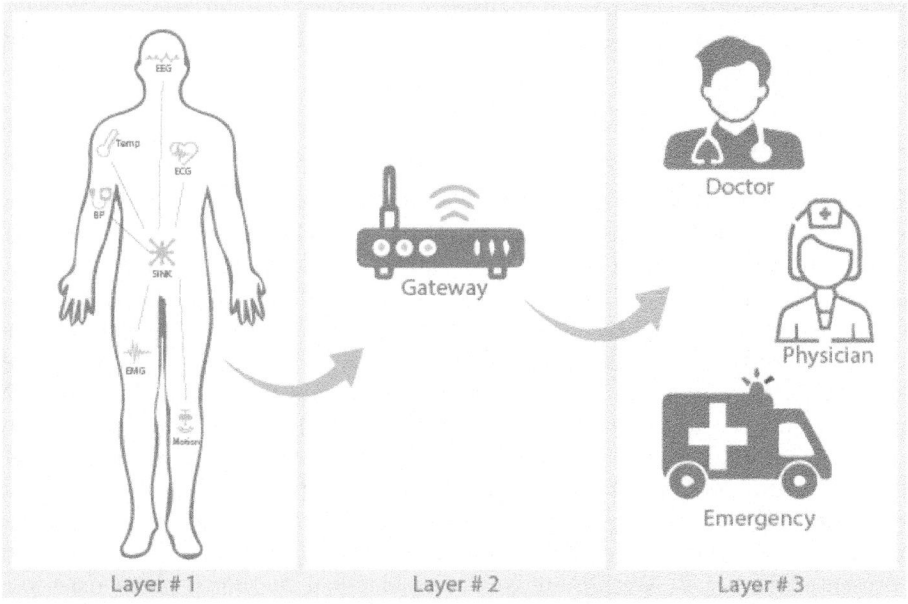

Fig. 1. WBAN Architecture

Sensors: The sensors within a Wireless Body Area Network (WBAN) are crafted to assess a range of physiological metrics, including heart rate, body temperature, blood glucose levels, and blood pressure. These sensors can be placed on the body or close to it, and they are typically low-power and miniaturized to minimize discomfort and interference with the user's daily activities.

Wireless Communication Channel: The wireless communication channel is used to convey the data collected by sensors to central monitoring station. The choice of wireless technology depends on the application requirements, such as the range, data rate, and power consumption. Common wireless technologies used in WBANs include Bluetooth, ZigBee, and Wi-Fi.

Central Monitoring Station: The central monitoring station is responsible for processing the information gathered by the sensors and providing feedback to the user or healthcare provider. The central monitoring station can be a dedicated device, a smartphone, or a tablet. The feedback can be in the form of alerts, notifications, or recommendations. The architecture of a WBAN can also include a gateway, which acts as an interface between the WBAN and other networks, such as the Internet. The gateway has the capability to transmit data to a distant monitoring center, enabling healthcare providers to oversee patients in real-time and offer timely interventions as needed. Overall, the architecture of a WBAN is designed to be low-power, unobtrusive, and comfortable for the user, while also providing accurate and continuous monitoring of physiological parameters. The sensors collect the physiological data, the wireless communication channel transmits the data, and the central monitoring station processes the data and provides feedback to the user or healthcare provider. The gateway can transfer data to remote monitoring centers, enabling real-time monitoring and timely interventions.

2   Related Work

In this section, we delve into research efforts focused on the optimal placement of nodes in Wireless Body Area Networks (WBANs). The placement of these sensors and nodes is critical to ensure accurate monitoring of the vital signs, and thus, the design of the WBAN must take into consideration the body postures of the person wearing the sensors. In a comprehensive review of WBAN, the authors noted that the positioning of the sensors on the body is influenced by the body postures of the person wearing them and that the design of the WBAN must take into account the possible changes in body postures. This is especially crucial for medical applications of WBANs, which require accurate and continuous monitoring of the patient's physiological indicators. Node localization can be categorized into two overarching categories. Classical methods and artificial intelligence methods. The classification of localization methodologies is visually represented in Fig. 2. Within the realm of classical methods, there exist two subcategories: Angle-based Techniques, encompassing Angle of Arrival (AOA), Triangulation, and Multiangulation; and Distance-based Techniques, comprising Time of Arrival (TOA), Received Signal Strength Indicator (RSSI), Trilateration, and Multilateration. On the other hand, artificial intelligence methods

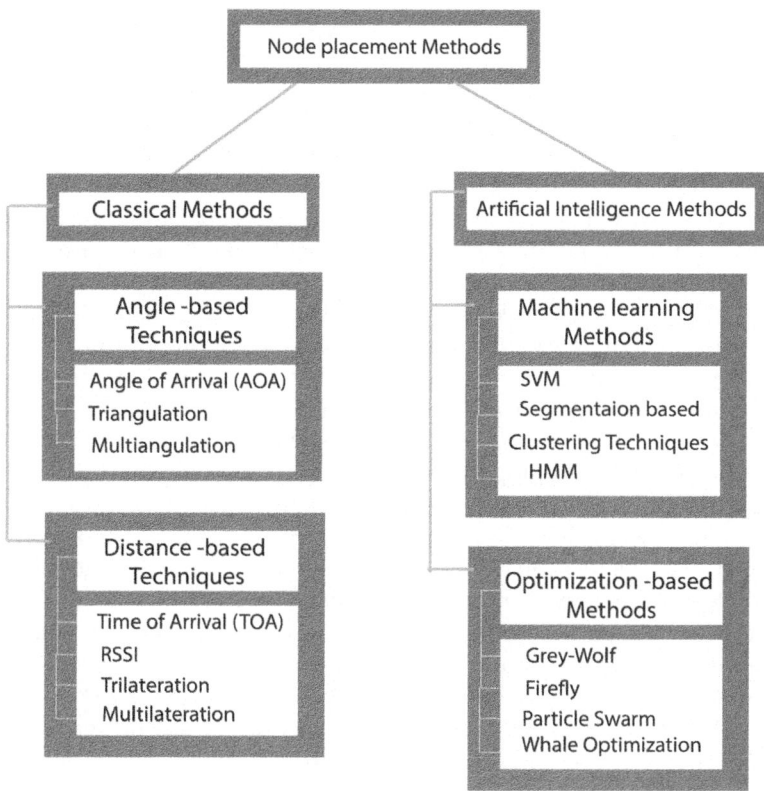

Fig. 2. Node placement Techniques

can be further categorized into Machine Learning methods, specifically Clustering and Segmentation-based approaches. Additionally, the second approach involves Optimization-based methods, such as Grey-wolf optimization, Firefly optimization, Particle Swarm optimization, and Whale optimization techniques. This taxonomy provides a structured framework for understanding the diverse approaches employed in node placement. Tamil et al. in [11] main focus is to increase the network lifetime of sensor nodes placed on the body, so MPAA (adjusted position-aware algorithm) was proposed as a flexible Body Node Coordinator (BNC), this is where the battery of each node is shared among all nodes. Hardeep et al. [14] compare two routing protocols (SIMPLE and ATTEMPT) with varying body posture mobility (head, leg, and arm movement). Results indicate that when the hub is positioned at the body's center without posture mobility performs better but more packets drop. Moreover, when a hub is placed on different body parts with posture mobility and when a node is fixed on a specific body position, both affect the performance of the SIMPLE protocol. Network lifetime is improved in the SIMPLE protocol. The authors Jasem et al. [4] evaluate the performance of three protocols i.e.; Ad Hoc on-demand Distance vector, Ad Hoc on-demand Multi-path Distance vector, and Destination sequence distance vector for different mobility models where the hub is placed at a fixed position [15] Multi-path destination distance outperforms regarding end-to-end delay, energy, and throughput. Patra and Kabat [16] challenge to reduce relay node cost, and energy usage and unevenly distribute loads among nodes. Researchers proposed an adaptive cuckoo search model that uses a fitness function for the placement of the relay node. 13 biosensors are fixedly positioned in two different body positions, and 50–100 node installations are also taken into consideration. In addition, we also tested the scalability of our method, 80 biosensors were randomly placed in a rectangle region comprising 50–300 potential locations. The simulation results demonstrate that the proposed algorithm not only consumes less energy compared to its alternatives but also distributes the load among the relay nodes in a fair manner. This work [17,18] offers a comprehensive data routing approach for WBAN that integrates a cluster routing protocol with a multi-criteria particle swarm optimization (MO-PSO) as a BNC placement technique. The suggested method makes use of a particle structure with three variables, the first two of which give the coordination of the BNC and the third of which specifies the node acting as the cluster head. The fitness of MO-PSO particles is estimated using a multi-criteria fitness evaluation operator using the average bit error rate (BER) and network energy consumption recorded within a single data transmission loop. The created model develops into an ideal BNC site that simultaneously reduces average BER and network energy consumption. Moreover, a lower BER results in a significant boost to the network throughput rate. Table 1 shows contributions related to Hub placement.

3   Proposed Work

For the health monitoring application of WBAN, sensors are placed on the body so that all of the patient's critical indications can be estimated and data can be communicated effectively. In our proposed framework, the Wireless Body Area Network (WBAN) is conceptualized as an undirected graph.
$G = \{S\_n, H\_n, D\_sh, L\}$ where;
$S\_n = (S\_n1, S\_n2, S\_n3, \ldots S\_nm)$: Set of Sensor Nodes.
H_n: Hub Node
L : link between S_n(sensor node) and H_n(Hub node).
D_s_h: distance from the hub to all sensors.

In the current research, we have attached six sensors to a patient's body i.e.; Temperature (Temp), EEG, Motion, Blood pressure (BP), ECG, and EMG. Figure 3 depicts where these sensors are located. The star stands for the sink node, whereas the circle represents the sensor nodes. It is presumed that each node possesses the ability to manage the same power. The initial energy and transmission range capacities of every sensor are the same.

Direct communication between the sink node and the nearby sensors is required. It is also expected that the sink node will have limitless power and the capability to process multiple packets simultaneously. An integrated framework

Table 1. Related Work Analysis

References	Methods	Performance Metrics
[19] (2022)	Grasshopper and DV-HOP algorithm was proposed for node localization	Localization error
[20] (2020)	The optimal placement for the central node is determined through the analysis of the Reflection Coefficient (S11) of an antenna situated on the body, along with the IEEE 802.15.6 CM3A path loss model between the communicating nodes.	Path loss & link quality metrics (SNR) & (BER), and (RSSI)
[21] (2022)	Whale Optimization Algorithm (WOA)-based hub placement scheme for wireless body area networks (WBANs) that aims to minimize node power consumption in data transmission, increase network stability, and improve network throughput and latency	Stability period & Residual Energy & Throughput & End-to-End Delay
[22] (2017)	locating the sink node between the hip and the chest. Assuming that the back, arms, and ankle have been implanted with transmitting sensor nodes	Network lifetime
[23] (2019)	A relay node algorithm based on adaptive cuckoo search, aiming to minimize relay node cost, energy consumption, and achieve uniform load distribution, particularly in challenging optimization problems.	Energy-Consumption & Computation Time
[24] (2014)	This paper proposes the Distance-aware BNC Placement Algorithm-Iterative (DBP-I), Distance-aware BNC Placement Algorithm-Fixed (DBP-F), and Position-aware BNC Placement Algorithm (PBP).	Energy efficiency & Depletion time

of HWOA(Humpback whale optimization algorithm) and D-RMS (Distance-based random mean shift clustering) the algorithm is presented as a central hub strategy for Wireless Body Area Network (WBAN) systems.

3.1 Distance-Based Random Mean Shift Clustering (D-RMS)

In the Distance-based random mean shift clustering (D-RMS) scenario, the body is in the standing position, and six sensors (eeg, ecg, temp, bp, motion, and EMG)are positioned on the human body this scenario to record electrical data that provide useful information of patient's physiological state are deployed at various locations across the body, and 10 to 15 random Sink node is placed on preset locations. Moreover, we have applied Shift Clustering algorithms to compute the average of sink nodes. The following factors were taken into account for:

Step 1: Sensor and Sink Node Placement

The proposed approach in this work is implemented using a WBAN made up of 6 biosensor nodes and 10 random sink node placements. Depending on the physiological parameters that need to be assessed, the patient's body may have one or several biosensor nodes implanted. To evaluate the performance of D-RMS, we take into account the WBAN topology as shown in Fig. 4.

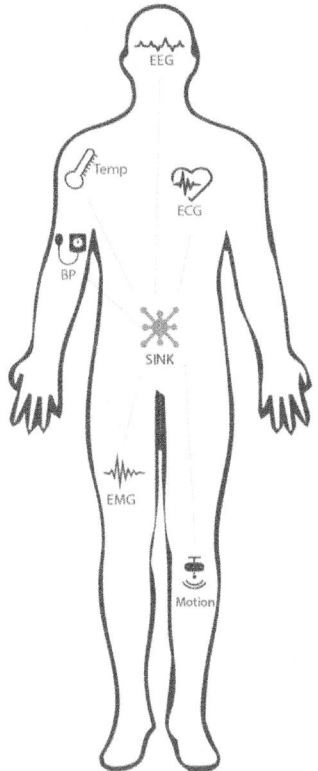

Fig. 3. Network Topology

The coordinates of each node's position are established once the nodes are implanted. The test subjects are always standing with their arms at their sides. Experiments demonstrate how wearable antenna performance is affected by different body locations.

Step 2: Apply Shift Clustering

After coordinator node placement, We perform the following steps:

a. Compute the mean shift vector for the current initial point. The mean shift vector indicates the direction of the most significant increase in the density of the data point, as follows:

$$m(x) = \frac{\sum_{i=1}^{N} K\left(\frac{x \cdot x_i}{h}\right) \cdot x_i}{\sum_{i=1}^{N} K\left(\frac{x \cdot x_i}{h}\right)} - x \tag{1}$$

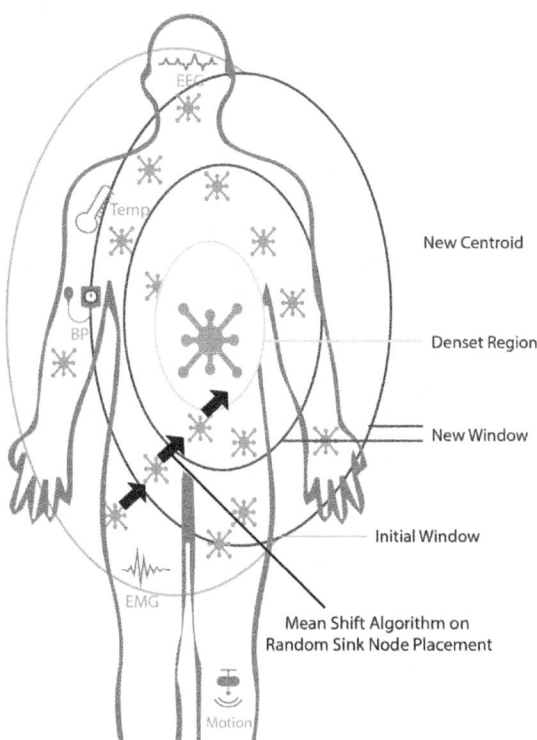

Fig. 4. D-RMS for sink placement

b. Update the initial point by shifting it in the direction of the mean shift vector.
c. Repeat steps a and b until the starting point approaches a local mode. (density peak) in the dataset.
d. Get the cluster centers, which represent the average positions of the combined nodes.
e. Display Sink Coordinates (x, y).

Step 3: Compute distance from SNP

The distance from d_node to d_sink can be measured as follows:

$$d_{\text{node-sink}} = \sqrt{(X_a - X_b)^2 + (Y_a - Y_b)^2} \qquad (2)$$

Here, (Xa, Ya) represents the coordinates of sensor nodes, whereas (Xb, Yb) denotes the coordinates of the sink node. Following is the Pseudo-code of DRMS.

3.2 Humpback-Based Sink Placement Technique

The Whale Optimization Algorithm is inspired by the social behavior of humpback whales during their hunting process. It leverages the concepts of exploration and exploitation to efficiently search for optimal solutions in a given problem space. In the Humpback whale optimization algorithm (HWOA), some whales perform an "encircling prey" behavior during exploration. This behavior involves random movements by a group of whales around the potential prey, trying to find better solutions. In the algorithm, the positions of these whales are updated using random coefficients and the distance to the current best solution found so far as shown in Fig. 5. Here, the Hump-based optimization method is described in detail as a potential remedy for the best placement of the sink node within the WBAN. The suggested procedure involves the following steps, which happen in the following order:

Algorithm 1 RMS for Sink-Node-Placement

Inputs:
S_n: Fixed node deployment.
C_n: Random node placement.
Outputs:
C_P: Coordinator Node Placement.
Procedure:
Import libraries: NumPy & MeanShift
Define Sensor node Positions: S_n
Define Random node Placement: C_n
Convert C_n list to array
Apply Mean Shift clustering on C_n
$meanshift \leftarrow MeanShift()$
$meanshift.fit(C_n)$
Get cluster centers ← average positions
$C_C \leftarrow meanshift.C_C$
Retrieve: C_P
$average_{CP} \leftarrow C_C$
Display result:
Print C_P
End of Algorithm
---

1) Define the number of iterations, population size, and dimensions.
2) Define the lower and upper bounds for the search space.
3) Define the positions of the fixed sensor nodes.
4) Define the fitness function (Mean Squared Error) The following equation of the mean square error (MSE), which is minimized by employing an efficient optimization algorithm:

$$MSE = \frac{1}{M} \left(\sum_{i=1}^{M} \sqrt{(x - x_i)^2 + (y - y_i)^2} - \widehat{d_i} \right)^2 \tag{3}$$

5) Initialize the population with random positions within the search space.
6) Initialize the best position and best fitness value.
7) Perform the Whale Optimization Algorithm.
   7.1) Update the a and b parameters.

$$\vec{D} = \left| \vec{C} \cdot \vec{X}_{\text{best}}(t) - \vec{X}(t) \right| \tag{4}$$

$$\vec{X}(t+1) = \vec{X}_{\text{best}}(t) - \vec{A} \cdot \vec{D} \tag{5}$$

where t denotes the current iteration, A and C denote the coefficient vectors, denotes the position vector of the best solution, and X is a position vector.

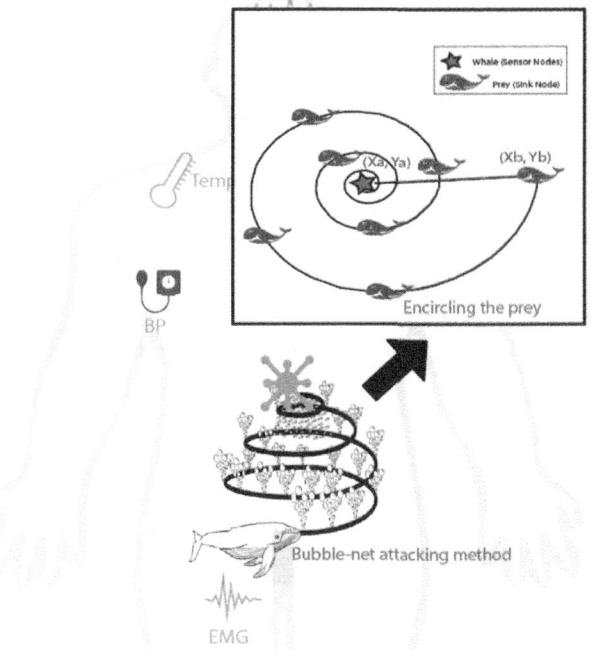

Fig. 5. Bubble-net search mechanism

$$\vec{A} = 2\vec{a}\vec{r_1} - \vec{a} \tag{6}$$

$$\vec{C} = 2\vec{r_2} \tag{7}$$

where $r1$ and $r2$ are random vectors in $[0, 1]$.

7.2) Update the position and fitness of each whale.

a) Generate a random whale.

b) Update the position of the current whale.

c) Clamp the position within the search space bounds.

d) Update the fitness of the current whale.

Algorithm 2 Humpback-Whale for Sink-Node-Placement

Inputs:

Define:

n_i: number of iterations

p_s & d: population size & dimensions

u_b & l_b: lower and upper bounds for search space

S_n: fixed sensor nodes

F_F: fitness function (MSE)

$P_S S$: Population within search space.

B_P: Best position for an optimal solution.

B_F: Best Fitness value.

Outputs:

C_P: Coordinator Node Placement. **for** $iter = 1$ to n_i **do**

Update a and $a2$ for SS

for $i = 1$ to p_s **do**

$position = population[i]$

Generate a random whale (R_W)

Update the position of the whale using WOA equation:

$d = |a \cdot R_W - position|$

$c = 2 \cdot R_{vector}(num\_dim)$

$distance\_to\_random\_whale = d \cdot \exp(b \cdot c) - 0.5 \cdot d$

$updated\_position = R_W - a2 \cdot distance\_to\_whale$

Clamp the position within the search space:

$updated\_position = \text{clamp}(updated\_position, l_b, u_b)$

Update fitness of current whale:

$fitness = F_F(updated\_position)$

Update the best position and best fitness if the current whale's fitness is better than the previous best: **if** $fitness < B_F$ **then**

$B_P = updated\_position$

$B_F = fitness$

Update the current whale's position:

$population[i] = updated\_position$

Display the B_F for current iteration:

print("Iteration:", $iter$, "Best Fitness:", B_F)

Display Final:

print("Final Best Position:", B_P)

print("Final Best Fitness:", B_F)

---

e) Update the best position and best fitness.

f) Update the current whale's position in the population.

7.3) Display the best fitness value for the current iteration.

8) Display the final best position and best fitness value.

Following is the pseudo-code of the Humpback Whale Optimization Algorithm (HWOA):

4   Results and Analysis

In this section, the general system model that was used to analyze the suggested methodology is briefly described. Network model configuration, the radio model, and the energy consumption model are all included in wireless data packet transmission. Table 2 shows the parameter values of all models used in our research.

Table 2. Model Parameters

Parameter	Value
d0(cm)	within 5 cm range
PL(do)	49.81 dB
n	4.22
X	6.81 dB
f	0.402–0.405 GHz
ETX_elec	18.75 nJ/bit
ERX_elec	18.75 nJ/bit
E_init	0.5 J
E_elec	100e−9
E_amp	50e−6
Overhead	80 bits
ACK/NACK	64 bits
Transmission power	−10 dBm
Noise power	−100 dB
Data Rate	800 kbps
R/BN	2 bps/Hz

4.1   Sink Coordinates of D-RMS(Proposed) and HWOA

Figure 6 and 7 show the Best Coordinator placement using D-RMS(Proposed), and HWOA technique. In Fig. 6(a), 6(b), 6(c), and 6(d), we have placed 25, 50, 75, and 100 random nodes according to sensor node location and applied the mean shift clustering algorithm on all data points and after 10 runs we compute the optimal position of 25 random points is (100.49, 106.19), best position of 50 points are (94.15, 134.30), for 75 points it is (98.80, 117.45) and 100 points best placement us (97.49, 115.76).

In Fig. 7, we have placed 25, 50, 75, and 100 whales and solved this for multiple iterations, and in all cases 7(a), 7(b), 7(c), and 7(d) figures best coordinator placement is (97.0, 100.0)

4.2   Energy Model

A radio model explains how much energy the sensor's electronic system uses. In our research, we selected the first-order radio model presented in [19], shown in Fig. 3. The radio model defined in Eqs. (11) and (12) explains The energy dynamics between the transmitter and receiver during the transmission of a data packet of size "n" across a distance of "d" (Fig. 8).

$$E_{TX}(n, d) = E_{TX\_Elec} * n + E_{TX\_Amp} * n * d^2 \tag{8}$$

$$E_{RX}(n, d) = E_{RX\_Elec} * n \tag{9}$$

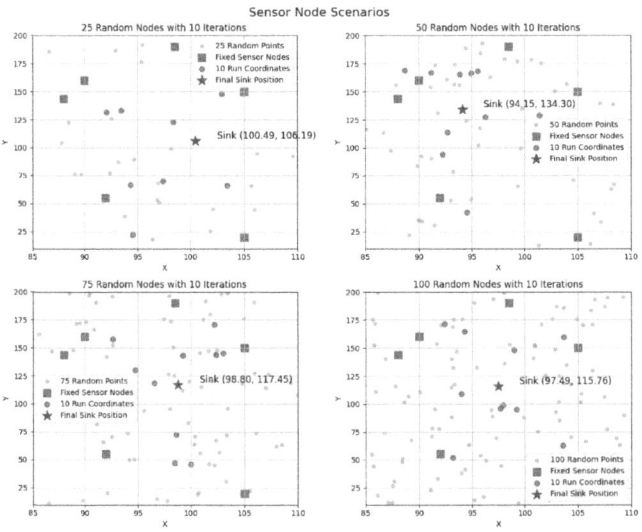

Fig. 6. Sink Node Best Position using D-RMS

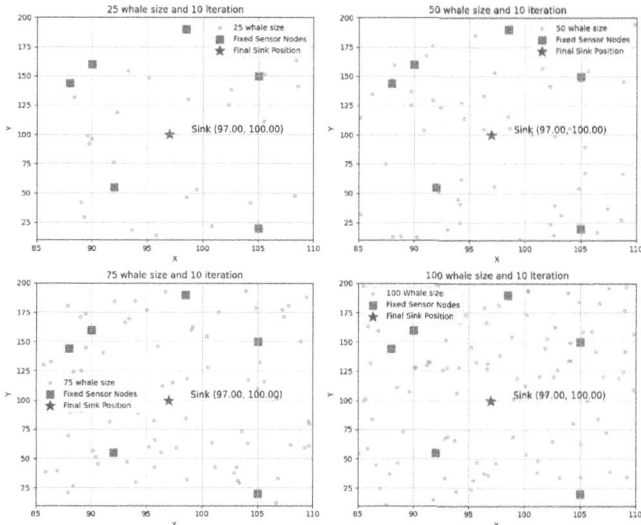

Fig. 7. Sink Node Best Position using HWOA

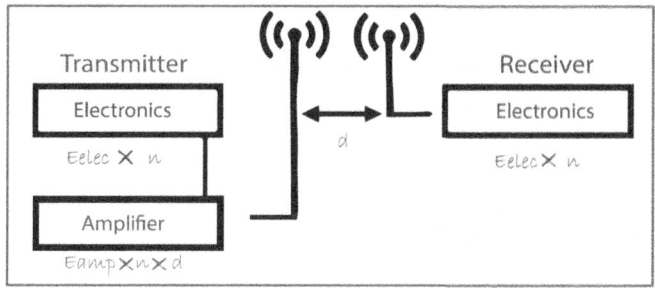

Fig. 8. First Order Energy Model

4.3   Residual Energy

Residual energy differs between a node's initial energy and the energy used to send packets. In essence, it is the energy that is left over after the operator. Figure 10 shows the Residual energy of D-RMS (Proposed) and HWOA. Out of the two sink node placement strategies, D-RMS offers the slowest energy depletion rate and provides the longest network lifetime. Table 3 presents the residual energy values across various iterations and for distinct population sizes in the context of D-RMS (Proposed) and the Humpback Whale Optimization Algorithm (HWOA).

Notably, D-RMS consistently outperforms the Humpback Whale Optimization Algorithm (HWOA) across nearly all scenarios. Specifically, the residual energy for the HWOA technique remains fixed at 90% throughout all iterations.

Table 3. Residual Energy

Iterations	HWA Residual Energy (%)	DRMS Residual Energy (%)
25	90%	91.49%
50	90%	91.70%
75	90%	92%
100	90%	92%

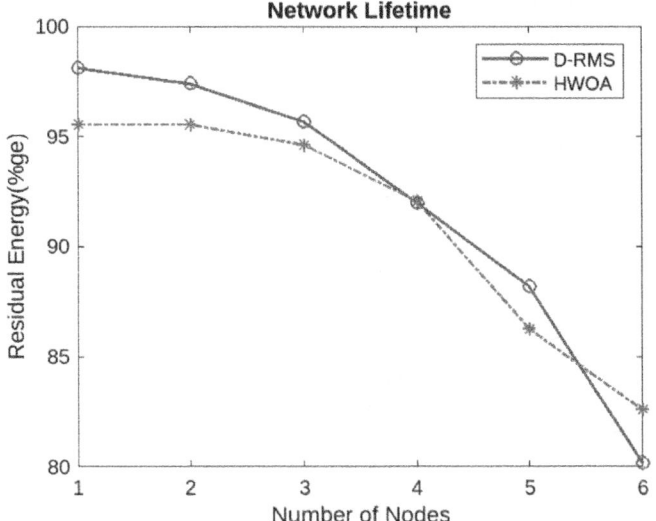

Fig. 9. Residual Energy

Conversely, DRMS initially registers a higher residual energy at 91.49%, which undergoes a gradual increment after 50 iterations and stabilizes at a commendable 92% (Fig. 9).

4.4 Energy Consumption

D-RMS demonstrates a notably efficient performance with an average energy consumption of 8%. The Humpback Whale Optimization Algorithm (HWOA) registers a comparatively higher average energy consumption level of 10% as shown in Fig. 10. These values reflect the varying degrees of energy efficiency achieved by each algorithm, with D-RMS showcasing the most favorable outcome in terms of lower energy consumption.

4.5 Energy Efficiency

Let PT denote the transmitted power output, and ETX_elec signify the energy expended by the transmitter electronics per bit. The expression ETX_DATA

is employed to denote the overall energy consumed by the transmitting node to transmit a data packet of size L bits.

$$E_{TX\_DATA} = \left(E_{TX\_elec} + \frac{P_T}{R}\right)(L + H) \tag{10}$$

In this context, R represents the data transmission rate. The energy expended by the receiver electronics to receive and decode one bit is represented by the variable ERX_elec. The quantity ERX_DATA, indicating the overall energy consumption by the receiving node for the reception and decoding of a data packet, can be expressed as follows:

$$E_{RX\_DATA} = (E_{RX\_elec})(L + H) \tag{11}$$

Energy efficiency is characterized by the proportion of the energy consumed that contributes to the effective operation in a communication link between the sender and receiver [25]. It quantifies the useful fraction within the total energy consumption. The method for determining this is outlined as follows:

$$\eta_{DC} = \frac{(1 - PER_{DC})\,xL}{x(L + H) + E_{TX\_ACK/NACK} + E_{RX\_ACK/NACK}} \tag{12}$$

The outcomes for the Energy Efficiency of both techniques are shown in Figs. 11-a, 11-b respectively. To compare the D-RMS(Distance-based random mean shift clustering) with HWOA (Humpback whale optimization algorithm) strategies,

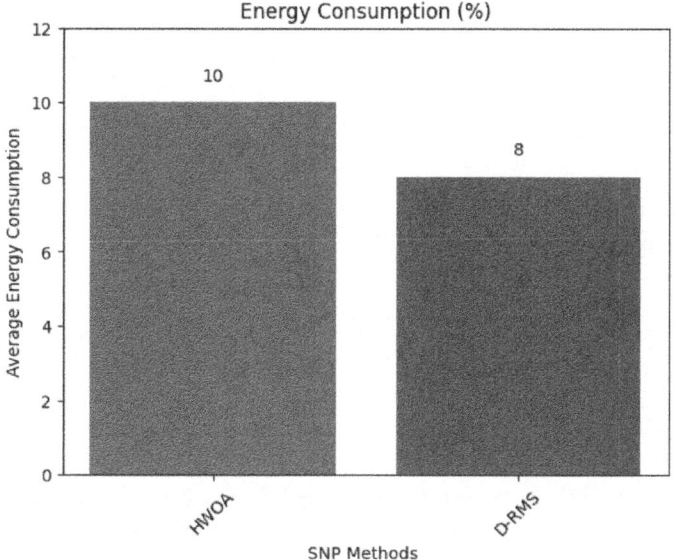

Fig. 10. Energy Consumption

EE is plotted against source-destination hop length. The results confirm that the energy efficiency of all six sensors declines as the source-destination distance increases. This is because a longer source-destination distance requires more energy to transmit the same amount of information bits compared to a shorter source-destination distance.

4.6   Minimum Localization Error

The disparity or difference between an object, device, or sensor's true or real position in a given coordinate system or geographic space is referred to as localization error, also known as positioning error or localization inaccuracy. It measures how precisely or accurately the location of an entity has been identified and computed using Eq. (16):

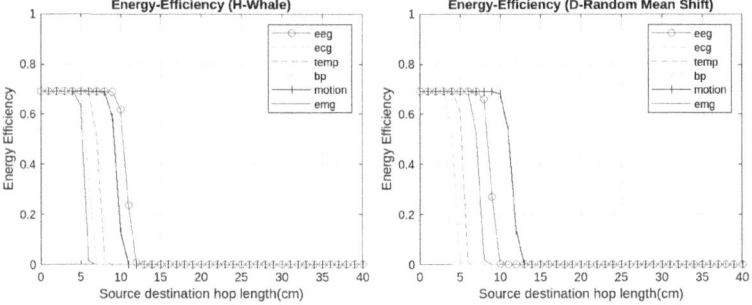

Fig. 11. Energy Efficiency (a) HWOA, (b) D-RMS

$$\text{MSE} = \frac{1}{w} \sum_{i=1}^{w} \left((x_{\text{est}_i} - x_{\text{act}_i})^2 + (y_{\text{est}_i} - y_{\text{act}_i})^2 \right) \tag{13}$$

The suggested algorithm's performance in terms of the minimum localization error (MLE) is illustrated in Fig 13. Finally, the Average Localization Error (ALE) is given in Eq. (17):

$$\text{ALE} = \frac{1}{N} \sum_{i=1}^{N} \sqrt{(x_{\text{est}_i} - x_{\text{act}_i})^2 + (y_{\text{est}_i} - y_{\text{act}_i})^2} \tag{14}$$

Figure 12 shows the localization error of all sensors for both techniques.

MLE of $D-RMS-eeg$ is 0.742 whereas $HWA-eeg$ is 0.900, $D-RMS-ecg$ is 0.349, whereas $HWA-ecg$ is 0.506, $D-RMS-temp$ is 0.449, and $HWA-temp$ is 0.604. MLE of $D-RMS-bp$ is 0.299, whereas $HWA-bp$ is 0.449, $D-RMS-motion$ is 0.960, whereas $HWA-motion$ is 0.803, $D-RMS-emg$ is 0.610, moreover, $HWA-emg$ is 0.452. Finally, the ALE of D-RMS is 0.568 m and HWOA is 0.619 m, respectively.

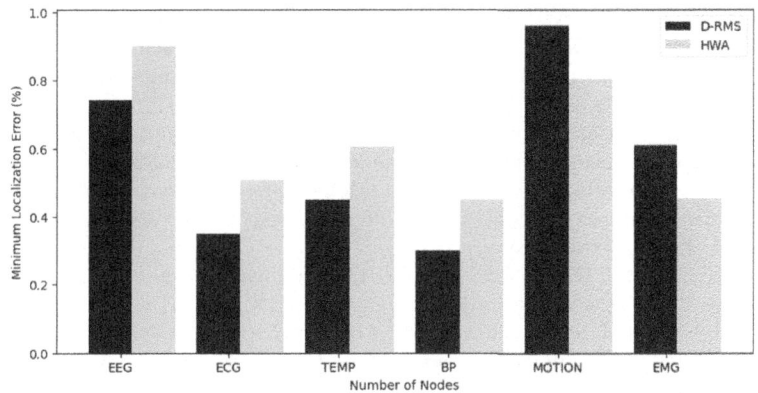

Fig. 12. Minimum Localization Error vs. Sensor Nodes

5   Conclusion

The sink node is strategically placed to provide sufficient coverage over the targeted body area. Adequate coverage ensures that all required data can be collected effectively and transmitted to the central monitoring system. In this paper, we have identified coordinator placement using $D - RMS$ and $HWOA$. The best position of Coordinator placement using D-RMS is *(97.9175, 115.76)* and HWOA is *(97, 100)*. Overall, the residual energy of D-RMS is *92*% and HWOA is *90*%. The ALE of D-RMS is *0.568* m and HWOA is *0.619* m.

Acknowledgement. This work is partly funded by Estonian research council research grant PRG424, and "Information and Communication Technologies (ICT) programme" was supported by the European Union through European Social Fund. ERDF in the framework of the Tallinn University of Technology Development Program 2016–2022.

References

1. Wu, H., Zhu, H., Gu, J., Peng, C., Han, X.: Efficient Health data transmission method in a wireless body area network for rural elderly. Electronics **11**(18), 2817 (2022)
2. Shahid, J., Ahmad, R., Kiani, A.K., Ahmad, T., Saeed, S., Almuhaideb, A.M.: Data protection and privacy of the internet of healthcare things (IoHTs). Appl. Sci. **12**(4), 1927 (2022)
3. Wu, T., Wu, F., Redoute, J.-M., Yuce, M.R.: An autonomous wireless body area network implementation towards IoT connected healthcare applications. IEEE Access **5**, 11413–11422 (2017)
4. Singh, S., Prasad, D., Rani, S., Singh, A., Alharithi, F.S., Almotiri, J.: Wireless body area routing protocols impact analysis on entity mobility models with static sink node. Appl. Sci. **12**(11), 5655 (2022)

5. Saboor, A., Mustafa, A., Ahmad, R., Khan, M.A., Haris, M., Hameed, R.: Evolution of wireless standards for health monitoring. In: 2019 9th annual information technology, electromechanical engineering, and microelectronics conference (IEMECON), pp. 268–272. IEEE (2019)

6. Panhwar, M.A., et al.: Energy-efficient routing optimization algorithm in WBANs for patient monitoring (2020). https://doi.org/10.1007/s12652-020-02541-7

7. Alam, M.M., Hamida, E.B., Berder, O., Menard, D., Sentieys, O.: A heuristic self-adaptive medium access control for resource-constrained WBAN systems. IEEE Access 4, 1287–1300 (2016)

8. Bilandi, N., Verma, H.K., Dhir, R.: PSOBAN: a novel particle swarm optimization-based protocol for wireless body area networks. SN Appl. Sci. 1, 1492 (2019)

9. Samal, T.K., Patra, S.C., Kabat, M.R.: An adaptive cuckoo search based algorithm for placement of relay nodes in a wireless body area networks. J. King Saud. Univ. - Comput. Inf. Sci. 14 (2019)

10. Choudhary, A., Nizamuddin, M., Zadoo, M.: Body node coordinator placement algorithm for WBAN using multi-objective swarm optimization. IEEE Sensors Journal 22(3), 2858–2867 (2021)

11. Pradeep, T., Vetrivelan, P., Latha, R.: Novel BNC placement strategy for wireless body area networks. Indian J. Sci. Technol. 9, 36 (2016)

12. Waheed, M., Talha, S., Ahmad, R., Kiani, A.K., Alam, M.M., Ahmed, W.: Network coding and hierarchical modulation for energy efficient cooperative WBAN. Int. J. Distrib. Syst. Technol. (IJDST) 10(3), 90–111 (2019)

13. Chen, G., Zhan, Y., Sheng, G., Xiao, L., Wang, Y.: Reinforcement learning-based sensor access control for WBANs. IEEE Access 7, 8483–8494 (2018)

14. Sharma, R., Ryait, H.S., Gupta, A.K.: Analyzing the effect of posture mobility and sink node placement on the performance of routing protocols in WBAN. Indian J. Sci. Technol. 9(40), 1–11 (2016)

15. Gupta, D., Wadhwa, S., Rani, S., Khan, Z., Boulila, W.: EEDC: an energy efficient data communication scheme based on new routing approach in wireless sensor networks for future IoT applications. Multidisciplinary Digital Publishing Institute (MDPI) (2023). https://doi.org/10.3390/s23218839

16. Samal, T.K., Patra, S.C., Kabat, M.R.: An adaptive cuckoo search-based algorithm for placement of relay nodes in wireless body area networks. J. King Saud Univ.-Comput. Inf. Sci. 34(5), 1845–1856 (2022)

17. Choudhary, A., Nizamuddin, M., Zadoo, M.: Body node coordinator placement algorithm for WBAN using multi-objective swarm optimization. IEEE Sens. J. 22(3), 2858–2867 (2021)

18. Abedi, F., et al.: Chimp optimization algorithm based feature selection with machine learning for medical data classification. Tech Science Press (2023). https://doi.org/10.32604/csse.2023.038762

19. Javaid, N., Ahmad, A., Nadeem, Q., Imran, M.A., Haider, N.: iM-SIMPLE: iMproved stable increased -through-put multi-hop link efficient routing protocol for wireless body area networks. Comput. Hum. Behav. 1003–1111 (2015)

20. Janabi, S.M.A., Kurnaz, S.: A new localization mechanism in IoT using grasshopper optimization algorithm and DVHOP algorithm. Wirel. Netw. 17(14), 4647–4660 (2023)

21. Shukla, S., Choudhary, A., Pandey, S.K., Sachan, V.K., Kumar, P.: WHOOPH: whale optimization-based optimal placement of hub node within a WBAN (2022)

22. Arora, N., Gupta, S.H., Kumar, B.: An approach to investigate the best location for the central node placement for energy-efficient WBAN. J. Ambient Intell. Humaniz. Comput. 1–12 (2020)

23. Razavi, A., Jahed, M.: Node positioning and lifetime optimization for wireless body area networks. IEE Sens. (2017)

24. Huque, M.T.I., Munasinghe, K.S., Jamalipour, A.: Body node coordinator placement algorithms for wireless body area networks. IEEE Internet Things J. 2(1), 94–102 (2014)

25. Waheed, M., Ahmad, R., Ahmed, W., Drieberg, M., Alam, M.M.: Towards efficient wireless body area network using two-way relay cooperation. Sensors 18(2), 565 (2018)

Ultrawideband On-Body Area Network for Navigational Support

Dilshan N. Wickramarachchi[✉], Robert Brown, Mohammad Ghavami, and Sandra Dudley

School of Engineering, London South Bank University, London SE1 0AA, UK
wickramw@lsbu.ac.uk

Abstract. The number of patients with blindness and partial sightedness has grown over time. These vision impairments significantly affect the quality of life, and navigation is one of the main challenges these patients face. Although assistive devices were introduced in the past, they have a low acceptance rate due to their limited usability, cost, portability, battery life and higher cost. This paper proposes an on-body area network based on ultra-wideband (UWB) technology and a novel algorithm to detect and classify the obstacles. The on-body radar network captures the backscattered UWB pulses and publishes them to an MQTT network at a rate of 5 frames per second. Then the algorithms unit obtains the UWB radar frame and generates a detection image. This image presents the position and features of the obstacles. At the final stage, detection images are fed to machine learning classifiers to identify the obstacles. The proposal system was experimentally validated and obtained a classification accuracy of 93% with the support vector machine utilising the radial basis function kernel.

Keywords: Ultra-wideband (UWB) · Body Area Networks (BAN) · Assistive Technologies

1 Introduction

The European Blind Union (EBU) estimated that there are more than 30 million people suffering from blindness or partially sightedness within the European region [1] and National Health Services (NHS) states that there are 340,000 registered blind or partially sighted patients [2]. EBU and NHS have predicted that these values will rapidly increase over time. These impairments can significantly affect the activities of daily living (ADL) of patients and reduce the quality of life.

Braille language-based magazines, displays, and keyboards support the reading and writing process. Also, machines such as ATMs and Kiosks provide audio guides to assist with human-machine interactions. A walking cane or guide dog is commonly recommended to assist with independent navigation [2]. The patients can use a walking cane to identify the obstacles in the part. These canes are limited to identifying obstacles below the waist level and can miss obstacles due to their shape, dimension, and location. Guide

M. Mizmizi et al. (Eds.): BodyNets 2024, LNICST 524, pp. 246–260, 2024.
https://doi.org/10.1007/978-3-031-72524-1_18

dogs are trained to provide navigation support, but the owners need to maintain proper communication when navigating and caring for the dog which could be challenging for a vision-impaired person [3].

Therefore, researchers have focused on introducing assistive technologies to address the challenges of using the walking cane or guide dogs. Although these systems provide navigation assistance, they have a low acceptance rate due to limited usability, portability, battery life and higher cost [4]. Therefore, there is a requirement for a system that can aid in indoor and outdoor navigation, lower cost, portable and ergonomic.

Therefore, this paper proposes an Ultra-wideband (UWB) Radar-based system to provide obstacle awareness. The contributions include a UWB Radar-based body area network architecture to capture the surrounding environment and a novel detection algorithm to detect the objects in the surrounding environment. This paper is structured as follows. The next section will describe related work, the underlying technologies, and their limitations, followed by the features of UWB which could address these limitations. The methodology section will explain the proposed system architecture, hardware, and algorithms. The next section will present the results obtained and the discussion followed by the conclusion and future work.

2 Background Study

The researchers have proposed assistive devices to support blind and partially vision loss people with navigation. These systems include technologies such as RGB camera systems, optical time of flight sensors, acoustic ultrasound sensors, radar sensors and hybrid sensor models. These sensors are integrated into wearable devices, hand-held devices, or mobile robot devices to identify the obstacles in the surroundings. Then actuators such as vibration motors, tactile motors or audio descriptions are used to communicate the information to the person.

Optical time-of-flight (ToF) sensors such as laser and infrared (IR) have been widely used for a long time for research related to smart guide devices such as canes [5, 6]. These technologies provide high-range resolution, low cost, and faster response time, but the usability of these technologies is limited as they are sensitive to ambient lighting conditions and limited to short-ranging applications [7].

Researchers have implemented acoustic ToF sensors such as sonar in smart shoes [8], glasses [9] or handheld devices [10] to describe the environment. These sensing technologies are low-cost and simple to operate, but they are sensitive to the ambient temperature, pressure and noise making them less robust for different terrains [11].

Camera-based systems are widely used in research to provide a guiding system for the visually impaired. Web cameras and mobile phone cameras are used as monocular systems to describe the surroundings. The images captured from these systems are used to extract features [12] for classifying different objects or used in deep-leaning models to detect the obstacles in the images [13]. The monocular systems are unable to provide depth information and therefore, lead to errors in identifying the dimensions of objects. Also, they often fail to separate foreground from background due to lighting conditions and clutter [11]. The stereo systems contain more cameras or depth cameras to provide RGBD images (depth images). M Poddi et al. used RGBD cameras and implemented a Convolutional Neural Network (CNN) on depth images to recognize the obstacles and calculate the distance [14]. Intel RealSense is a stereo depth camera system widely used with deep learning algorithms to detect objects in the environment to provide audio feedback to the person [9]. Stereo and depth camera systems utilise deep learning and machine learning techniques to provide an accurate and detailed description of the surroundings, but they are sensitive to lighting conditions and require a lot of energy, computational power, and memory [11]. Therefore, these technologies are yet to provide a guide device that is usable in different terrains and environmental conditions, has a low cost and is portable.

UWB is a radar technology introduced for short-range communication applications. This Federal Communication Commission (FCC) has allocated the frequency band 3.1 – 10.6 GHz with a power spectral density (PSD) limitation of −41.3 dBm/MHz [15]. The PSD limitation makes UWB technology safer for medical applications. The high bandwidth of UWB radar is obtained by transmitting extremely narrow pulses. These narrow pulses provide high temporal and spatial resolution. Furthermore, these systems are robust to jamming and interferences. Due to the architecture of these systems, they consume very little power, and they are available in small System-on-Chip [16]. Furthermore, Yan et al. have conducted a review of state-of-art UWB antenna technologies and identified the potential of the latest research on UWB antenna for wireless body area networks [17].

3 Methodology

The proposed system is implemented using an MQTT Network [18] which consists of on body radar network, an MQTT broker, a data logger, a data visualiser, and a signal processor unit, as shown in Fig. 1.

3.1 System Architecture

The radar network consists of two UWB mono-static radar sensors used to capture the backscattered radar signals and a control unit to control UWB sensors and transmit the

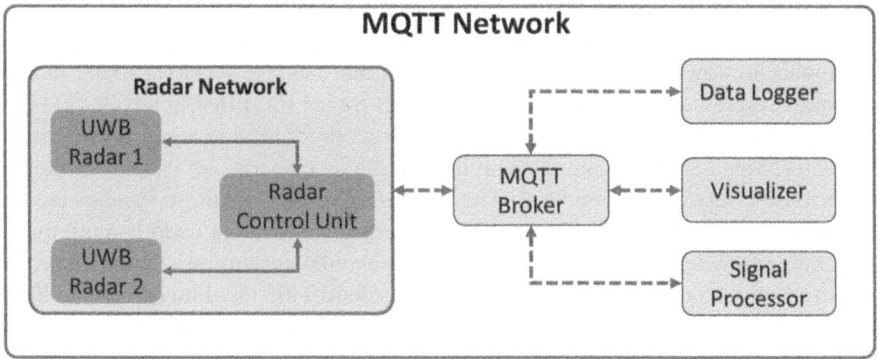

Fig. 1. System Architecture

signals. The radar publishes a data packet containing the radar frames from UWB radar 1, UWB radar 2, a timestamp and a message-id. The data logger is a subscriber which reads the radar packets received by the MQTT network and saves them into a log file. The visualizer is a subscriber which can be configured to visualise the raw radar data packets or radar signals processed using the algorithms. The signal processor subscribes to the MQTT broker, accesses the radar packets, processes them, and identifies the obstacles.

3.2 Algorithm

The X4M300 modules function as mono-static radars and consist of a transmitter, receiver, and a system control unit. The transmitter sends narrow UWB pulses, and these pulses are backscattered by the obstacles in the surroundings. The receiver captures these backscattered pulses and generates a radar frame. This section will describe the key steps of the algorithm and the underlying intuition.

Radar Frame.

The radar frame R_f obtained is a discrete 1-dimensional array each element representing the amplitude a_r of the backscattered signal at the range bin r. Therefore, R_f obtained at the time t can be shown as

$$R_f(r, t) = (a_{r,t}), r \in [0, rbin] \tag{1}$$

where *rbin* is the number of range bins covering the maximum range r_{max} and r is the range bin number. Range bins can be converted to distance by multiplying the range bin number r with the range resolution of the radar system.

Motion Filter

As the person moves, obstacles both stationary and dynamic relative to the environment, will have a motion relative to the person. Therefore, a modified version of the moving target indicator filter is used to detect the obstacles in the surroundings. This modified Moving Target Indicator (mMTI) filter with window length 2, can be shown as

$$mMTI\left(R_f(r|t = t_i)\right) = |R_f(r|t = t_i) - R_f(r|t = t_{i-1})|$$
$$= (|a_{r,t_i} - a_{r,t_{i-1}}|)r \in [0, rbin] \tag{2}$$

Calibration

The calibration process is used to generate a reference signal R_{ref} to generate a detection threshold for different environments so that the system functions across different terrains. This process includes collecting w radar frames, applying an mMTI filter and averaging to obtain a baseline reference signal. This process can be shown as

$$R_{ref}(r) = \frac{1}{w}\sum_{j=1}^{w} mMTI\left(R_f(r|t = t_j)\right)$$
$$= \frac{1}{w}\sum_{j=1}^{w}(|a_{r,t_j} - a_{r,t_{j-1}}|)r \in [0, rbin] \tag{3}$$

Detection Filter

After the calibration process ends, the person can start to walk. While walking the radar network generates the radar frames. These frames undergo motion filtering using mMTI filter and detection filter. The detect filter uses the reference signal as a threshold and calculates the probability of a detection as follows,

$$p(D_{r_i}|t = t_j) = \begin{cases} 1; & mMTI\left(R_f\left(r_i|t = t_j\right)\right) > R_{ref}\left(r_i\right) \\ 0; & otherwise \end{cases} \tag{4}$$

2-Dimensional Detection Image

The 2-D detection image is created to represent the horizontal position of the obstacle with respect to the radar network position.

Consider a detection zone of origin $O(0,0)$ covered by two monostatic directional radars R_1 and R_2 placed at (x_{R1}, y_{R1}) and (x_{R2}, y_{R2}) respectly, as shown in the Fig. 2. At time $t = t_i$, consider a point $P(x_p, y_p)$, at a distance represented by the range bins r_1 of the radar R_1 and r_2 of the radar R_2. The relationship between the positions of the R_1, R_2 and P is given by the equation,

$$OP - OR_1 = R_1P \text{ and } OP - OR_2 = R_2P \tag{5}$$

$$\therefore r_1 = \sqrt{\left(x_p - x_{R1}\right)^2 + \left(y_p - y_{R1}\right)^2} \text{ and } r_2 = \sqrt{\left(x_p - x_{R2}\right)^2 + \left(y_p - y_{R2}\right)^2} \tag{6}$$

Since the detection events of the two radars R1, R2 are mutually exclusive, we can calculate the probability of a detection at P as,

$$p_P\left(D_{r_i}|(x_p, y_p), t = t_j\right) = p_{R1}\left(D_{r_i}|r = r_1, t = t_j\right) \times p_{R2}\left(D_{r_i}|r = r_2, t = t_j\right) \tag{7}$$

The 2-Dimensional Detection Image is obtained by iterating the Eq. (7) over each point in the detection zone. This undergoes erosion and dilation operations with a 3×3 kernel to remove the noise. Then detection image is downsampled and flatten to generate the feature vector for the machine learning classifier. The main stages of the algorithms are shown in the Fig. 3.

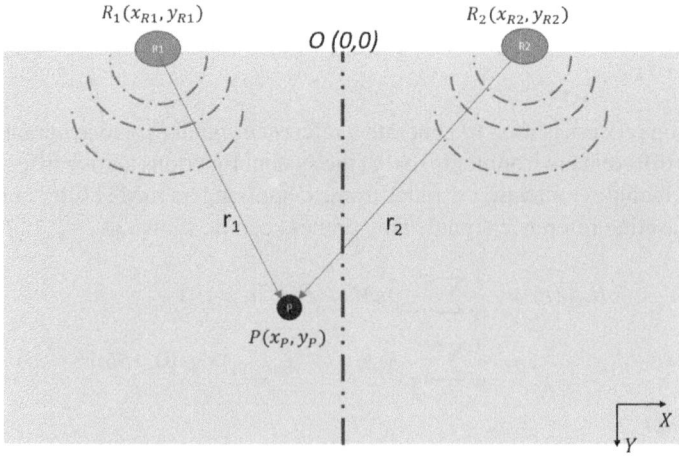

Fig. 2. Position of a point P relative to the radars R_1 and R_2

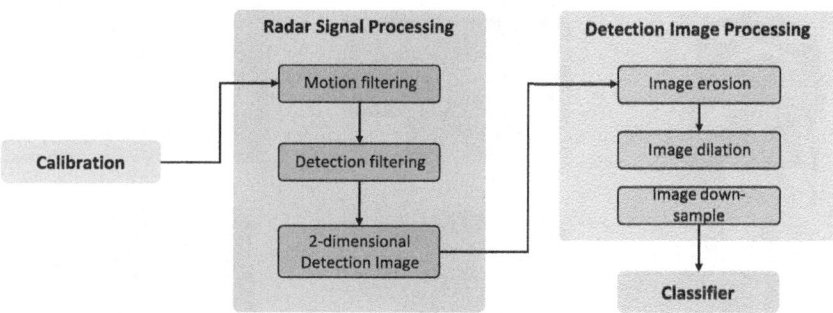

Fig. 3. Block diagram of the algorithm

4 Results and Discussion

The proposed system was implemented, and an experimental analysis was conducted to evaluate the performance of the system. The experimental analysis included a qualitative analysis on radar signal processing and novel detection image processing followed by a quantitative analysis on the classifier performance.

4.1 Hardware Implementation

Novelda X4M300 UWB radar modules (Table 1) are used as sensors to capture information about the surroundings. They are attached to the chest as shown in Fig. 4. The Raspberry Pi 3B + is used as the Radar control unit. Each X4M300 is configured to provide raw signals and the detection zone is adjusted to 2.075m. Each radar is controlled by a single process and the main process is used for synchronising radars, creating data packets and publishing to the MQTT network. The complete radar network is powered by a 10,000mAh power bank and has a frame rate of 5 frames per second. MQTT broker and other subscriber units are implemented in a desktop computer with Intel i9-13900 and the signal processor uses Nivida GeForce RTX 3060 to accelerate the matrix operations.

Table 1. Features of X4M300 UWB Radar

Radar configuration	Ultra-wideband Impulse Radio
Centre frequency	7.29 GHz
Bandwidth	1.4 GHz
Range	0.4–9.87 m
Range Bin Resolution	0.6 cm
Typical power consumption	120 mW

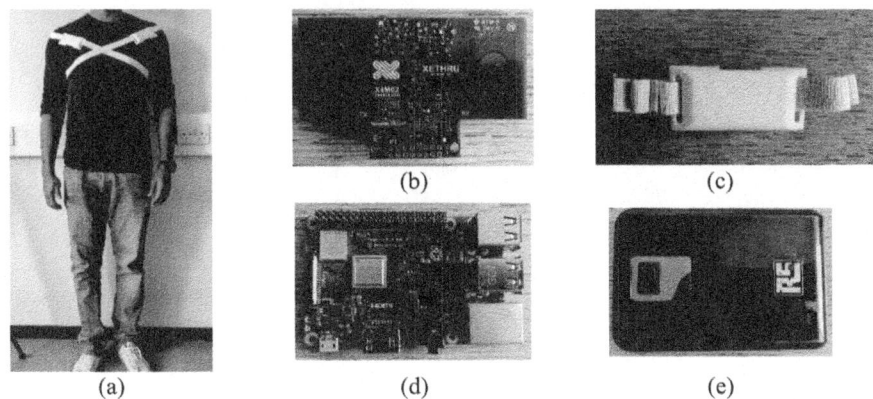

Fig. 4. Hardware setup, a) A person wearing the radar network, b) X4M300 UWB radar, c) The 3D printed brackets to contain X4M300, d) Raspberry Pi 3B + and e) Power bank

4.2 Experimental Data Collection

A data collection session was carried out to analyse the performance of the proposed system and algorithms. This consists of a subject wearing the system and,

1. Another person walking towards and away from the subject (Person).
2. Walking towards a flat wall (Wall)
3. Walking along a clear straight corridor (Open Corridor)

10 data collection was carried out for each scenario. The duration of each session was 2 min where the first minute was allocated for the calibration and the remaining duration for the test. The dataset was manually reviewed and labelled to create the dataset for the machine learning classifier. This pre-processed dataset included 600 detection images, 200 per class. The detection image is 33 × 15 pixels with each pixel having a value of 1 or 0 and is flattened to create a feature vector of 495.

4.3 Radar Signal Processing Algorithm Analysis

The qualitative analysis was conducted to develop and evaluate the radar signal processing algorithms and detection image processing algorithms.

The Fig. 5 represent the raw radar frames (Fig. 5a and c) and the output signal of the mMTI filter (Fig. 5b and d) when a person steps in the detection zone of the radar network. The orange colour line represents the average reference signal obtained after the calibration process. The Fig. 5b and d clearly shows that output of mMTI filter significantly high global peak representing the position of the person relative to the system. Similar pattern is observed in the Fig. 6 which represents the subject moving towards the wall. Compared to the Fig. 5, mMTI filter output of the Fig. 6 has significant number of local peaks which represents the multipath reflections from the wall. The mMTI filter output obtained for the open corridor shown in the Fig. 7 is similar to that of the wall shown on Fig. 6. But the local peaks of the mMTI output of the open corridor scenario are more spread from the global peak.

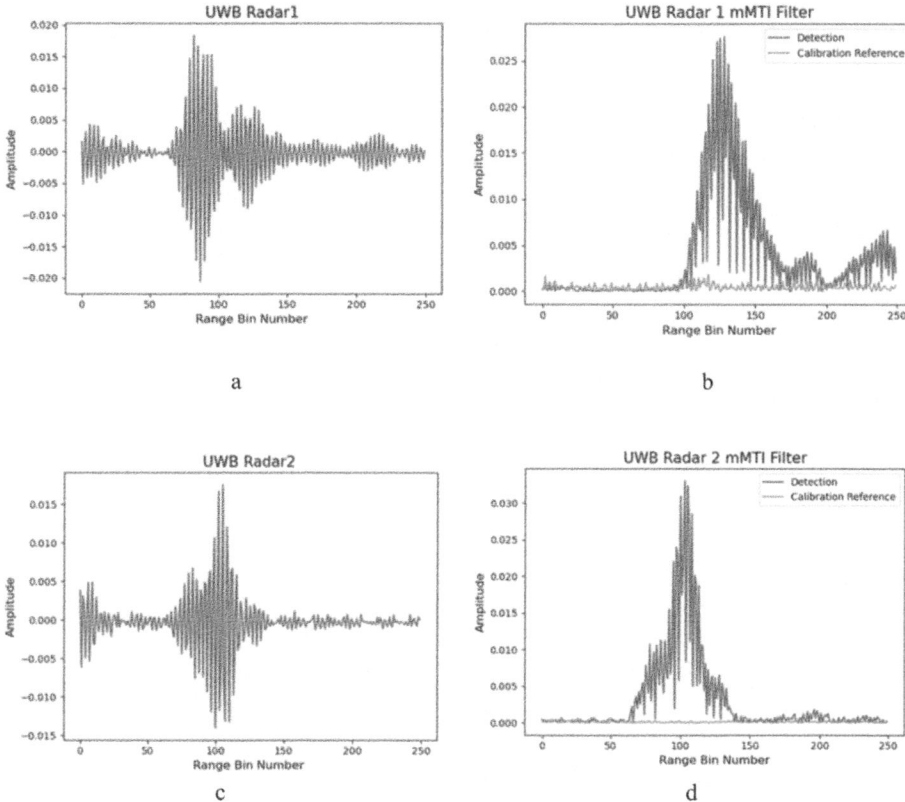

Fig. 5. Plots obtained when another person enters the detection zone of the radar network. a) Raw radar signal obtained by radar 1, b) Respective mMTI filter output for radar 1, c) Raw radar signal obtained by radar 2, d) Respective mMTI filter output for radar 2. (**orange**– reference signal obtained after calibration vs **blue**- mMTI filter output when detection occurred) (Color figure online)

4.4 Detection Image Processing Algorithm Analysis

In the last stage of radar signal processing, radar frames are combined to create the detection image. The detection images undergo image erosion and dilation morphological operations. Then images are down sampled to 33 × 15. The morphological are used to remove multipath noise and image down sampling is used to reduce the size of the feature vector.

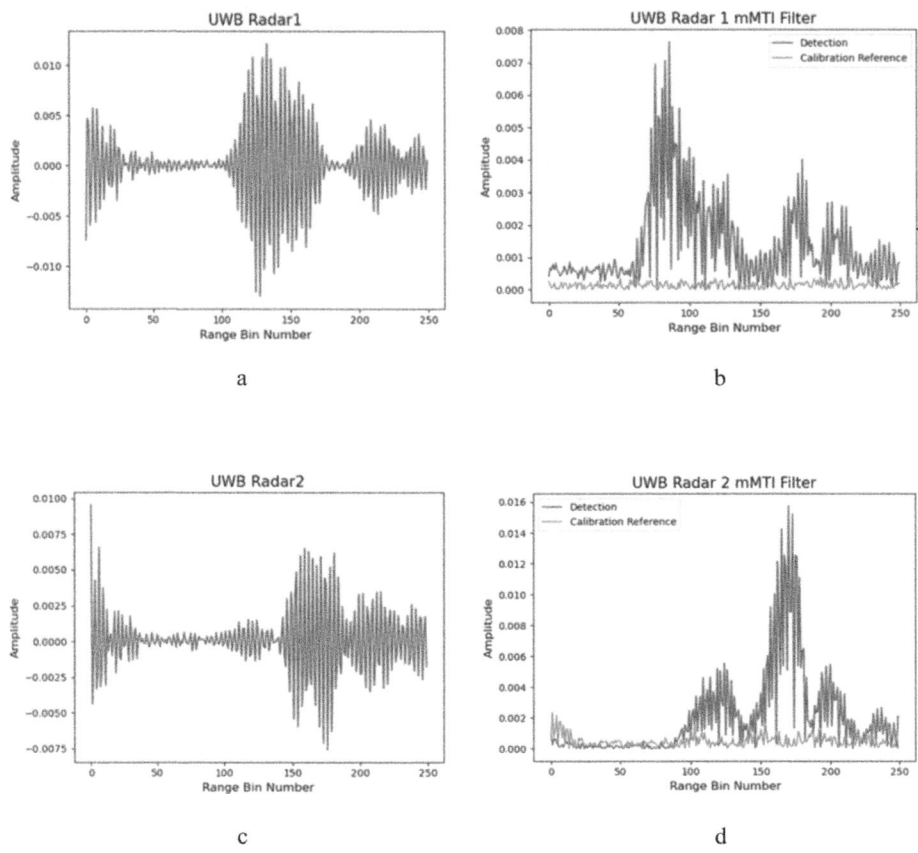

Fig. 6. Plots obtained when the subject wearing the radar system move towards a wall. a) Raw radar signal obtained by radar 1, b) Respective mMTI filter output for radar 1, c) Raw radar signal obtained by radar 2, d) Respective mMTI filter output for radar 2. (**orange**– reference signal obtained after calibration vs **blue**- mMTI filter output when detection occurred (Color figure online)

The Fig. 8 shows the variation of detection images as a person walk towards the radar system. The Fig. 8a) show a detection image obtained during the calibration process. The white blob represents the other person, and as the other person comes closer to the subject, in appears to increase in size as shown in Fig. 8b and c. Compared to the mMTI filter output, detection images can identify the direction of the other person.

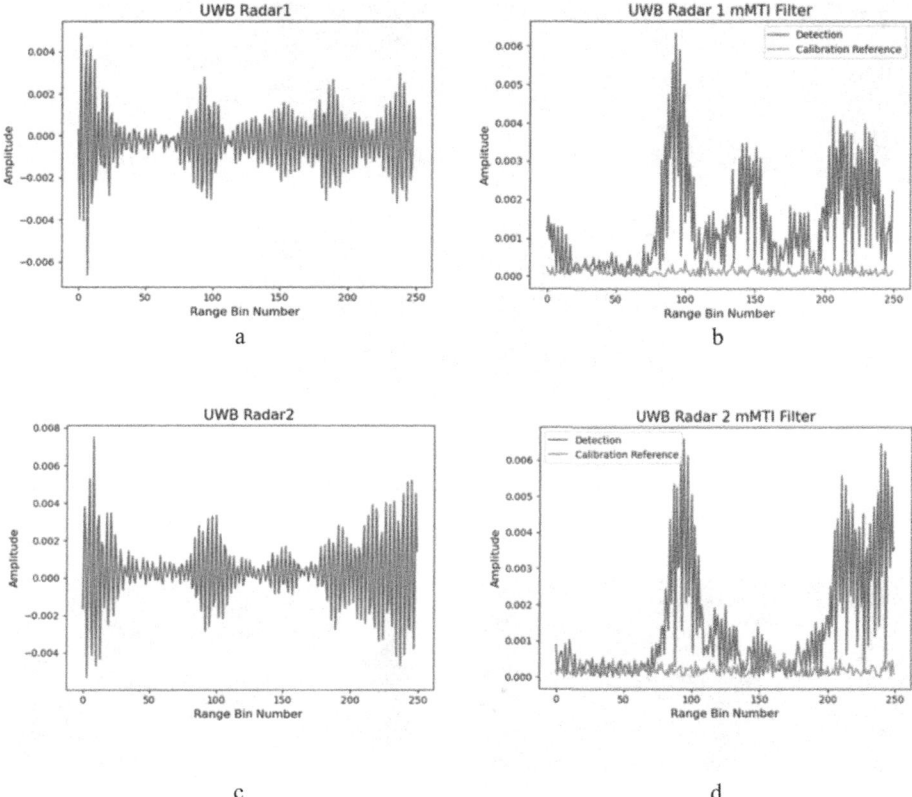

Fig. 7. Plots obtained when the subject walks through an open corridor wearing the radar network. a) Raw radar signal obtained by radar 1, b) Respective mMTI filter output for radar 1, c) Raw radar signal obtained by radar 2, d) Respective mMTI filter output for radar 2. (**orange**– reference signal obtained after calibration vs **blue**- mMTI filter output when detection occurred (Color figure online)

The detection images for the Wall Fig. 9 shows that as a subject move towards the wall the arc appears closer to the subject and thickness of the arc increases to represent the larger number of multipath reflections appears when subject move towards the wall. The detection images obtained for the open corridor (Fig. 10) scenario are somewhat similar to the wall Fig. 8, due to the presence of the side walls but arc is presented at the same distance. As the subject reaches the wall at end of the corridor similar pattern to the wall can be observed Fig. 9d, e.

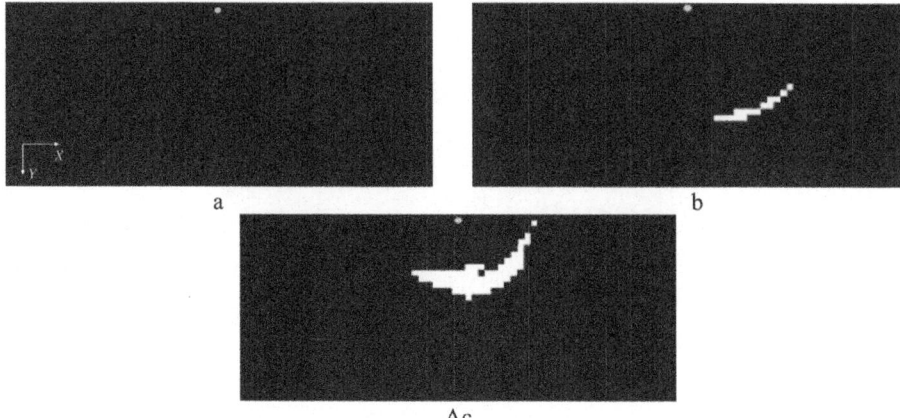

Fig. 8. Detection Images obtained when another person enters the detection zone of the radar network. a) The other person is outside the detection zone b) The other person inside the detection zone, c) The other person moves closer to the subject wearing the radar network.

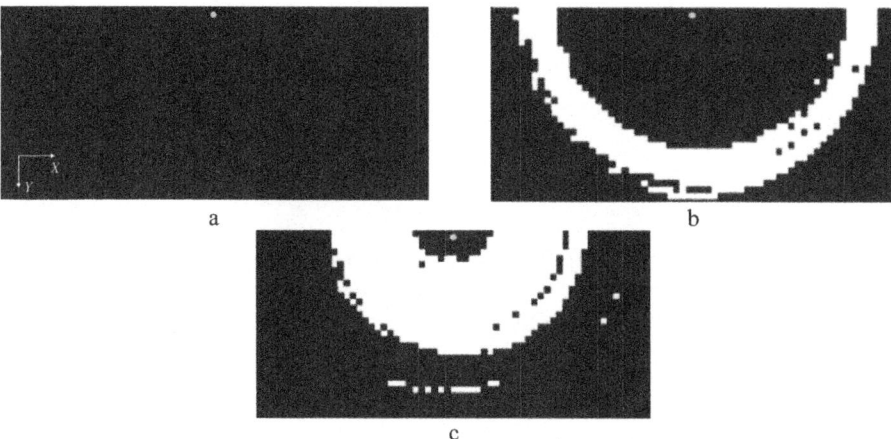

Fig. 9. Detection images obtained when the person moves towards a wall. a) The wall is outside the detection zone of the radar network, b) The wall appears in the detection zone, c) The subject moves closer to the wall.

4.5   Results of the Machine Learning Classifiers

The databases created using the detection images are used in classical machine learning models to identify the obstacles detected by the radar system. The dataset was randomly split into training and test sets according to a 7:3 ratio respectively. Then training dataset was used to train the classifiers and the testing dataset was used to validate the results. The summary of the configurations of the machine learning classifiers are shown in the Table 2. According to the results, Support Vector Machine with Radial basis function (RBF) based kernel has the highest performance followed by the random forest model. The Fig. 11 shows the confusion matrix generated for each classifier.

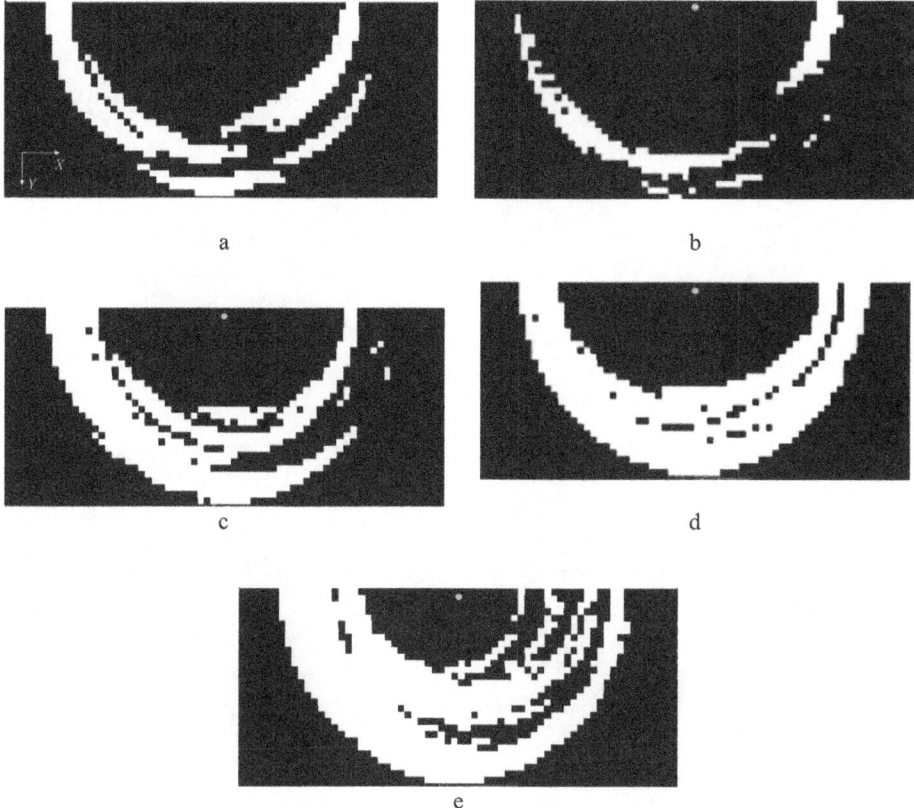

Fig. 10. Detection images obtained when the subject wearing the radar network moves through a corridor. a–c) subject moves through the corridor d–e) The wall at the end of the corridor appears in the detection zone as subject reaches the end of the corridor

The qualitative analysis of the proposed algorithms and quantitative analysis of proposed system and algorithms shows great potential to use UWB as a wearable body area network for assistive technologies. The although the proposed algorithm is implemented using two UWB radars, it can be extend simply extended to include more radars. When the number of radars increases, the effective detection zone converges to a small region, which is the intersection of radar antenna lobes. This can be address by creating different radar clusters and obtaining the union of detection images of each cluster.

It is important to note that the proposed system primarily focus on the obstacle in the horizontal plane and extending the proposed algorithm for 3-dimensions can increase the usability. Furthermore, using advance deep learning methods on the proposed detection images can improve the accuracy. Finally, the proposed algorithms heavily depend on the position of the antennas. Therefore, future research needs to focus on wearable antenna or integrating motion sensors to address the change of the antenna positions.

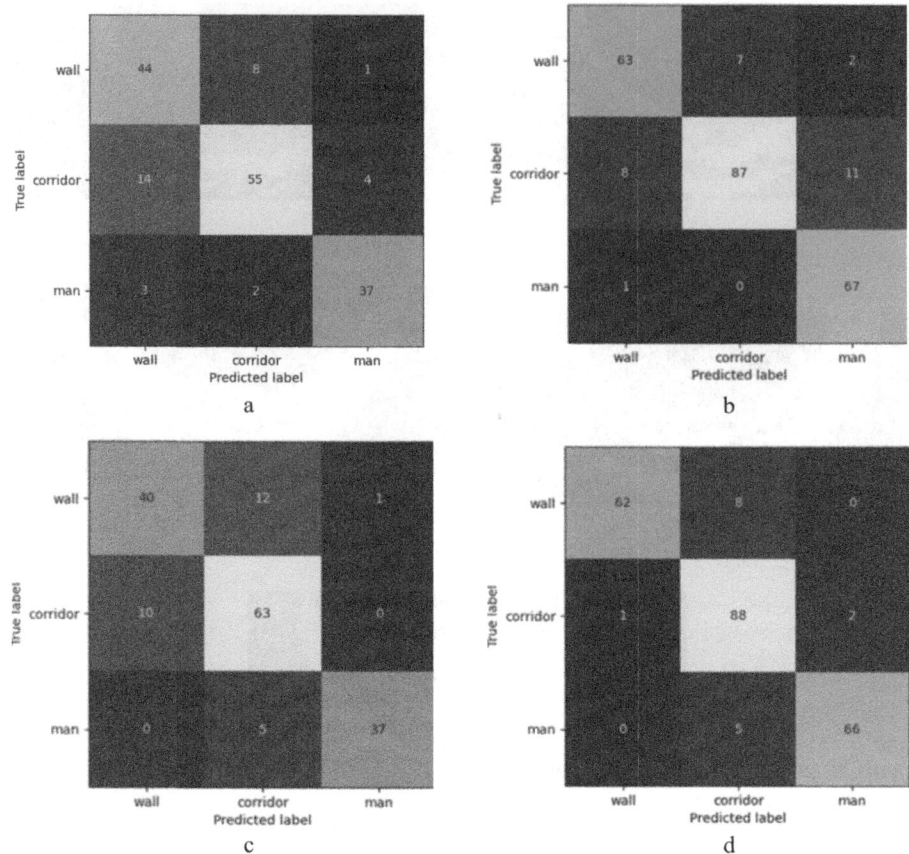

Fig. 11. Confusion Matrices. a) KNN, b) Random Forest, c) SVM using linear kernel, and d) SVM using RBF kernel

Table 2. Accuracies obtained for the machine learning classifiers

Model	Configuration	Average Accuracy
K-Nearest Neighbours (KNN)	5 nearest neighbours	80.95%
Random Forest	100 estimators	88.21%
Support Vector Machine (SVM)	Linear Kernel	83.34%
Support Vector Machine (SVM)	RBF Kernel	93.10%

5   Conclusion

This paper proposes a novel UWB Radar-based on body area network system to assist the blind and partially sighted patients with the navigation. This method utilises the novel UWB technology, body area networks and probability-based detection algorithm to identify the obstacles in the surroundings. This was tested experimentally and obtained an average accuracy of 93% for classifying obstacles. Although the proposed system was tested with two UWB radars, the algorithms are expandable to any number of radar units, limited by the processing power of the radar controller.

References

1. Facts and figures | European Blind Union. https://www.euroblind.org/about-blindness-and-partial-sight/facts-and-figures. Accessed 12 Sept 2023
2. Blindness and vision loss. https://www.nhs.uk/conditions/vision-loss/. Accessed 12 Sept 2023
3. Pereira, A., Nunes, N., Vieira, D., Costa, N., Fernandes, H., Barroso, J.: Blind guide: an ultrasound sensor-based body area network for guiding blind people. Procedia Comput. Sci. **67**, 403–408 (2015). https://doi.org/10.1016/j.procs.2015.09.285
4. Han, Y., Beheshti, M., Jones, B., Hudson, T.E., Seiple, W.H., Rizzo, J.-R.: Wearables for persons with blindness and low vision: form factor matters. Assist. Technol. 1–4 (2023). https://doi.org/10.1080/10400435.2023.2205490
5. Villanueva, J., Farcy, R.: Optical device indicating a safe free path to blind people. IEEE Trans. Instrum. Meas. **61**, 170–177 (2012). https://doi.org/10.1109/TIM.2011.2160910
6. Nada, A.A., Fakhr, M.A., Seddik, A.F.: Assistive infrared sensor based smart stick for blind people. In: 2015 Science and Information Conference (SAI), pp. 1149–1154 (2015). https://doi.org/10.1109/SAI.2015.7237289
7. Joseph, A.M., Kian, A., Begg, R.: State-of-the-art review on wearable obstacle detection systems developed for assistive technologies and footwear. Sensors. **23**, 2802 (2023). https://doi.org/10.3390/s23052802
8. Nanduri, S., Umamaheswari, E., Kishore, R., Ajaykumar, M.: Smart Bottine for autistic people. Mater. Today: Proc. **62**, 4788–4794 (2022). https://doi.org/10.1016/j.matpr.2022.03.344
9. Zhang, Z., Xiang, C., Zhao, Z., Liang, W., Cui, D., Liu, H.: ISEE: a wearable image-sound translation system for partially sighted people. IEEE Sens. J. **23**, 13585–13597 (2023). https://doi.org/10.1109/JSEN.2023.3266793
10. Zhang, L., Jia, K., Liu, J., Wang, G., Huang, W.: Design of blind guiding robot based on speed adaptation and visual recognition. IEEE Access. **11**, 75971–75978 (2023). https://doi.org/10.1109/ACCESS.2023.3296066
11. Madake, J., Bhatlawande, S., Solanke, A., Shilaskar, S.: A qualitative and quantitative analysis of research in mobility technologies for visually impaired people. IEEE Access **11**, 82496–82520 (2023). https://doi.org/10.1109/ACCESS.2023.3291074
12. Sivan, S., Darsan, G.: Computer vision based assistive technology for blind and visually impaired people. In: Proceedings of the 7th International Conference on Computing Communication and Networking Technologies, pp. 1–8. Association for Computing Machinery, New York (2016). https://doi.org/10.1145/2967878.2967923
13. Chang, W.-J., Chen, L.-B., Sie, C.-Y., Yang, C.-H.: An Artificial intelligence edge computing-based assistive system for visually impaired pedestrian safety at zebra crossings. IEEE Trans. Consum. Electron. **67**, 3–11 (2021). https://doi.org/10.1109/TCE.2020.3037065
14. Poggi, M., Mattoccia, S.: A wearable mobility aid for the visually impaired based on embedded 3D vision and deep learning. In: 2016 IEEE Symposium on Computers and Communication (ISCC), pp. 208–213 (2016). https://doi.org/10.1109/ISCC.2016.7543741
15. Federal Register, Tuesday, October 12, 2010. https://www.govinfo.gov/content/pkg/FR-2010-10-12/xml/FR-2010-10-12.xml. Accessed 14 Sept 2023

16. Wickramarachchi, D.N., Rana, S.P., Ghavami, M., Dudley, S.: Comparison of IR-UWB Radar SoC for non-contact biomedical application. In: 2023 IEEE 17th International Symposium on Medical Information and Communication Technology (ISMICT), pp. 01–06 (2023). https://doi.org/10.1109/ISMICT58261.2023.10152276

17. Yan, S., Soh, P.J., Vandenbosch, G.A.E.: Wearable ultrawideband technology—a review of ultrawideband antennas, propagation channels, and applications in wireless body area networks. IEEE Access. **6**, 42177–42185 (2018). https://doi.org/10.1109/ACCESS.2018.286 1704

18. MQTT - The Standard for IoT Messaging. https://mqtt.org/. Accessed 14 Sept 2023

Healthcare Data Governance, Privacy, and Security - A Conceptual Framework

Amen Faridoon[1,2]([⊠])(iD) and M. Tahar Kechadi[1,2]

[1] University College Dublin, Dublin, Ireland
tahar.kechadi@ucd.ie
[2] The Insight Centre for Data Analytics, Dublin, Ireland
amen.faridoon@ucdconnect.ie

Abstract. The abundance of data has transformed the world in every aspect. It has become the core element in decision-making, problem-solving, and innovation in almost all areas of life, including business, science, healthcare, education, and many others. Despite all these advances, privacy and security remain critical concerns of the healthcare industry. It's important to note that healthcare data can also be a liability if it is not managed correctly. This data mismanagement can have severe consequences for patients and healthcare organisations, including patient safety, legal liability, damage to reputation, financial loss, and operational inefficiency. Healthcare organisations must comply with a range of regulations to protect patient data. We perform a classification of data governance elements/components in a manner that thoroughly assesses the healthcare data chain from a privacy and security standpoint. After deeply analysing the existing literature, we propose a conceptual privacy and security-driven healthcare data governance framework.

Keywords: Healthcare Data Governance · Electronic Health Record Governance · Medical Data Protection · Conceptual Health Data Governance Framework

1 Introduction

Digital data collection has undergone a transformative journey since its inception. It started with manual data entry and simple electronic databases in the mid 20th century. Since then, the process has gained momentum with the proliferation of computers and the internet. The 21st century has witnessed an explosion in data sources, from social media and IoT devices to advanced sensors and machine-generated data. This influx prompted the development of advanced data collection techniques, including big data analytics, machine learning, and AI-driven insights. Similarly, healthcare data collection spans several centuries, evolving from rudimentary record-keeping to sophisticated digital systems. The 20th century saw the rise of electronic health records (EHRs), allowing for more efficient patient information storage and retrieval. With the advent of the 21st

© ICST Institute for Computer Sciences, Social Informatics and Telecommunications Engineering 2024
Published by Springer Nature Switzerland AG 2024. All Rights Reserved
M. Mizmizi et al. (Eds.): BodyNets 2024, LNICST 524, pp. 261–271, 2024.
https://doi.org/10.1007/978-3-031-72524-1_19

century, technological advancements enabled the integration of various data sources, such as wearable devices and mobile apps, contributing to the growth of comprehensive and real-time healthcare data collection. This evolution has significantly enhanced healthcare delivery, research, and policy-making by providing insights into disease patterns, population health trends and treatment effectiveness.

However, this evolution has also raised concerns about privacy, security, and ethical considerations, leading to stringent data protection regulations to balance innovation with individual rights. Healthcare data often contains sensitive and personal patient information, including medical history, diagnoses, treatments, prescriptions, test results, social security numbers, and home addresses, making it highly valuable and vulnerable to misuse and theft. Table 1 represents the types of information stored in the electronic health records and their sensitivity level. Data privacy and security are essential for protecting patient rights,

Table 1. Types of Information Present in Electronic Health Records and Their Sensitivity Level

Common Features	Description	Sensitivity Level
Entity Identifiers	Personal identification information such as; name, address, email, phone number etc.	Identifiable
Demographic Information	Classification of a person in a specific group such as; age, education, gender, area etc.	Quasi-Identifiable
Clinical Records	Patient's medical history include treatments, diagnoses, medication, n etc.	Quasi-Identifiable and sensitive
Medical Biometrics	Patient's physical health-related information such as; blood pressure, heart rate, X-Ray, test reports etc.	sensitive
Mental Health Information	Patient's psychological related information such as; sleep problems, dietary information, psychosocial issues etc.	sensitive
Activities and lifestyle	Person's physical activities and their lifestyle-related information such as; physical activities, nutrition, exercise plans, etc.	sensitive
Financial Information	Person's financial data such as; health insurance, billing, reimbursements, financial class etc.	Quasi-Identifiable and sensitive
IoT and Wearable Data	Person's wearable and monitoring data include healthcare wearable devices, healthcare IoT devices, sensors data, etc.	Quasi-Identifiable and sensitive

preventing identity theft and cyber-attacks, maintaining trust in the healthcare system, ensuring continuity of care, and complying with legal and ethical standards. Unfortunately, healthcare organizations remain a popular target for hackers due to the sensitive nature of the data they possess. For instance, in 2020, there were 616 reported data breaches affecting healthcare organizations in the United States, according to the HIPAA Journal. Recently, in January 2023, LifeBridge Health in Maryland exposed the personal and medical information of approximately 1.4 million patients, including names, birth dates, medical diagnoses, and treatment information. These data breach cases demonstrate the insufficient implementation and management of security and privacy measures.

Inadequate management of data can lead to potential legal responsibilities. Healthcare organizations need to proactively safeguard patient information through solid security and privacy protocols to counter various risks. Considering the sensitivity, usability, and multiple access to electronic health records, healthcare institutions should adopt preemptive data governance frameworks. These frameworks ensure operational efficiency without compromising the confidentiality of data, even from internal individuals with authorised system access who might have malicious intent. The concept of Electronic Health Record (EHR) Governance was first introduced by the Institute of Medicine (IOM) in their 2003 report titled "Key Capabilities of an Electronic Health Record System" [4]. This report emphasized the necessity of a systematic approach to managing EHR systems, including the requirement of governance structures that could supervise the development, implementation and maintenance of these systems. Similarly, the report "Nationwide Privacy and Security Framework for Electronic Exchange of Individually Identifiable Health Information" was issued by the US Department of Health and Human Services (HHS) in 2008[1]. This report accentuates the need for governance frameworks to guarantee the secure and efficient utilisation of Electronic Health Records. Organisations like the Office of the National Coordinator for Health Information Technology (ONC) have created guidelines and frameworks to assist EHR governance. These resources concentrate on aspects such as data privacy, data security, data quality, and data interoperability. Data governance encompasses the comprehensive administration of data within an organization. It entails assigning roles and duties for data management, establishing regulations and protocols for ensuring data accuracy, confidentiality, protection, and adherence to regulations, and setting up mechanisms to uphold these regulations. The primary goal of data governance is to establish well-defined principles/guidelines for gathering, retaining, accessing, and utilizing data to optimize its usefulness while minimising potential hazards like data breaches and legal violations.

Contributions: We have managed to conduct a wide review of the concerns related to data privacy and security by focusing on or analysing data governance activities in the healthcare industry. After deeply analyzing the literature, we

---

[1] https://digital.ahrq.gov/health-it-tools-and-resources/health-it-bibliography/privacy-and-security/nationwide-privacy-and.

categorised data governance activities presented in Sect. 3. The primary goals of this critical evaluation are as follows:

- Study the existing state-of-the-art healthcare data governance models/systems.
- Categorize the data governance activities/elements in such a way that deeply analyses the healthcare data chain with the privacy and security perspective.
- Propose a privacy and security-driven conceptual healthcare data governance framework.

2   Existing Healthcare Data Governance Models

Delving into Helen Nissenbaum's approach (explains privacy as more than just a right to secrecy or control; instead, it is about the suitable flow of private information within specific social contexts) to privacy (2010), the study [24] presenting a fascinating work for accessing data governance in a specific context of private health data. This study examines the use scenario involving the Royal Free Trust and Alphabet's AI Venture DeepMind Health initiative. It sheds light on the clashes among the partners concerning crucial aspects, particularly the governance systems, objectives and gain attained via initiative. Researchers emphasize the intricacies of governing PHI data to foster healthcare innovation and advancement while safeguarding privacy and serving the public benefit. In a study [23], the authors discovered six interconnected yet distinct models for governing Personal Health Information (PHI) by focusing on what types of value are possibly afforded by PHI beyond the fundamental concerns of data privacy and security. Five analytical aspects should be used to administer data governance in the realm of Personal Health Information (PHI): the field of data, those who are engaged, the significance or utilization of the PHI, the governance objective, and the governance platform.

In [13], the authors examined the fundamental model of contemporary data governance and emphasised five crucial data decision fields: data postulates, metadata, accuracy, access management, and information management cycle. Whereas a composite synthesis of research paper [1] evaluates 145 academic and practitioner papers related to data governance, encompassing the period from 2001 to 2019. The second one suggests a pyramidal governance system that uses governance mechanisms to balance data, realm, and organizational capacity. These mechanisms are all structured by organizational ethical and technological "antecedents" pre-data ingestion and impacted by risk control and performance-driven "consequences" post hoc. A comparative data governance activities examination found in academic and practitioner articles is conducted in [3]. The analysis explored a total of 120 information management elements that are classified as domains of governance, action, and decision areas. Authors [6] constructed an organization governance model derived from a case study, the proposed framework includes three levels and their interconnections with one another. At the strategic level of an organization, a data governance council's responsibilities include approving guidelines, coordinating business and data projects, and assessing budget requests for data-related projects. In addition, significant roles are played by data custodians and data stewards on the tactical level. The significant data stakeholders from various categories (user groups) operate at the lowest level. This model aids in comprehending what organisational layer data governance duties should work on; but, it does not provide a way to set up data governance.

Furthermore, the study [21] determines the condition, factors influencing, and potential obstacles to data governance in Kenyan health professional regulating entities. The primary focus of this paper is to construct a framework which can be applicable to develop an official data governance initiative at these healthcare governing bodies. This particular work determined the quality of data maintenance, attaining customer satisfaction, safeguarding security and control of the data, and reaching a state of operational effectiveness as the driving force behind data governance in the governing authorities. These bodies encounter challenges such as insufficient knowledge of data governance, lack of management ownership and backing, and constrained distribution of funds and resources, each functioning as a barrier to efficient data administration. The scholarly article [15] suggested a comprehensive layout for the governance of big data drawn from an analysis of ten representative case studies of medical information exchange organizations in China. The framework was condensed into the following three domains: drive domain, capability domain and support domain. It also incorporates a total of 12 elements, such as massive data strategy formation, legal and regulatory aspects, business actions practices, assistance, big medical data maintenance authority, collection of data, preservation, process and analysis, usage, resource utilization, quality management, and data protection safeguards that pertain to each respective domain.

However, other studies [2,8,9,11,12,17,18] are also considered which are not directly investigate the healthcare data governance activities, frameworks or elements but highlight the needs and importance of data governance frameworks or activities focusing on privacy and security perspective, challenges and risks associated with data governance regarding big data, involvement of IoT devices, data access controls or ownership, regulating multiple data actors, data quality dimension in healthcare etc. These studies provide the basic elements or activities that should be part of the healthcare data governance frameworks

3   Healthcare Data Privacy and Security Framework

These studies provide comprehensive data governance frameworks/elements/activities via which we categorised them into three distinct pillars: (1) Data Governance Organization, (2) Data Communication, and (3) Data Privacy and Security by Design, as shown in Fig. 1. This categorisation underscores healthcare data's security and privacy concerns throughout the chain, from records collection to sharing analysed results or data. However, existing state-of-the-art healthcare data governance frameworks treated privacy as an afterthought or an add-on feature, but instead as an integral part of the entire design process.

3.1   Data Governance

Data governance is critical to a successful data governance program. It provides a structured approach to managing data by defining policies, rules, regulations, and procedures. The framework outlines the roles and responsibilities of various stakeholders, including owners, stewards, custodians, and users of data. Moreover, employees' training and accountability are also necessary and challenging components of the data governance organization pillar in healthcare.

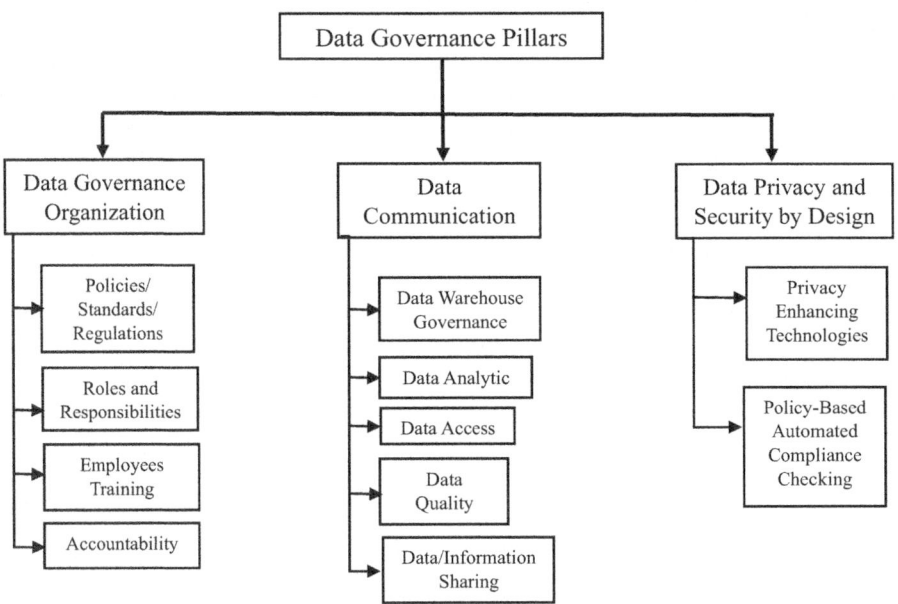

Fig. 1. Healthcare Data Protection Governance - A Conceptual Framework

Policies, Standards, Regulations: Fair Information Practice Principles (FIPPs)[2] are a set of principles that form the basis of modern data protection laws and regulations. These principles were first established by the United States in 1970s and have since been adopted by many countries worldwide. The FIPPs provide a framework for gathering, utilizing, and revealing individual information fairly and transparently. In healthcare, the principles of FIPPs are reflected in various regulations and acts, including the General Data Protection Regulation (GDPR) [14,19] in the European Union, in the United States, the Health Insurance Portability and Accountability Act (HIPAA) [7], the Personal Information Protection and Electronic Documents Act (PIPEDA)[3] in Canada,

---

[2] https://www.ftc.gov/sites/default/files/documents/reports/privacy-online-report-congress/priv-23a.pdf.

[3] "Office of the Australian Information Commissioner (OIAC)", https://www.cdr.gov.au/.

etc. Additionally, healthcare organizations must establish internal policies and regulations that provide a framework for data privacy, security, consent management, and other critical aspects of healthcare compliance.

Roles and Responsibilities: Data governance requires collaboration and communication among various stakeholders to ensure data is managed effectively, efficiently and securely. The roles and responsibilities in data governance may differ according to the size of the organization, structure, and industry. Data Governance organisational structure describes typical roles: 1) the composition, charter, and leadership of the Data Governance Committee; 2) the tasks of other relevant Data Governance committees 3) positions in huge organisations; links to other groups and entities and 4) top-level funding. In addition, the structure demonstrates how the Data Governance process gives supervision to owners of data, administrators, guardians, IT staff, compliance officers, and users of data, who are typically involved in the data warehouse management.

Employees Training: Healthcare workers are less tech-savvy and have less understanding of the safety of data, and technologies related to healthcare lag well behind those of the financial sector. Consequently, an understanding of data protection concerns requires education and training. Staff training works well for handling low-tech breaches of data. Keeping end-users informed about medical provider policies and fundamental security precautions is a part of preserving the privacy of data. Accidental interference can be prevented by teaching staff members about security risks including tapping on email links, pressing the computer desk login credentials, and visiting unapproved web pages.

Accountability: Systems for evaluation and surveillance must be put in place by healthcare businesses to make certain that staff members are abiding by the regulations of the company. They create guidelines to prevent security lapses and specify precisely how infractions will be handled. Healthcare data is ideal for the identity thief. Being proactive and putting plans into action is essential. Reactive actions, like playing catch-up after a security breach happens, are not an effective approach.

3.2   Data Communication

Organizing or listing data elements with their description and other valuable information (metadata) enables numerous insights into the core data or business concepts and terminologies. Everyone implicated in the data management cycle uses the same terms to discuss the same things, making communication easy. Effective communication reduces operational friction and minimises data misuse due to inaccurate understanding. We further categorise this pillar into five components to keenly analyse the security and privacy situation in the healthcare industry.

Data Warehouse Governance (DWG): Data Warehouse Governance gives guidelines, rules and practices to guarantee gain, utility, significance and risk management. Strategic choice-making and monitoring should ideally be the main concern of data warehouse governance, with secondary objectives including resource distribution, value of investment, and minimizing risk. Nevertheless, DWG could be more concerned regarding security and confidentiality, compliance, and risk prevention in healthcare settings given the delicate nature of protected health information.

Data Analytic: Since the end of the 1950s, interest in artificial intelligence (AI) has cycled through periods of hope and disappointment due to unsatisfactory performance of algorithms and computing infrastructure [20]. While, the development of big data, machine learning, deep learning algorithms, and suitable computing infrastructure has rekindled interest in artificial intelligence (AI) technology and expedited its uptake across a number of industries. Even though modern AI techniques like machine learning have just recently been used in the healthcare industry, the prospects for better healthcare outcomes are encouraging [22]. Analyzing, or mining, the data without disclosing personally identifying or delicate private data about specific persons is known as privacy-preserving data analytics.

Data Access: Institutions and people are both impacted by breaches of data and fraud. To safeguard patients' confidential information, the majority of healthcare organizations have developed sophisticated security protocols [10]. While, software flaws, phishing, identities being stolen, and fraudulent attempts allow cyber criminals to get access and capture private information, which can lead to theft of identity, financial loss, anxiety, depression, prejudice, humiliation, assault, and other issues [5,16]. Insider dangers, however, are far more challenging to identify and stop than external ones. *Insider threat* is any harm carried out by users with authorized access to an organization's network, apps, or data repositories. Therefore, strong security management structures are needed to guard against unauthorized access to healthcare information by outside parties and malevolent insider threats.

Data Quality: Healthcare data quality is critical for delivering safe, efficient, and effective patient care, driving medical research and innovation, informing healthcare policies, facilitating quality improvement initiatives, ensuring interoperability, and complying with legal and regulatory requirements. Governing bodies should design a data quality management framework composed of six key dimensions: accuracy, completeness, consistency, uniqueness, timelessness and validity because privacy and security compliance can only be achieved with accurate and consistent data.

3.3   Data Privacy and Security by Design

The third pillar of the proposed data governance framework focuses on data forti-fication by design. Data Privacy and Security by Design (PSbD) is an approach to developing systems, products, and services with a strong focus on privacy and security. Integrating privacy and security considerations into any system's design, development, and implementation stages. After reviewing the legal per-spective through law articles, the privacy-by-design framework has been defined. By doing so, medical data privacy risks can be minimized, and individuals can have more control over their personal and sensitive data.

Privacy Enhancing Technologies: Privacy-enhancing technologies (PETs) are tools, techniques, and systems designed to protect and enhance privacy in the digital realm. They aim to safeguard sensitive information, limit data collection and sharing, and give individuals greater control over their data. PETs can be applied in various contexts of the data life-cycle and help healthcare providers meet their legal and ethical obligations regarding data protection.

Policy-Based Automated Compliance Checking: Automated compliance checking involves leveraging technology, such as software applications or plat-forms, to systematically evaluate the organization's activities, processes, and behaviour to comply with the established policies. To identify deviations or vio-lations, these automated systems can analyze various data sources, including logs, records, and transactions. As regulations and policies evolve, the systems can be updated with new rules and requirements. This adaptability can enable healthcare providers to stay compliant with the latest industry standards and regulations, even in a rapidly changing healthcare landscape.

4   Conclusion

The proliferation of data has brought about profound changes across various domains. Likewise, using cutting-edge technology for Electronic Medical Records not only transforms illness treatment but also benefits insurance, law enforce-ment, pharmaceutical, and other product-selling businesses. However, the health-care industry is still grappling with persistent concerns related to data protec-tion. It is noteworthy that mishandling healthcare data can lead to significant lia-bility, impacting patients and organisations. Healthcare entities must adhere to a multitude of regulations to safeguard patient data. After thoroughly examining the literature, we have determined that the previously established cutting-edge healthcare data governance frameworks often regarded privacy as a secondary consideration rather than an inherent and essential component integrated into the design process. We have conducted an in-depth review of existing studies and proposed a conceptual healthcare data governance framework with a pri-mary focus on data privacy and security.

References

1. Abraham, R., Schneider, J., Vom Brocke, J.: Data governance: a conceptual framework, structured review, and research agenda. Int. J. Inf. Manage. **49**, 424–438 (2019)
2. Al-Badi, A., Tarhini, A., Khan, A.I.: Exploring big data governance frameworks. Procedia Comput. Sci. **141**, 271–277 (2018)
3. Alhassan, I., Sammon, D., Daly, M.: Data governance activities: a comparison between scientific and practice-oriented literature. J. Enterp. Inf. Manag. **31**(2), 300–316 (2018)
4. Aspden, P., Corrigan, J.M., Wolcott, J., Erickson, S.M., et al.: Key capabilities of an electronic health record system: letter report. In: Patient Safety: Achieving a New Standard for Care. National Academies Press (US) (2004)
5. Chabot, Y., Bertaux, A., Nicolle, C., Kechadi, T.: An ontology-based approach for the reconstruction and analysis of digital incidents timelines. Digit. Investig. **15**, 83–100 (2015)
6. Cheong, L.K., Chang, V.: The need for data governance: a case study. In: ACIS 2007 Proceedings, p. 100 (2007)
7. HHS Office for Civil Rights: Standards for privacy of individually identifiable health information. Final rule. Federal Register **67**(157), 53181–53273 (2002)
8. Dasgupta, A., Gill, A., Hussain, F.: A conceptual framework for data governance in IoT-enabled digital is ecosystems. In: 8th International Conference on Data Science, Technology and Applications. SCITEPRESS–Science and Technology Publications (2019)
9. Fleissner, B., Jasti, K., Ales, J., Thomas, R.: The importance of data governance in healthcare.: 1–11. [White Paper] (2014)
10. Greenaway, K.E., Chan, Y.E., Crossler, R.E.: Company information privacy orientation: a conceptual framework. Inf. Syst. J. **25**(6), 579–606 (2015)
11. Juddoo, S., George, C., Duquenoy, P., Windridge, D.: Data governance in the health industry: investigating data quality dimensions within a big data context. Appl. Syst. Innov. **1**(4), 43 (2018)
12. Kariotis, T., et al.: Emerging health data platforms: from individual control to collective data governance. Data Policy **2**, e13 (2020)
13. Khatri, V., Brown, C.V.: Designing data governance. Commun. ACM **53**(1), 148–152 (2010)
14. Lea, N.C.: How will the general data protection regulation affect healthcare? Acta Med. Port. **31**(7–8), 363–365 (2018)
15. Li, Q., et al.: A framework for big data governance to advance RHINs: a case study of china. IEEE Access **7**, 50330–50338 (2019)
16. Van der Meulen, N.: The challenge of countering identity theft: recent developments in the united states, the united kingdom, and the European union. Report Commissioned by the National Infrastructure Cyber Crime program (NICC). Retrieved May **20**, 2007 (2006)
17. Paparova, D., Aanestad, M., Vassilakopoulou, P., Bahus, M.K.: Data governance spaces: the case of a national digital service for personal health data. Inf. Organ. **33**(1), 100451 (2023)
18. Perez-Pozuelo, I., Spathis, D., Gifford-Moore, J., Morley, J., Cowls, J.: Digital phenotyping and sensitive health data: implications for data governance. J. Am. Med. Inform. Assoc. **28**(9), 2002–2008 (2021)

19. Regulation, G.D.P.: General data protection regulation (GDPR). Intersoft Consulting, Accessed in October **24**(1) (2018)
20. Salathé, M., Wiegand, T., Wenzel, M.: Focus group on artificial intelligence for health. arXiv preprint arXiv:1809.04797 (2018)
21. Were, V., Moturi, C.: Toward a data governance model for the Kenya health professional regulatory authorities. TQM J. **29**(4), 579–589 (2017)
22. Whittlestone, J., Nyrup, R., Alexandrova, A., Dihal, K., Cave, S.: Ethical and societal implications of algorithms, data, and artificial intelligence: a roadmap for research. Nuffield Foundation, London (2019)
23. Winter, J.S., Davidson, E.: Investigating values in personal health data governance models. In: 23rd Americas Conference on Information Systems (AMCIS) (2017)
24. Winter, J.S., Davidson, E.: Big data governance of personal health information and challenges to contextual integrity. Inf. Soc. **35**(1), 36–51 (2019)

Towards Robust IoT Defense: Comparative Statistics of Attack Detection in Resource-Constrained Scenarios

Zainab Alwaisi[1]([✉]) and Simone Soderi[1,2]

[1] IMT School for Advanced Studies, Lucca, Italy
{zainab.alwaisi,simone.soderi}@imtlucca.it
[2] CINI Cybersecurity Laboratory, Rome, Italy

Abstract. Resource constraints pose a significant cybersecurity threat to IoT smart devices, making them vulnerable to various attacks, including those targeting energy and memory. This study underscores the need for innovative security measures due to resource-related incidents in smart devices. In this paper, we conduct an extensive statistical analysis of cyberattack detection algorithms under resource constraints to identify the most efficient one. Our research involves a comparative analysis of various algorithms, including those from our previous work. We specifically compare a lightweight algorithm for detecting resource-constrained cyberattacks with another designed for the same purpose. Notably, the latter employs TinyML for detection. In addition to the comprehensive evaluation of the proposed algorithms, we introduced a novel detection method for resource-constrained attacks. This method involves analyzing protocol data and categorizing the final data packet as normal or attacked. Subsequently, the attacked data is further analyzed in terms of the memory and energy consumption of the devices to determine whether it's an energy or memory attack or another form of malicious activity. We compare the suggested algorithm performance using four evaluation metrics: accuracy, probability of detection, probability of false alarm, and probability of misdetection. Notably, the proposed dynamic techniques dynamically select the classifier with the best results for detecting attacks, ensuring optimal performance even within resource-constrained IoT environments. The results indicate that the proposed algorithms outperform the existing works with accuracy for algorithms with TinyML and without TinyML of 99.3%, 98.2%, a probability of detection of 99.4%, 97.3%, a probability of false alarm of 1.23%, 1.64%, a probability of misdetection of 1.64%, 1.46 respectively. In contrast, the accuracy of the novel detection mechanism exceeds 99.5% for RF and 97% for SVM.

Keywords: Smart Home · Internet of Things (IoT) · resource constraints · detection · smart devices · security · machine-learning

M. Mizmizi et al. (Eds.): BodyNets 2024, LNICST 524, pp. 272–291, 2024.
https://doi.org/10.1007/978-3-031-72524-1_20

1   Introduction

The Internet of Things (IoT) facilitates the connection of numerous devices, enabling data exchange and updates for various applications across smart city infrastructure, smart homes, smart vehicles, advanced healthcare systems, and other intelligent environments. The IoT network requires swift communication with low latency to avoid delays and high throughput to accommodate the vast number of devices through wireless or wired connections. IoT devices can connect directly to the Internet using technologies like cellular connections or Wi-Fi or indirectly via specific IoT protocols. In the latter case, the devices initially communicate with a base station or a gateway, and then the gateway acts as a bridge to connect to the internet [11]. The complexity of IoT models is steadily increasing [16,17]. People are becoming increasingly accustomed to data-driven infrastructure, driving the research of more Machine Learning-based applications in conjunction with IoT. IoT and Machine Learning (ML) techniques are currently being applied in virtually every facet of human life. IoT devices utilize wireless communication, making them susceptible to potential security breaches [13]. Unlike typical communication attacks in local networks, which are often limited to local nodes or small local domains, attacks on IoT systems can extend over a broader area, causing significant disruptions to IoT installations [18]. As energy efficiency demands in IoT applications rise, the need for low latency, enhanced reliability, and strengthened security also increases. Particularly crucial in applications like smart cities, digital healthcare, and Industry 4.0 [10]. Integrating edge and fog computing into conventional IoT networks provides substantial advantages by placing computational resources closer to devices and data sources. Incorporating Artificial Intelligence (AI) and other advanced technologies enables automated and expedited data processing, analysis, and decision-making. In prior research [1–4], we extensively investigated resource-constrained attacks on smart devices, developing lightweight detection mechanisms for timely monitoring. Emphasizing energy and memory attack analysis, these solutions focus on detecting and monitoring attacks effectively.

Subsequently, recognizing the potential of TinyML as an additional approach to detect resource-constrained attacks on smart devices, we explored the integration of TinyML as an innovative solution to address resource constraints more effectively. Leveraging TinyML in this context significantly enhances the cybersecurity posture of smart devices. It enables real-time attack detection and the capacity to predict future attacks through ML, which learns from resource-based attacks in their nascent stages. The statistical analysis to show the best detection mechanism to detect resource constraint attacks is proposed to address the challenges arising from the increased utilization of IoT devices, which generate substantial volumes of data overwhelming security providers. This statical analysis advocates for cybersecurity providers to effectively detect resource constraints and cyber attack problems and understand the best mechanisms to tackle this security issue. Advanced analytics and ML algorithms play a crucial role in achieving this objective, enabling the identification of patterns and trends in the data and prioritization of the most pertinent information for clinicians.

By leveraging the potential of IoT data through these approaches, cybersecurity providers can enhance the security outcomes of IoT smart devices and elevate the overall quality of detecting such attacks.

Moreover, this paper proposes a resource constraints attack detection method based on ML techniques. Based on the previous research papers [1–4], through the analysis of the principle of resource constraints attack, the three common attack packets obtained by operating the energy and memory attacks tool are grouped in the feature extraction stage. The characteristics of attack flow are obtained through the analysis of normal flow data. The attack traffic characteristics obtained in the model detection phase are trained in the training model based on the Random Forest (RF) algorithm. Finally, the test model is validated by the resource constraints attack, and the Support Vector Machines (SVM) method in ML is compared in terms of detection accuracy. The results show that the resource constraints attack detection method based on ML proposed in this paper has a reasonable detection rate for the current popular energy and memory attacks. In addition, this method involves analyzing protocol data and categorizing the final data packet as normal or attacked. Subsequently, the attacked data is further analyzed in terms of the memory and energy consumption of the devices to determine whether it's an energy or memory attack or another form of malicious activity. To specify the type of attack, we used ML techniques to compare the fetched attacked data with the stored data related to energy and memory.

1.1   Organization of the Paper

This paper is organized as follows: Sect. 2 provides related works. Section 3 outlines the architecture of our previous studies, while the detection mechanism of the novel study is presented in Sect. 4. Sections 5 present the results and evaluations. Finally, Sect. 6 concludes with some final remarks and suggestions for future work.

1.2   Motivation and Contribution

IoT represents an interconnected network that links smart objects to the Internet. While a multitude of IoT devices are connected to the Internet, a significant portion of them lack robust security measures, rendering them vulnerable to various cybersecurity threats. These devices are often resource-constrained, making the application of conventional security protocols challenging. To address this, many researchers have proposed the implementation of intrusion detection systems at IoT gateways. However, the vulnerability of IoT devices persists if these gateway-based security mechanisms prove insufficient.

Therefore, there is a growing need for innovative solutions that can effectively safeguard IoT devices against resource-constrained attacks, particularly those aimed at depleting energy and memory resources. To enhance the security of IoT systems and services and defend against cyber threats that exploit the resource constraints of smart devices, an additional layer of protection specifically designed for resource-constrained IoT devices and networks is imperative. Our primary contribution lies in conducting a comprehensive statistical analysis of the algorithms we've introduced in our previous studies [1–3]. This analysis serves to determine the most effective algorithms for detecting resource-constraint attacks. We achieve this by calculating various critical variables, including the probability of detection, probability of misdetection, probability of false alarm, and overall accuracy. This in-depth statistical examination allows us to provide valuable insights into the performance and effectiveness of these algorithms in defending against resource-constraint attacks. Furthermore, we introduce a novel method for detecting resource constraint attacks. This innovative approach involves the analysis of captured packets at the protocol level, segmenting them into two categories: normal packets and attacked packets. Subsequently, ML techniques are employed to classify the nature of the attacked packet on the protocol, whether it involves an energy or memory-related attack. The classification process relies on comparing the extracted information from the attacked packets with our existing energy and memory attack pattern datasets. Furthermore, we concurrently monitor energy and memory metrics during the attack detection phase to determine the presence of an energy attack, memory attack, or both on the targeted smart devices. The calculation of accuracy and detection attack rate is also involved.

2   Related Work

Several researchers have proposed methods to identify attacks on energy consumption. Valentina *et al.* [7] emphasized the significance of energy efficiency, promoting the use of smarter devices for sustainability. Efficient home automation control is crucial for minimizing energy losses, optimizing consumption based on specific needs, and ensuring effective system operation [8]. This investigation [12] evaluated established home energy management systems, highlighting differences in functionality and quality to identify opportunities for energy conservation, considering both behavioural and operational aspects. It's noteworthy that factors such as comfort, convenience, and security often influence the adoption of energy-efficient scenarios. In another approach proposed by Shi *et al.*, [20], a detection framework for IoT systems relies on energy consumption analysis. This method involves scrutinizing smart devices' energy usage, and categorising monitored devices' attack status, encompassing both cyber and physical attacks. The proposed two-stage process involves a short time window for initial attack detection and a longer time window for more refined attack identification. Similarly, various authors have addressed the issue of detecting memory attacks. For instance, Mosli *et al.* [14] introduced a technique to detect malware by extracting three key features from memory images: Application Programming Interface (API) calls, registry activities, and imported libraries. These experiments were carried out on each feature separately, and the highest accuracy, reaching 96%, was achieved using the SVM classifier with the registry activities feature. In a subsequent work [15], the same authors utilized process handles available in memory to detect malware. Their research found that malware typically employs process handles, mutants, and section handles. However, their approach achieved a modest accuracy when employing the RF classifier, slightly exceeding 91%. Duan et al. [6] also introduced an approach for extracting live Dynamic-Link Library (DLL) features from memory, which was used to detect malware variants that employed the same DLLs. Their experiments resulted in an accuracy of 90%, achieved through the hidden naïve Bayes classifier. Furthermore, Dai et al. [5] proposed a malware detection and classification approach based on extracting memory images and converting them into fixed-size greyscale images. Features were extracted from these images using a gradient histogram, and these features were used for malware classification. An accuracy of 95.2% was achieved using a neural network classifier. In a previous work by the same authors, API calls from behaviour analysis and memory analysis were combined into a single vector to represent each sample. They employed a dataset consisting of 1200 malware and 400 benign files to train the SVM classifier. The research demonstrated that memory analysis could mitigate the limitations of behaviour analysis [21]. Indeed, the application of TinyML is indispensable in ensuring the security of smart devices against resource-constrained attacks. TinyML, which has effectively expanded the domain of ML to encompass low-power microcontrollers [22], is a vital component in addressing the evolving landscape of IoT. As IoT devices become increasingly sophisticated in their analytical capabilities, networking, security, and decision-making challenges become more complex.

The existing constraints, including power, memory, and computational capacity limitations, are significantly impeding the creation of robust connections, the implementation of stringent security measures, and the fine-tuning of systems. In this context, TinyML necessitates the development of models capable of autonomous operation on edge nodes, ensuring both low-latency response and resilience in the face of these challenges. While the studies presented in this paper have made substantial strides in resource-constraint attack detection for smart devices, the critical task of selecting the most effective detection mechanism remains. This study presents a comprehensive statistical analysis to address the limitations inherent in existing works. In addition to algorithmic comparisons, we further contribute to the field by introducing a novel detection mechanism designed to identify attacks on smart devices. This mechanism involves real-time monitoring of packets, categorizing them into normal and attacked packets. Subsequently, ML algorithms are applied exclusively to the attacked packets, allowing us to precisely specify whether the attack is related to energy consumption or memory usage. Through this innovative approach, we aim to enhance the overall security posture of smart devices. The comprehensive statistical analysis not only evaluates existing algorithms but also introduces a novel mechanism to bolster the detection capabilities, providing a more holistic understanding of the effectiveness of these techniques against resource-constraint attacks on smart devices.

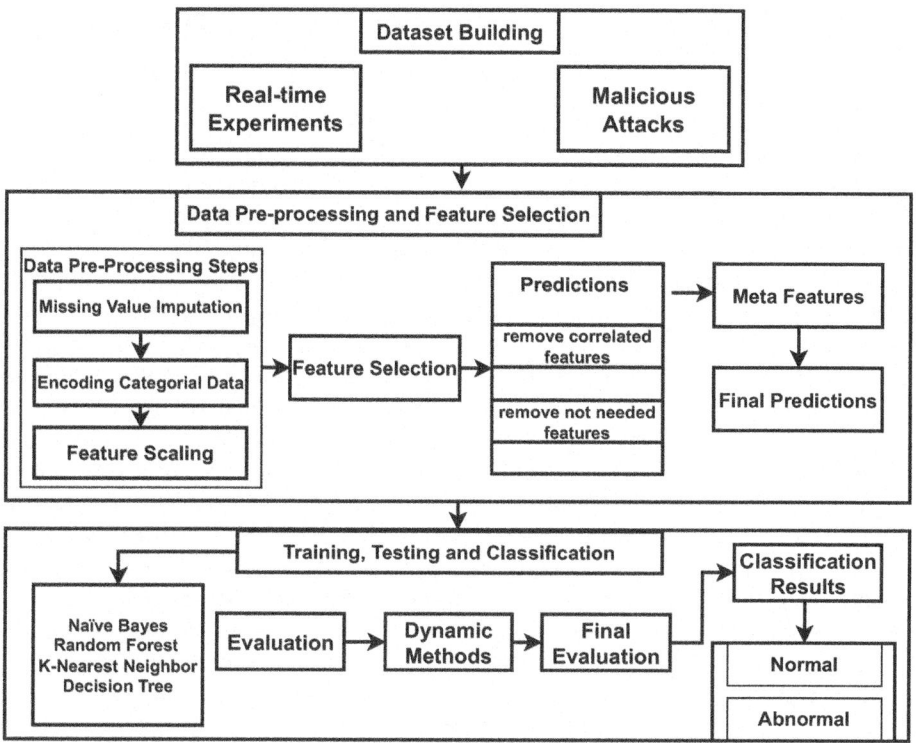

Fig. 1. Proposed Architecture.

3 Proposed Architecture and Dataset Selections

The proposed system architecture for both techniques used to detect resource constraint attacks is described as follows and shown in Fig. 1:

The first technique encompasses a monitoring system to observe the energy consumption and memory usage of smart devices in various system states, such as *Idle*, *Normal*, and *Abnormal*. Subsequently, the detection mechanism compares the normal energy consumption and memory usage behaviour with abnormal behaviour to identify potential attacks. The second algorithm primarily employs the TinyML technique to distinguish between normal and abnormal behaviour in the context of resource constraints within smart devices. This system follows four key phases: dataset creation, data pre-processing, feature selection, and resource constraint attack detection. During dataset creation, real-time experiments are conducted to collect data on energy consumption and memory usage in the presence and absence of attacks. Features are extracted from the recorded energy consumption, memory usage readings, and simulated attack signals. These features, representing all samples, are included in a dataset for further pre-processing. The second phase involves data pre-processing and feature selection, focusing on extracting energy and memory values from the dataset. TinyML techniques, such as Naive Bayes (NB), Decision Tree (DT), K Nearest Neighbor (K-NN), and RF, are employed for dataset training.

A classifier is utilized to analyze normal behaviour in these devices to detect resource constraint attacks on smart devices. It then compares this behaviour with abnormal patterns, enabling the detection of anomalies. Incoming signals are subjected to a classification process to determine their authenticity or whether they may be considered potentially spoofed. The probabilities associated with these signals are evaluated during the protection phase.

For the dataset and data pre-processing. This study leverages a dataset developed in our prior work [4]. Real-time experiments were conducted on authentic smart devices to gauge resource metrics such as energy consumption and memory usage, facilitating the creation of a dataset representing normal and abnormal behaviours. Energy consumption was measured using a smart circuit [3], while memory usage was monitored through various Python and C language libraries [2]. Abnormal behaviour was induced for dataset collection, including Distributed Denial-of-Service (DDoS) and Energy Consumption-Distributed Denial-of-Service (EC-DDoS) attacks. Extracted features from the energy consumption dataset include device information, ports, protocols, and energy consumption values. Similarly, features extracted from memory monitoring encompass device details, ports, protocols, and memory usage metrics. For pre-processing the dataset the dataset underwent meticulous pre-processing, entailing the identification and elimination of null, unknown, and noisy values during the missing value identification step.

4   Resource Constraints Detection Method Based on Machine Learning

This section delves deeper into our ML approach, a pivotal element in our paper. Our objective is to detect attacks on the protocols of smart devices effectively. To achieve this, we meticulously categorise protocol data into two distinct classes: normal and abnormal. The abnormal data is then subjected to a thorough analysis, with a primary focus on resource usage, particularly memory and energy consumption. The aim here is to precisely identify the nature of the attack, whether it involves energy, memory, or falls into another category of malicious activity. In this context, the choice of ML algorithms plays a pivotal role in the effectiveness of our approach. We have opted for two highly regarded algorithms: RF and SVM [9,19]. Both have proven their worth in various domains, and their application offers several significant advantages.

To achieve this, we employ a packet capture tool to perform a comparative analysis between the captured attack packets and the regular data packets. This process involves identifying patterns and rules within the attack data and translating them into distinctive features. Through the analysis of the protocol data, we sent malicious attacks that affect the energy consumption and memory usage of the smart devices, e.g., DDoS attacks. Then, we collect the normal and abnormal packet data for further analysis. These extracted data are then utilized as inputs for training the ML model to specify whether there is an energy or memory attack on the smart devices (Fig. 2).

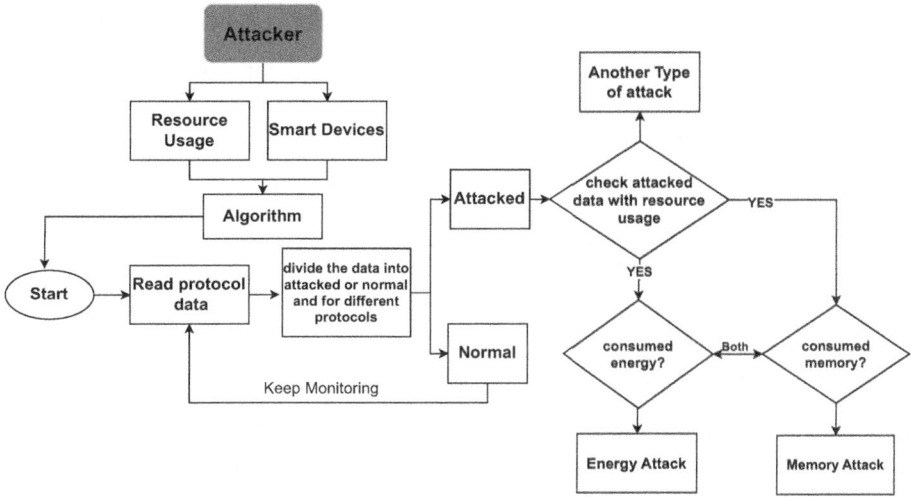

Fig. 2. Testing Environment and a technique to detect resource usage attacks in smart devices.

The packet capture tool takes advantage of tcpdump, and Wireshark, a robust network data analysis tool well-regarded among internet system administrators. Tcpdump offers extensive flexibility, allowing users to create custom filters for packet analysis. For example, using a straightforward command like (tcpdump -i en1 -v tcp), users can capture Transmission Control Protocol (TCP) protocol network packets from the *en1* network interface. Once it accumulates sets of attack packets related to resource constraint attacks, the tool initiates a comparative analysis by juxtaposing these attack packets against regular traffic for TCP and User Datagram Protocol (UDP). This analytical process reveals distinct characteristics associated with each attack mode. Notably, variations emerge between attacked data packets and normal data packets across different protocols. For instance, in the case of the TCP protocol, differences manifest in the packet sequence-regular for normal cases and random during attacks. Similarly, IP sources exhibit regular patterns for normal scenarios, with multiple destination IPs, while abnormal cases present confusion and a single destination IP. Furthermore, Packet Identification in normal cases features varying bits, whereas in attacked cases, the identification aligns with packets sent by the attacker. Contrastingly, in the UDP protocol, deviations are observed in the port number—normal cases display a specific port number, while abnormal behaviour involves random ports. Additionally, packet length demonstrates irregularities in normal scenarios, whereas abnormal cases exhibit consistent lengths.

In summary, based on the comparative analysis of regular protocol data and protocol attack data, the general characteristics of protocols can be summarized as follows:

$$PROT_{protocol} = (NUM_{packet}, LEN_{packet}, IDEN_{packet}, PORT) \qquad (1)$$

For the TCP protocol, the characteristics will be as follows:

$$TCP_{protocol} = (TCP_{NUM}, TCP_{LEN}, TCP_{IDEN}) \qquad (2)$$

For the UDP, the characteristics will be defined as follows:

$$UDP_{protocol} = (UDP_{NUM}, UDP_{LEN}, UDP_{port}) \qquad (3)$$

After dividing the protocol packet into normal and attacked data packets, we then use ML on the attacked packets to specify whether there is an energy or memory attack on the smart devices by comparing the fetched data with the energy and memory of the smart devices. Thus, RF represents a crucial ensemble learning technique built upon the Bagging framework, primarily designed for addressing classification and regression challenges. Decision trees serve as the base model for the Bagging process. RF offers notable advantages, including straightforward parallelization and enhanced prediction accuracy, all achieved without substantially increasing computational overhead. In contrast, SVM is a versatile classification and regression tool known for its proficiency with linear and non-linear data. It excels in high-dimensional spaces, a trait particularly valuable in our analysis of intricate protocol data. SVM's ability to determine optimal hyperplanes for distinguishing between different classes provides an effective means of identifying abnormal data patterns.

$$\text{Decision} = \begin{cases} \text{Attacked} & \text{if } \sum_{i=1}^{n} w_i x_i + b > \text{Threshold} \\ \text{Normal} & \text{otherwise} \end{cases}$$

w_i represents the weights assigned to each feature (x_i) in the feature vector, b is the bias term, n is the number of features, and the threshold is a decision boundary separating attacks from normal packets. Therefore, the normal packets and the feature (X_i) are learned during the training phase of the ML model. The features (x_i) include various characteristics of the packet data, such as packet length, source/destination IP addresses, protocol type, etc.

The combined use of RF and SVM in our training and evaluation processes enhances the reliability of our results. These algorithms work in synergy to handle the complexities of resource-constrained attacks. RF's adaptability and SVM's proficiency in classifying data types play a vital role in our approach. Therefore, based on the categorization of attack protocols, the attack detection models are categorized into three distinct groups: the TCP attack detection model, the UDP attack detection model, and a general attack detection model. The specific training model steps are outlined as follows:

1. Execute feature extraction, data format conversion, and dimensional reconstruction on the acquired attack data to create efficient datasets, retaining the relevant feature values.
2. Partition the training dataset into K subsets of equal size, using K-1 subsets for model training and the one designated for cross-validation.
3. Reiterate the model using various K values and determine the number of decision trees compared to the highest average accuracy among the different K values as the number of decision trees in the RF algorithm.

4.1   Data Collection Process

In our pursuit of a comprehensive security solution, we extend our methodology by not only evaluating algorithms but also by conducting an in-depth analysis of the collected data. The data collection process involves capturing information from the protocols commonly used by smart devices, including TCP and UDP. This approach allows us to curate datasets that serve as the foundation for both our statistical analysis and ML model training. Our system distinguishes between normal and abnormal behaviour through the collected data. In the abnormal behaviour scenario, we intentionally expose smart devices to various malicious attacks, simultaneously collecting data. This process facilitates a robust evaluation of the system's response to attacks under different conditions. Subsequently, the attacked data is meticulously compared with the energy and memory usage of the smart devices. This comparative analysis aids in precisely specifying whether the attack pertains to energy consumption or memory usage, offering insights into the nature of the threat. For data collection, we employ specialized tools, such as tcpdump, to capture packets from TCP and UDP protocols. Tcpdump operates from the command line, providing the capability to capture and display detailed packet information, making it suitable for scripting and automation. Additionally, we utilize Wireshark, a widely-used network protocol analyzer with a graphical user interface, to monitor and capture further information, enhancing our understanding of the network traffic and facilitating more nuanced analysis. By leveraging real-world scenarios and intentional exposure to attacks, our approach ensures a holistic understanding of smart device security, paving the way for effective defences against resource-constrained attacks.

1. Dataset preparation: During this phase, the dataset has been acquired. The initial step involves gathering data on normal activities, ensuring their integrity without any associated attacks. This phase encompasses subphases focusing on IoT sensor devices, packet analysis, and subsequent data.
2. Data collection: At this stage, the data for the different protocols are collected for normal and abnormal behaviours. The analysis of attacks took place at various time intervals every 2, 3, 5, and 10 s, respectively. The data collection involved gathering information both before and after the occurrence of the two specified types of attacks. This data was meticulously formatted and structured in CSV format to calculate further information. Subsequently, the

data pre-processing phase commences, involving the capture and analysis of network packets using Wireshark. This process aims to extract attributes such as timestamp, source IP address, destination IP address, source port, destination port, protocol, and bytes. Additionally, IP addresses are converted into numerical values.

3. Data cleaning and parsing: In this phase, we grapple with a substantial volume of data, necessitating thorough cleaning and extraction of distinct features from the dataset. We remove duplicate entries and eliminate superfluous information to ensure data quality. Subsequently, the refined data is stored in the database, poised for further computational analysis. Clean$(D) \rightarrow \{D_i \mid D_i \in D, i = 1, 2, \ldots, N\}$ this indicates that the cleaned data is a set of elements D_i for each index i from $1 to N$, where each D_i is selected from the original array D and contains non-redundant data.

$$D' = \text{Clean}(D) \tag{4}$$

where D' is the cleaned array.

4. Feature extraction: the information collected for this experiment encompasses diverse data attributes, including packet sequence, IP sources, packet identification, port numbers, and packet length. These data play a pivotal role in the initial stages of distinguishing between normal and abnormal behaviours. Additionally, they provide essential insights into energy and memory usage patterns.

5   Experimentation and Discussion

5.1   Test Results and Discussions

Determining whether the detection data corresponds to a resource constraints attack constitutes a classification problem. To assess the experimental outcomes, we utilize evaluation criteria such as the false positive rate, true positive rate, false detection rate, and accuracy.

The accuracy (ACC) calculation pertains to the ratio of correct predictions (Attack traffic and Normal traffic) to the total number of observations, and it is computed as follows:

$$ACC = \frac{TP + TN}{N} \tag{5}$$

Moreover, it is important to calculate some important variables. For example, the false positive rate (FPR) denotes the percentage of normal behaviour inaccurately recognized as attack data, and it is defined as:

$$FPR = \frac{FP}{(FP + TN)} \tag{6}$$

The true positive rate (TPR), also known as sensitivity or recall, is the proportion of true positives to the total number of observations predicted as positive.

$$TPR = \frac{TP}{TP + FN} \tag{7}$$

The false detection rate (FDR) is defined as $(1 - ACC)$, and it is defined as follows:

$$FDR = \frac{FP + FN}{N} \tag{8}$$

TP (True Positive) denotes instances where the model correctly predicts attack traffic as an attack. TN (True Negative) indicates instances where the model correctly predicts normal traffic as normal. FP (False Positive) occurs when the model incorrectly predicts normal traffic as an attack. FN (False Negative) represents instances where the model incorrectly predicts attack traffic as normal. Finally, N is the number of samples. After the RF model is trained using the training dataset, we proceed to create the test dataset by integrating the remaining attack data packets with normal traffic. This involves systematically combining normal and attack traffic samples, determining the classification of each sample, and carefully controlling the flow to maintain the desired ratio of normal to attack traffic. Simultaneously, we utilize the LIBSVM library for processing data using the SVM algorithm, and these outcomes are subsequently compared with the results obtained from the RF model. Therefore, after detecting if there is an attack across the mentioned protocol, we then take the attacked data to specify the main reason behind such a type of attack; we will compare the fetched attacked data from a protocol and then compare its values with energy or memory measurements to specify if the attack is on memory or energy or effect both energy consumption and memory usage of the smart devices. Table 1 presents the findings for detecting if there is an attack across the different mentioned protocols:

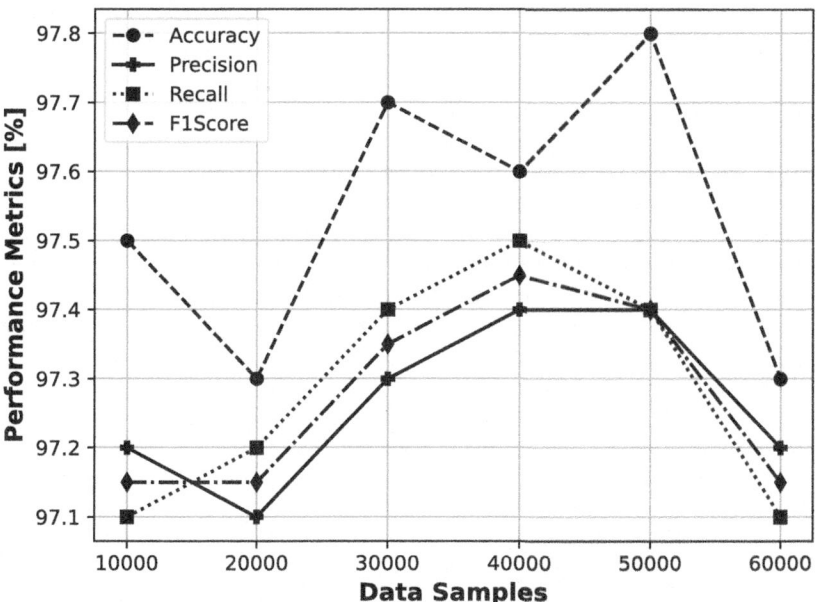

Fig. 3. Accuracy, Precision, Recall, F1Score of the proposed models.

Table 1. Comparison of Detection Performance Metrics for SVM and RF Algorithms across TCP and UDP Protocols.

Algorithm	Protocol	ACC [%]	TPR [%]	FPR [%]	FDR [%]
SVM	TCP	94.5	93.75	5.70	5.5
	UDP	98.8	95.7	0.04	0.05
RF	TCP	99.50	95.83	0	0.50
	UDP	99.12	91.17	0	0.01

The RF algorithm consistently exhibits higher accuracy across all protocol types compared to the SVM technique, as illustrated in Table 1. Specifically, RF achieves an accuracy of approximately 99.50% for TCP and 99.12% for UDP. In contrast, SVM yields an accuracy of 94.5% for TCP and 98.8% for UDP. Examining false positive rates, the SVM algorithm registers 5.70 for TCP and 0.04% for UDP. Conversely, the RF algorithm demonstrates lower false positive rates, recording values of 0% for both protocols. Simultaneously, the False Discovery Rate (FDR) for RF is 0.50% for TCP and 0.01% for UDP. In comparison, the SVM algorithm achieves an FDR of 5.5% for TCP and 0.05% for UDP. Finally, considering the True Positive Rate (TPR), RF attains 95.83% for TCP and 91.17% for UDP, while SVM records TPR values of 93.75% for TCP and 95.7% for UDP.

Furthermore, Fig. 3 depicts a comprehensive analysis of performance metrics, encompassing accuracy, recall (formulated as $TP/(TP + FN)$), precision (expressed as $TP/(TP + FP)$), and F1 score (calculated as $2 \times \frac{\text{Precision} \times \text{Recall}}{\text{Precision} + \text{Recall}}$). This analysis spans multiple models evaluated across varying data sample sizes, specifically $10,000$, $20,000$, $30,000$, $40,000$, $50,000$, and $60,000$ instances.

5.2 Statistical Analysis Results

We conducted our simulation on an Intel Core i7-10750H CPU, operating at 2.60 GHz, with 16.0 GB of memory.

We employed four evaluation metrics to appraise the effectiveness of the proposed model. These metrics include the Probability of Detection (P_d), Probability of False Alarm (P_{fa}), Probability of Misdetection (P_{md}), and Accuracy (ACC). The calculations for these metrics were carried out using the following formulas:

$$P_d = \frac{T_P}{T_P + F_N} \tag{9}$$

$$P_{fa} = \frac{F_P}{T_F + F_N} \tag{10}$$

$$P_{md} = \frac{F_N}{T_N + F_P} \tag{11}$$

$$ACC = \frac{T_P + T_N}{T_P + T_N + F_P + F_N} \tag{12}$$

In the context of our evaluation, we used the following notation: TP represents the count of correctly predicted malicious flows, TN corresponds to the count of accurately predicted normal flows, FP stands for the count of erroneously predicted malicious flows, and FN represents the count of improperly predicted normal flows. To assess the performance of the proposed dynamic methods, we conducted a simulation analysis and compared the results against those of the different devices chosen and the different techniques used in our previous studies.

Figure 4 presents the results of the proposed methods and two different algorithms applied to various smart devices, focusing on accuracy. Notably, the proposed algorithm for detecting resource-constrained attacks using TinyML in

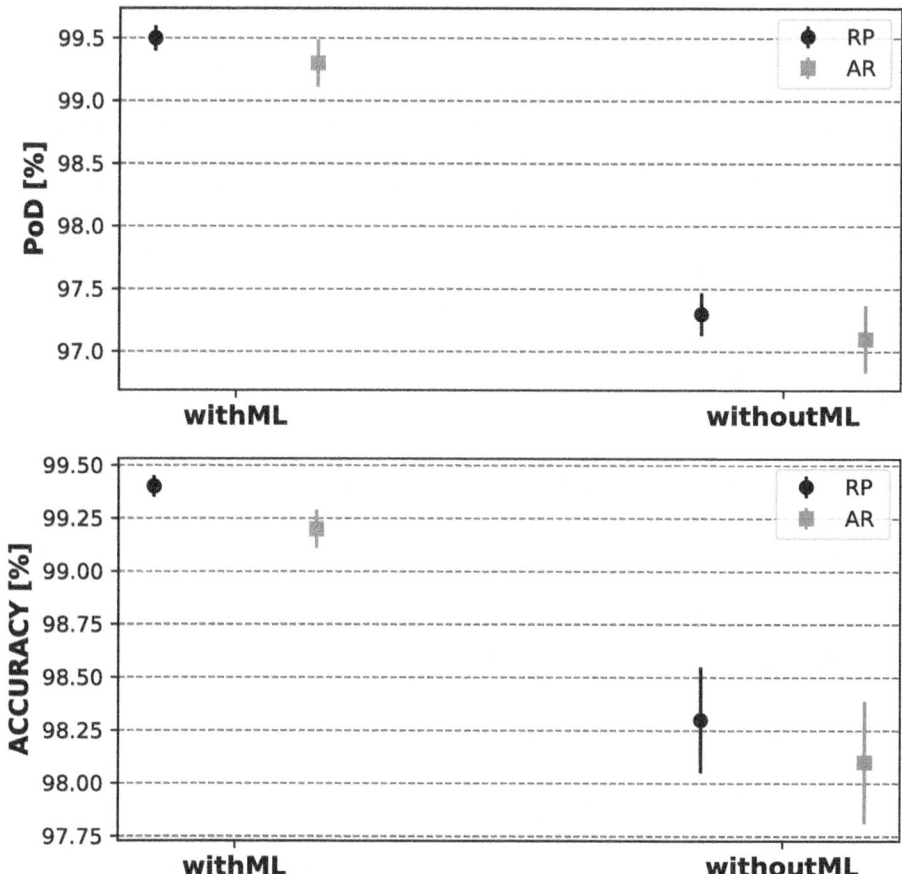

Fig. 4. Evaluation Results in terms of Accuracy and Probability of Detection (PoD).

Raspberry Pi (RP) and Arduino (AR) devices showcases superior accuracy compared to the other algorithms. As evident from the data, the resource-constrained attack detection using RP and AR devices with Tiny ML achieved an impressive accuracy of 99.4% and 99.2%, respectively. In contrast, the algorithms for detecting resource-constrained attacks without the utilization of Tiny ML yielded accuracies of 98.3% for RP and 98.1% for Arduino. The latter represents the lowest accuracy among the considered algorithms. Moreover, we employed k-fold cross-validation to provide a more detailed analysis of the algorithmic performance. Given the constraints of small datasets related to smart devices, we employed 5-fold cross-validation independently for each algorithm, a total of ≈66000 samples divided between these five folds. This approach helps robustly assess our algorithms' accuracy across different subsets of the data, as shown in Fig. 5.

The accuracy across the folds was consistently good, with values of 98.6% 98.3%, 99.3%, 99.1%, and 98.9%, respectively, for the algorithm that uses TinyML, and 97.1% 97.9%, 98.8%, 98.6%, and 98.4% for the other algorithm, respectively. This enhanced accuracy contributes to the reliability and generalizability of our models, which is particularly crucial when dealing with limited data on smart devices.

Figure 4 also presents the results of the proposed methods and two different algorithms applied to various smart devices, focusing on the probability of detection. As can be seen, the proposed algorithm for detecting resource-constrained attacks using TinyML in RP and AR in terms of probability of detection has a slight difference. TinyML has the highest probability of detection of 99.4% for the RP and 99.2% for the AR. The other algorithm has a probability of detection of 97.3% for the RP and 97.1% for the AR.

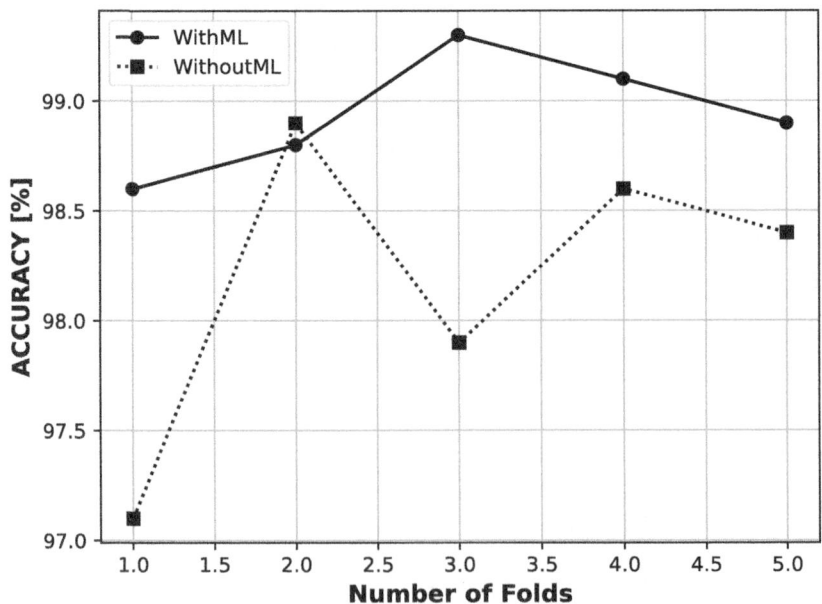

Fig. 5. The accuracy for various numbers of folds.

Figure 6 depicts the outcomes of PoFA and PoM for detecting resource constraint attacks. We utilized TinyML for the RP and AR models, while the other approach did not employ TinyML techniques. Specifically, this analysis examines the probability of misdetection (PoM). As one can observe, the PoM of the RP and AR using TinyML have an acceptable probability of misdetection; however, the lowest probability of misdetection belongs to the other algorithm. The proposed methods have a probability of misdetection of 1.60% for both smart devices by using TinyML to detect resource constraint attacks, while the other algorithm for both device models has a probability of misdetection of 1.46%. We also examine these results in terms of the probability of false alarms. It is clear that RP and AR, utilizing TinyML, achieve superior performance in terms of the probability of false alarms compared to the alternative algorithm, which does not employ TinyML.

To be precise, methods used TinyML yield a probability of false alarm of 1.23%. For RP and AR, specifically, these values stand at 1.2% and 1.23%, respectively. In contrast, the other algorithms, when not utilizing TinyML, yield higher probabilities of false alarms for AR and RP, which are 1.6% and 1.64%, respectively, as shown in Table 2. The count of false positive predictions (f_p) is a crucial metric in algorithm evaluation, as depicted in Table 2. This metric

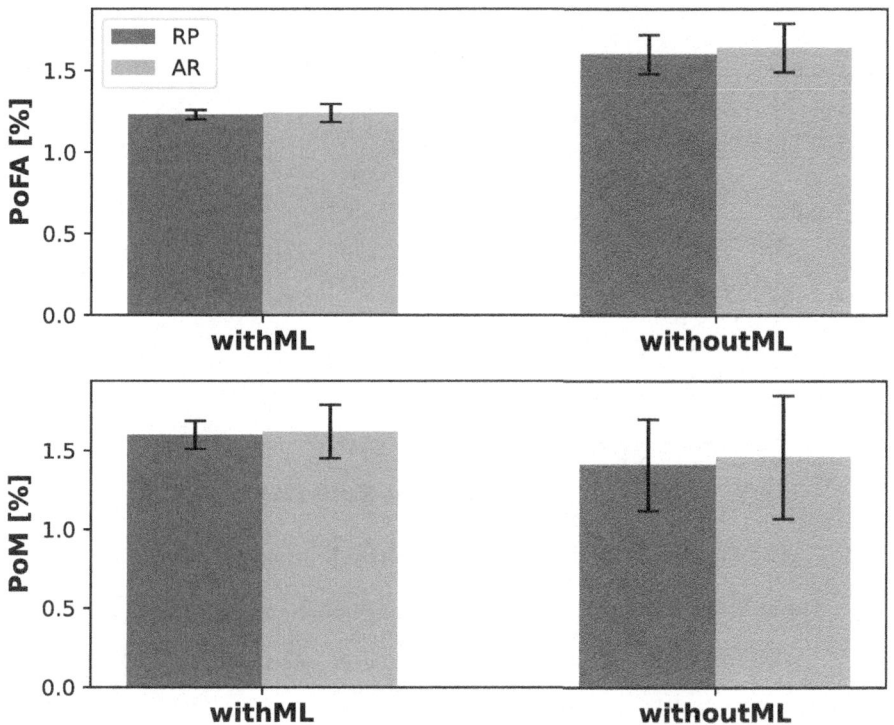

Fig. 6. Evaluation Results in terms of PoF and PoM.

compares the instances where the algorithm wrongly predicts a positive outcome to the total number of samples predicted as negative. In our proposed algorithm utilizing TinyML, the false positive rate is 10.9 per second. In contrast, the alternative algorithm records a higher rate of 16 false positives per second. Moreover, achieving a balance between the detection and false positive rates necessitates a trade-off. With an increase in the false positive rate, there is a corresponding rise in the detection rate. Hence, the false positive rate becomes a key metric for evaluating the system's effectiveness. As presented in Fig. 7 the provided information includes the detection rate corresponding to various false positive rates for both the algorithms, namely withML and withoutML. The presented results show different instances when resource-constraint attacks flooded smart devices. The threshold for normal cases was shown in different instances to show the effect of the threshold on the final results of FPR and DR. The first algorithm outperforms the second one. The results reveal two discernible trends: the detection rate is influenced by the false positive rate, and the proposed system consistently exhibits notable improvements in the detection rate.

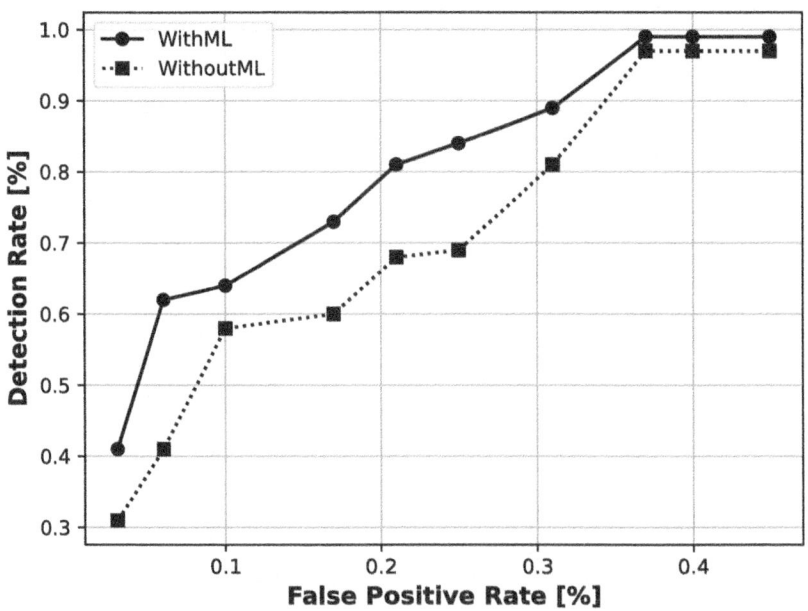

Fig. 7. Comparative Analysis of False Positive Rate and Detection Rate.

Table 2. Evaluation Results of the Proposed Detection Algorithms.

Methods	Devices	ACC (%)	PoD (%)	PoMD (%)	PoFA (%)	FP (s)
With TinyML	RP	99.4	99.5	1.60	1.23	10.9
	AR	99.2	99.3	1.64	1.24	
Without TinyML	RP	98.3	97.3	1.46	1.60	16
	AR	98.1	97.41	1.46	1.64	

6   Conclusion and Future Work

In recent years, the escalating interest in the IoT and the security of its smart devices has given rise to significant technological advancements. These innovations have paved the way for many techniques and methods designed to identify and mitigate vulnerabilities within IoT systems. Yet, despite the progress, this field continues to grapple with formidable challenges and limitations, notably marked by the persistence of high rates of misdetection and false alarms. Interest in detecting resource-constraint attacks in IoT systems has significantly increased in the last decade, leading to notable technological advancements. Several techniques and methods have been proposed to identify and address these vulnerabilities. However, this field of study still grapples with certain challenges and limitations, including high misdetection rates and false alarms. This work addresses this gap by proposing a novel detection mechanism for resource-constraint attacks in smart devices. Our approach involves calculating various variables on the protocol, such as fetching the protocol data and dividing them into normal or attacked packets. We then apply ML techniques to specify if it's an energy or memory attack by comparing the attacked data with real measurements of energy and memory. The final results demonstrate a very high accuracy using RF and SVM. Specifically, the accuracy for RF exceeds 99.7%, while for SVM, it surpasses 98.8%. These results hold true across different protocols.

As a comparative reference for our previous works and detection mechanisms in our previous algorithms, the first algorithm employed for detecting resource-constraint attacks with TinyML achieves an accuracy of 99.4% and 99.2%, a probability of detection of 99.5% and 99.3%, a probability of misdetection of 1.62%, and a probability of false alarm of 1.23%. Conversely, the other algorithm, which does not utilize TinyML, exhibits an accuracy of 98.3% and 98.1%, a probability of detection of approximately 97.4%, a probability of misdetection of about 1.46%, and a probability of false alarm of approximately 1.64%. These findings underscore the effectiveness of our proposed detection mechanism in addressing the challenges associated with resource-constraint attacks in IoT systems. In future work, we will delve deeper into utilizing ML techniques to detect other types of attacks that affect the resources of smart devices.

References

1. Al-Waisi, Z., Soderi, S., De Nicola, R.: Detection of energy consumption cyber attacks on smart devices, vol. 12, p. 1927. EAI-SPRINGER (2023)
2. Alwaisi, Z., Soderi, S., De Nicola, R.: Mitigating and analysis of memory usage attack in IOE system. In: Vo, N.S., Tran, H.A. (eds.) INISCOM 2023. LNICST, vol. 531, pp. 296–314. Springer, Cham (2023). https://doi.org/10.1007/978-3-031-47359-3_22
3. Alwaisi, Z., Soderi, S., Nicola, R.D.: Energy cyber attacks to smart healthcare devices: a testbed. In: Chen, Y., Yao, D., Nakano, T. (eds.) BICT 2023. LNICST, vol. 512, pp. 246–265. Springer, Cham (2023). https://doi.org/10.1007/978-3-031-43135-7_24

4. AlWaisi, Z.A.: Optimized monitoring and detection of internet of things resources-constraints cyber attacks (2023). https://e-theses.imtlucca.it/392/

5. Dai, Y., Li, H., Qian, Y., Lu, X.: A malware classification method based on memory dump grayscale image. Digit. Investig. **27**, 30–37 (2018)

6. Duan, Y., Fu, X., Luo, B., Wang, Z., Shi, J., Du, X.: Detective: automatically identify and analyze malware processes in forensic scenarios via DLLs. In: 2015 IEEE International Conference on Communications (ICC), pp. 5691–5696. IEEE (2015)

7. Fabi, V., Spigliantini, G., Corgnati, S.P.: Insights on smart home concept and occupants' interaction with building controls. Energy Procedia **111**, 759–769 (2017). https://doi.org/10.1016/j.egypro.2017.03.238, https://www.sciencedirect.com/science/article/pii/S1876610217302680. 8th International Conference on Sustainability in Energy and Buildings, SEB-16, 11–13 September 2016, Turin, Italy

8. Ford, R., Pritoni, M., Sanguinetti, A., Karlin, B.: Categories and functionality of smart home technology for energy management. Build. Environ. **123**, 543–554 (2017). https://doi.org/10.1016/j.buildenv.2017.07.020

9. Hussain, F., Hussain, R., Hassan, S.A., Hossain, E.: Machine learning in IoT security: current solutions and future challenges. IEEE Commun. Surv. Tutor. **22**(3), 1686–1721 (2020)

10. Kamaldeep, Dutta, M., Granjal, J.: Towards a secure internet of things: a comprehensive study of second line defense mechanisms. IEEE Access **8**, 127272–127312 (2020)

11. Khor, J.H., Sidorov, M., Woon, P.Y.: Public blockchains for resource-constrained IoT devices-a state-of-the-art survey. IEEE Internet Things J. **8**(15), 11960–11982 (2021). https://doi.org/10.1109/JIOT.2021.3069120

12. Kumar, A., Sharma, S., Goyal, N., Singh, A., Cheng, X., Singh, P.: Secure and energy-efficient smart building architecture with emerging technology iot. Comput. Commun. **176**, 207–217 (2021)

13. Liu, X., Liu, Y., Liu, A., Yang, L.T.: Defending on-off attacks using light probing messages in smart sensors for industrial communication systems. IEEE Trans. Industr. Inf. **14**(9), 3801–3811 (2018). https://doi.org/10.1109/TII.2018.2836150

14. Mosli, R., Li, R., Yuan, B., Pan, Y.: Automated malware detection using artifacts in forensic memory images. In: 2016 IEEE Symposium on Technologies for Homeland Security (HST), pp. 1–6. IEEE (2016)

15. Mosli, R., Li, R., Yuan, B., Pan, Y.: A behavior-based approach for malware detection. In: DigitalForensics 2017. IAICT, vol. 511, pp. 187–201. Springer, Cham (2017). https://doi.org/10.1007/978-3-319-67208-3_11

16. Pahl, M.O., Aubet, F.X.: All eyes on you: distributed multi-dimensional IoT microservice anomaly detection. In: 2018 14th International Conference on Network and Service Management (CNSM), pp. 72–80. IEEE (2018)

17. Pahl, M.O., Aubet, F.X., Liebald, S.: Graph-based IoT microservice security. In: NOMS 2018 - 2018 IEEE/IFIP Network Operations and Management Symposium, pp. 1–3 (2018). https://doi.org/10.1109/NOMS.2018.8406118

18. Pajouh, H.H., Javidan, R., Khayami, R., Dehghantanha, A., Choo, K.K.R.: A two-layer dimension reduction and two-tier classification model for anomaly-based intrusion detection in IoT backbone networks. IEEE Trans. Emerg. Top. Comput. **7**(2), 314–323 (2016)

19. Rana, V.K., Suryanarayana, T.M.V.: Performance evaluation of MLE, RF and SVM classification algorithms for watershed scale land use/land cover mapping using sentinel 2 bands. Remote Sens. Appl.: Soc. Environ. **19**, 100351 (2020)

20. Shi, Y., Li, F., Song, W., Li, X.Y., Ye, J.: Energy audition based cyber-physical attack detection system in IoT. In: Proceedings of the ACM Turing Celebration ConferenceChina, ACM TURC 2019. Association for Computing Machinery, New York (2019). https://doi.org/10.1145/3321408.3321588
21. Sihwail, R., Omar, K., Zainol Ariffin, K.A., Al Afghani, S.: Malware detection approach based on artifacts in memory image and dynamic analysis. Appl. Sci. **9**(18), 3680 (2019)
22. Tsoukas, V., Gkogkidis, A., Kampa, A., Spathoulas, G., Kakarountas, A.: Enhancing food supply chain security through the use of blockchain and TinyML. Information **13**(5), 213 (2022)

Author Index

GPSR Compliance

The European Union's (EU) General Product Safety Regulation (GPSR) is a set of rules that requires consumer products to be safe and our obligations to ensure this.

If you have any concerns about our products, you can contact us on ProductSafety@springernature.com

In case Publisher is established outside the EU, the EU authorized representative is:

Springer Nature Customer Service Center GmbH
Europaplatz 3
69115 Heidelberg, Germany

The manufacturer's authorised representative in the EU is Springer
Nature Customer Service Centre GmbH, Europaplatz 3, 69115 Heidelberg,
Germany. If you have any concerns regarding our products, please
contact ProductSafety@springernature.com

Printed and bound by CPI Group (UK) Ltd, Croydon, CR0 4YY
27/04/2026
02097851-0003